AF770775

CARDIOLOGY RESEARCH AND CLINICAL DEVELOPMENTS

PIONEER OF THE HOMOCYSTEINE THEORY

Cardiology Research and Clinical Developments

Additional books in this series can be found on Nova's website under the Series tab.

Additional e -books in this series can be found on Nova's website under the e-book tab.

Cancer Etiology, Diagnosis and Treatments

Additional books in this series can be found on Nova's website under the Series tab.

Additional e -books in this series can be found on Nova's website under the e-book tab.

CARDIOLOGY RESEARCH AND CLINICAL DEVELOPMENTS

PIONEER OF THE HOMOCYSTEINE THEORY

KILMER SERJUS MCCULLY

New York

Copyright © 2013 by Nova Science Publishers, Inc.

All rights reserved. No part of this book may be reproduced, stored in a retrieval system or transmitted in any form or by any means: electronic, electrostatic, magnetic, tape, mechanical photocopying, recording or otherwise without the written permission of the Publisher.

For permission to use material from this book please contact us:
Telephone 631-231-7269; Fax 631-231-8175
Web Site: http://www.novapublishers.com

NOTICE TO THE READER

The Publisher has taken reasonable care in the preparation of this book, but makes no expressed or implied warranty of any kind and assumes no responsibility for any errors or omissions. No liability is assumed for incidental or consequential damages in connection with or arising out of information contained in this book. The Publisher shall not be liable for any special, consequential, or exemplary damages resulting, in whole or in part, from the readers' use of, or reliance upon, this material. Any parts of this book based on government reports are so indicated and copyright is claimed for those parts to the extent applicable to compilations of such works.

Independent verification should be sought for any data, advice or recommendations contained in this book. In addition, no responsibility is assumed by the publisher for any injury and/or damage to persons or property arising from any methods, products, instructions, ideas or otherwise contained in this publication.

This publication is designed to provide accurate and authoritative information with regard to the subject matter covered herein. It is sold with the clear understanding that the Publisher is not engaged in rendering legal or any other professional services. If legal or any other expert assistance is required, the services of a competent person should be sought. FROM A DECLARATION OF PARTICIPANTS JOINTLY ADOPTED BY A COMMITTEE OF THE AMERICAN BAR ASSOCIATION AND A COMMITTEE OF PUBLISHERS.

LIBRARY OF CONGRESS CATALOGING-IN-PUBLICATION DATA

ISBN: 978-1-62257-723-1

Library of Congress Control Number: 2012944806

Published by Nova Science Publishers, Inc. † New York

To members of the younger generation who aspire
to the calling of medical science.

CONTENTS

Chapter 1

INTRODUCTION: A CHANCE DISCOVERY CONCERNING THE CAUSE OF HEART DISEASE

This personal scientific memoir describes how a chance observation concerning artery disease in children with rare inherited abnormalities of metabolism, often called experiments of Nature, led to the discovery of a new theory of heart disease, cancer and diseases of aging. As explained in subsequent chapters, this new theory places the amino acid homocysteine at the heart of altered metabolism of diseases of aging. Not only does this theory illuminate and explain the origin of these diseases, development of this theory logically leads to a novel and revolutionary metabolic and nutritional program for disease prevention and treatment, potentially benefiting individuals and populations.

At the age of 34, having completed an exciting and arduous educational and scientific program of training in chemistry, biochemistry, medicine, molecular biology, genetics and pathology, I had reached a critical juncture in my chosen career as a medical investigator. My childhood aspirations to become a medical scientist had finally been realized. I was fortunate to have been awarded a research grant from the National Institutes of Health (NIH) to study how constituent amino acids are selected in the process of building cellular proteins. One of my mentors and supporters, Benjamin Castleman, had offered me a research laboratory and a position as Assistant Pathologist in his Department of Pathology at Massachusetts General Hospital (MGH), giving me a wonderful opportunity to investigate an exciting area of medical science of my own choosing.

My previous training and experience in scientific research were concerned mainly with how transfer ribonucleic acid (tRNA) selects and organizes amino acids for assembly in the proper sequence, as dictated by the sequence of nucleotides in deoxyribonucleic acid (DNA), thus transmitting the genetic code of DNA into the nucleotide sequences of messenger RNA (mRNA) and ultimately into the amino acid sequences of protein molecules. Many biochemists and molecular biologists, including several of my scientific mentors, had made important discoveries in the previous two decades explaining many of the molecular details of this fundamental process of biology. My own contributions concerning the structure of t-RNA had a minor impact on aspects of this field. Yet my life long ambition to use my understanding of basic science to discover the nature of disease processes had not yet been realized in 1968.

Having completed my research training and my Board Certification examinations in Anatomic and Clinical Pathology, I decided that attending the newly founded Human Genetics program at MGH would provide an opportunity to use my knowledge of pathology, biochemistry, molecular biology and genetics in the study of inherited diseases. John Littlefield, the new Director of Human Genetics, encouraged my participation because he was familiar with my interests, training, and previous research publications. The most challenging aspect of scientific investigation is the choice of a significant and meaningful scientific question that can be addressed by current concepts and methods. The study of pathological changes in tissues of persons with inherited diseases seemed a logical way to choose a promising field of investigation.

A fascinating presentation at one of the Human Genetics conferences that I attended in 1968 concerned a 9 year old girl with a newly discovered inherited disease of metabolism called homocystinuria [1]. As explained in detail in Chapter 3, this new disease involves abnormal metabolism of the amino acid homocysteine, caused by an inherited abnormality of a key enzyme, cystathionine synthase. In my previous experience as a Research Associate at the NIH, I had learned a great deal about homocysteine and its precursor in metabolism, the essential amino acid methionine. The conference explained that children with homocystinuria are susceptible to thrombosis of arteries and veins. I immediately became interested in understanding how this inherited disease could affect blood coagulation and what role, if any, the amino acid homocysteine played in their blood clotting abnormality.

Many years previously the 8 year old uncle of this child with homocystinuria had died of thrombosis of the carotid artery and a massive stroke, and the pediatricians had located a description of the clinical and autopsy findings of this child in the Clinical Pathological Conferences published in the *New England Journal of Medicine* in 1933 [2]. Because this new genetic disease seemed amenable to investigation by methods and concepts that I had experienced during my fellowship years, I decided to restudy this case, using the original autopsy protocol, the pathological slides, and the tissues that had survived since publication in 1933. In reading the case report, I was astonished to find that the pathologist Tracey Mallory had demonstrated arteriosclerosis of the carotid artery with thrombosis and massive stroke as the cause of death. My own study of these surviving materials from 1933 confirmed these published findings.

By reading the published medical literature about homocystinuria, I found that my former colleague at NIH, Harvey Mudd, and his team of investigators had discovered an inherited abnormality of the enzyme, cystathionine synthase, as the cause of homocystinuria [3]. This enzyme is responsible for the normal metabolism of homocysteine from the essential amino acid methionine, and blockage of this pathway by the abnormal enzyme causes accumulation of homocysteine in the cells, tissues, and fluids of children with homocystinuria. This discovery and other published articles about homocystinuria, however, failed to explain why and how this obscure amino acid could cause the carotid arteriosclerosis and stroke that had killed the child in 1933 and others like him, as reported by other investigators.

It was my good fortune that another case of homocystinuria was discussed at a subsequent Human Genetics conference several months later. This 2 month old boy was desperately ill, suffering from failure to gain weight and pneumonia, when he was referred for care at MGH. The pediatricians caring for this baby boy discovered the presence of the amino acid homocysteine in his urine, as well as large quantities of the related amino acid cystathionine. Study by pediatricians at MGH, by Harvey Mudd at NIH, and by the biochemist Robert Abeles at Brandeis University demonstrated that the child suffered from a previously unrecognized abnormality of vitamin B12 metabolism, later called cobalamin C disease [4]. Unlike the abnormality of cystathionine synthase in previously studied cases of homocystinuria, this abnormality resulted in failure to convert excess homocysteine to methionine, causing accumulation of homocysteine and cystathionine in cells, tissues and body fluids.

Despite the best efforts of the pediatricians to treat this baby with cobalamin C disease with vitamins, supplements, and antibiotics, the child died and an autopsy was conducted. The doctors at the Human Genetics conference asked me to comment on the autopsy findings. Knowing the crucial significance of this case, because the homocystinuria was caused by a different enzyme abnormality than previous cases, I immediately returned to the Pathology Department to read the autopsy report of this case that had been completed, filed away and forgotten. I had expected that the report would contain a description of arterial plaques, thrombosis, and stroke similar to the findings in the previous case of homocystinuria that I had recently studied. Instead, there was only a lengthy discussion of the metabolic findings in the new disease causing homocystinuria and cystathioninuria. In the description of the pathological changes, there were findings of fatty liver, aspiration pneumonia, and metaplastic changes of the lining cells of the stomach, but there was no mention of the arteries.

Although I was disappointed because the completed autopsy had failed to confirm my prediction of arterial plaques and thrombosis, I decided to re-study the organs and tissues from this case, which had fortunately been saved in a jar of preservative. In examining the pathological slides from these tissues, I discovered rapidly progressing and severe arteriosclerosis in arteries throughout the major organs! From this discovery I concluded that this new observation provided evidence that the amino acid homocysteine caused arterial plaques by a direct effect on cells and tissues of the arteries. I could draw this conclusion because elevation of blood homocysteine was the only metabolic abnormality in common with these two inherited diseases causing homocystinuria.

Because of this critical new observation, I was confident that this interpretation could explain the origin of arteriosclerotic plaques in children with homocystinuria caused by different inherited enzymatic abnormalities. Because of my previous experiences with research on cholesterol biosynthesis and with steroid hormone research, I realized that this conclusion was of significance to understanding the origin of the most important disease of aging, namely heart disease, stroke and arteriosclerosis in the population.

In the 1950s and 1960s the prevailing view of the medical establishment was that high blood cholesterol in some way was responsible for arterial plaques and other abnormalities found in heart disease, stroke and arteriosclerosis. Yet in these children with homocystinuria and arteriosclerosis, there was no elevation of blood cholesterol. Furthermore, except for the absence of cholesterol and fats, the arterial plaques in these children exhibited most of the characteristic features of arteriosclerotic plaques found in patients with arteriosclerosis. My hypothesis then suggested that elevated blood homocysteine levels are capable of causing arterial plaques without apparent participation of fats and cholesterol in the most important degenerative disease of aging and the leading cause of mortality in mid 20th century America.

In a short 6 months in 1968, my research program and interests had taken an exciting new turn – I had found an important and highly significant field of study for which my previous training and research experience had prepared me! As explained in detail in Chapter 3, I carefully prepared my findings for publication, checking with knowledgeable colleagues about the characteristic features of arterial plaques in the cases of homocystinuria. I also confirmed the plausibility of the conclusions concerning the relation of abnormal homocysteine metabolism to the process of arteriosclerosis, experimental demonstration of vitamin B6 deficiency as a cause of arteriosclerosis in monkeys, and the implications of the observation for understanding the origin of an important disease of aging in the general population. In preparing the final draft of my article, I was careful to describe my hypothesis that homocysteine is somehow involved as the inciting cause of plaques, placing blood cholesterol as a secondary factor in the disease process [5].

My feeling of excitement and exhilaration with my new discovery and hypothesis concerning the most important disease in the population could hardly be contained. It was difficult for me to sleep through the night for two to three weeks. New ideas crept into my analysis of the new research finding. How was an amino acid with a sulfur atom able to play such an important role in arterial plaque formation? Were there other metabolic derivatives related to homocysteine that mediated plaque formation? What is the role of homocysteine in the aging process? Was there an important role for homocysteine in the normal growth process? Did cancer cells have abnormal homocysteine metabolism? The new questions seemed to be endless, and reading the related scientific and medical literature seemed to confirm my conclusions and to suggest new pathways for investigation. My wife, Annina, reported that I spouted chemical formulas and ideas while sleeping during this period.

After completing my manuscript describing my discovery for publication in the *American Journal of Pathology* in 1969, as explained in Chapter 3, I suspected that some investigators in the heart disease field would be interested in a new approach. I realized that placing blood cholesterol in a secondary role might engender criticism, but I was confident of my discovery and was positive in my suggestion that the effects of homocysteine on cells and tissues of arteries are the primary events in causation of heart disease in the general population. Rapid acceptance of the manuscript for publication and receipt of hundreds of reprint requests after publication confirmed my conjecture about the importance of my discovery for the medical science community worldwide.

At first, the publication of the homocysteine theory of arteriosclerosis had a positive impact on my chosen career of medical research. As explained in Chapter 4, I was given a research laboratory at MGH, one of the most coveted pieces of academic real estate anywhere. I was appointed Assistant Professor of Pathology at Harvard Medical School. For 11 years I was encouraged to conduct homocysteine research, to teach general pathology to medical students in the Harvard-MIT Program in Health Sciences and Technology, and to practice anatomic pathology in the Pathology Department of MGH. My discoveries of arterial plaque formation and thrombosis in animals given homocysteine, growth hormone promotion of normal and growth hormone-deficient animals by homocysteic acid, discovery of a new pathway for conversion of the sulfur atom of homocysteine to sulfate, and discovery of the blockade of this new pathway in cancer cells, all provided solid scientific evidence for the validity of the homocysteine theory of disease. Many invitations for presentation of my findings at local and national meetings soon followed.

After the retirement of my Department Chairman, Benjamin Castleman, in 1974, a distinct change occurred in support of my homocysteine research program. At first, in 1975 my laboratory was transferred out of the Pathology Department into a palatial laboratory space in the main research building tower at MGH. An article about my research program was published in the MGH Newsletter in 1976, featuring a photograph of me at my microscope. Soon thereafter, another investigator in heart disease research from the Cardiology Section of Medicine demanded my laboratory space, and I had no choice but to transfer my operation to a tiny, dreary, windowless, temporary laboratory space created in the basement of the Bulfinch Building, the original MGH building, which first opened in 1821.

All of these disastrous changes in my status as a medical investigator came without warning and without any explanation of the reasons for the change in political climate. It was very clear that the Harvard and MGH elders had decided to withdraw support of the medical establishment for continuation of my program of homocysteine research. Appeals to the Director of the MGH, Charles Sanders, the new Pathology Department Chairman, Robert McCluskey, and my former scientific mentors were without avail. It became obvious that continuation of my chosen career in medical research, despite all of my interesting discoveries, must continue, if at all, at another institution, as explained in detail in Chapter 5.

The medical establishment had rejected the importance of homocysteine research with a denial of tenure and punishment for a "crazy theory" which is a "hoax and errant nonsense," as described in an article in the *Boston Globe* quoting a rival investigator of the cholesterol theory of heart disease. This drastic rejection of my research discoveries jeopardized my research career and called into question my skepticism about the primacy of cholesterol in causing arteriosclerosis, my skepticism of the primacy of genetic changes in causing cancer, and my views on the origin of abnormal oxygen metabolism in aging. My personal reaction had changed from exhilaration and excitement over my discoveries to dejection and despair over my research career, despite a decade of enthusiastic and productive effort.

Medical science is an inherently conservative and cautious field of endeavor because so much is at stake, namely, understanding of the origin of disease and the health of individuals and populations. Those medical scientists who seek to understand the origin of disease by making new observations and explanations inevitably encounter the conservative opinions of the medical establishment defending traditional explanations of the origin of diseases. In the history of medical science, the reaction of the medical establishment to new concepts has often taken the form of ridicule, disbelief, and ostracism for new ideas.

Galen was an influential and prolific Greek physician and writer whose theories of the origin of diseases held sway from 200 AD until the birth of modern medicine in the Renaissance during the 15th and 16th centuries. The anatomical dissections of the human body that were conducted by Leonardo da Vinci and others at this time prepared the way for publication of the anatomical treatise, *Fabrica Corporis*, in 1543 by the Belgian physician Andreas Vesalius. His great work, based on surreptitious dissections of the human body at the University of Padua, helped to found modern medicine and to discard many of Galen's ideas as obsolete, overturning many of the ancient concepts of the origin of disease. A century later, William Harvey introduced the concept of circulation of the blood, and he, like Vesalius before him, suffered ridicule and ostracism for his new concept.

While my own observation concerning the origin of arterial disease in children with abnormal homocysteine metabolism could hardly be considered as momentous as the observations of Vesalius or Harvey in the history of medical science, nevertheless my story of discovery, rejection and ridicule, ostracism and eventual redemption seemed to follow these early examples. To me the reaction of the medical establishment against my ideas was perplexing because it seemed out of proportion to the cautious references to the importance of dietary fats and blood cholesterol that I had included in my 1969 article in the *American*

Journal of Pathology. My new ideas did not seem to me to be a threat to the multi-billion dollar pharmaceutical industry, the food and nutrition industry, or the cancer industry. Yet my expulsion from Harvard medicine suggested to some that my ideas were perceived as a threat to these powerful financial interests.

In his important analysis, *The Structure of Scientific Revolutions*, Thomas Kuhn points out that new paradigm shifts in science are accompanied by a pattern of discovery, ridicule and rejection, and ultimate acceptance by practitioners of science [6]. According to Kuhn, "a scientific theory is declared invalid only if an alternate candidate is available to take its place." Was my hypothesis capable of providing an alternative to the cholesterol hypothesis of the origin of arteriosclerosis? Was my discovery of such importance that it merited this treatment by the medical establishment? Would development of homocysteine research yield a medical revolution in understanding of the origin of arteriosclerosis, cancer and diseases of aging? Could investigation of this obscure amino acid, homocysteine, be of such importance that it would ultimately take its place as a milestone in the history of medical science?

References

[1] Shih VE, Efron ML. Pyridoxine unresponsive homocystinuria. Final diagnosis of MGH case 19471. *New England Journal of Medicine,* 1970;283:1206-1208. This case report describes the diagnosis of homocystinuria in the 9 year old niece of the case of her uncle with homocystinuria, as first published in 1933.

[2] Case Record of the Massachusetts General Hospital, Case 19471. Marked cerebral symptoms following a limp of three months' duration. *New England Journal of Medicine,* 1933;209:1063-1066. This is the first case of homocystinuria published in the medical literature. Although the disease homocystinuria was first discovered and described in 1962, this case was identified as the 8 year old uncle of a child diagnosed with homocystinuria in 1965.

[3] Mudd SH, Finkelstein JD, Irrevere F, Laster L. Homocystinuria: an enzymatic defect. *Science,* 1964;143:1443-1445. This study established deficiency of cystathionine synthase as the cause of the most common form of the inherited disease of methionine metabolism, homocystinuria.

[4] Mudd SH, Levy HL, Abeles RH. A derangement in the metabolism of vitamin B12 leading to homocystinuria, cystathioninuria, and methyl malonic aciduria. *Biochemical and Biophysical Research Communications,* 1969;35:121-126. This case report is the first in the medical literature describing cobalamin C disease.

[5] McCully KS. Vascular pathology of homocysteinemia: implications for the pathogenesis of arteriosclerosis. *American Journal of Pathology,* 1969;56:111-128. This report describes the discovery of arteriosclerotic plaques in the arteries of two different patients with homocystinuria, one with cystathionine synthase deficiency, and one with cobalamin C disease. The study concludes that homocysteine causes arteriosclerotic plaques in homocystinuria by a direct effect of the amino acid on the cells and tissues of the arteries. The hypothesis is presented regarding the importance of elevation of blood homocysteine in arteriosclerotic disease occurring in the general population without these rare inherited enzymatic abnormalities.

[6] Kuhn TS. *The Structure of Scientific Revolutions.* Chicago: University of Chicago Press, 1952. This important study of the philosophy of scientific revolutions emphasizes the shift in scientific paradigms by observation of new facts that cannot be explained by previous scientific theories.

Chapter 2

ORIGINS: FROM PIONEER ANCESTRY TO MEDICAL SCIENCE AT HARVARD

Harvard College 1951 fulfilled the aspiration of this 17-year-old boy to attend college at a diversified and prestigious institution that offered a strong liberal arts and science education. On a warm, sunny day in September, my first impression of the famous Harvard Yard revealed bustling activity of students like myself bringing personal necessities for their first year in college. I was assigned to one of the historic brick dormitories, Thayer Hall, opposite Memorial Church and Widener Library. My room-mate in our Spartan room was Lawrence Fane, who became a close friend during four years of college and later a prominent abstract sculptor at Queens College in New York [1].

There were several reasons for my arrival at Harvard College. An important reason was my knowledge that James Bryant Conant, President of Harvard, was a prominent chemist and scientific advisor to the Manhattan Project for construction and use of the atomic bomb as a weapon in World War Two. Conant had written a textbook *Practical Chemistry* for high school students with his teacher Newton Henry Black at Roxbury Latin School in Boston [2]. During my experiences as a boy scientist and chemist in Denver and Memphis, I had read a copy of the book and tried several of their simple experiments, focusing my interest on explosives and magnesium flares. It was not long before I met President Conant himself at a reception for Freshmen and during an encounter on a walkway in Harvard Yard. Conant was an intellectually exciting scientist. He had written a case study of the phlogiston theory for one of his courses, in which he explained how this theory of combustion was overturned when the discovery of oxygen and its properties by Priestly and Lavoisier became known to scientists in the late 18th century. The philosophical concept of paradigm shift in acceptance of scientific theories, as pointed out by Conant, was developed by a protégé, Thomas Kuhn, in his important study, *The Structure of Scientific Revolutions* [3]. Kuhn was a Junior Fellow at Harvard working with Conant while I was an undergraduate.

Another reason for attending Harvard was my interest in poetry, music and the visual arts. My interest in the arts was encouraged in my early years by my parents. My father, Cyrus Harold McCully, was a descendent of the Kilmer family, one of whom, Joyce Kilmer, was a prominent journalist and poet in New York in the early 20th century [4]. My father, the fourth child in a family of pioneers, was born on a ranch in Sheridan, Wyoming in 1906 (Figure 1) and attended Seventh Day Adventist schools in Colorado and Nebraska. He and my mother enjoyed poetry reading, singing, and music at home in the days before radio and television. My father also played the oboe and the violin in community orchestras in small town Nebraska in the 1920s.

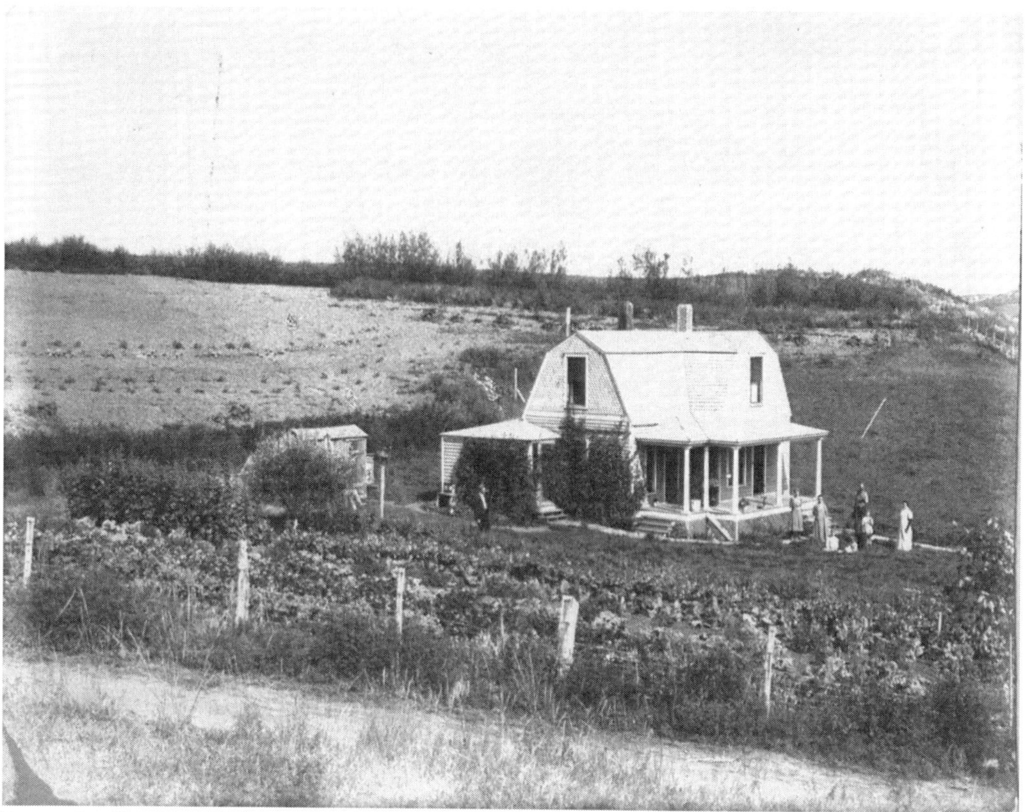

Personal collection of Kilmer McCully.

Figure 1. The 1902 Jim Creek Ranch of Sanford and Lily McCully is located near Sheridan, Wyoming. The photo is from 1910, showing the McCully family outside the home with the watermelon patch and garden in the foreground. Personal collection of Kilmer McCully.

My mother, Ludmilla (Lulu) Viola Litwinenco, was born in 1905 in a sod house on the pioneer family farm in Herreid, South Dakota (Figure 2)[5]. She was the eighth of nine children born to Ukrainian Russian immigrants who homesteaded the pioneer farm in 1890. Her interest in music and art was encouraged by my grandparents, Juda and Maria Litwinenco, during her childhood on the farm and at school in the Adventist Union College in Lincoln, Nebraska.

After my birth on December 23, 1933 in Daykin, Nebraska, my father enrolled in the Colorado State College of Education in Greeley during the Great Depression to complete his undergraduate and master's degrees in education. My parents had little money, and my father held teaching positions in small town Colorado, eventually becoming Dean of Students at Denver University in 1939. My mother had given me piano lessons as a young child in Denver, and after returning to Denver from Memphis, where my father served in the Navy in the 1940s, I started violin lessons, using a spare violin belonging to my father. My mother later became an artist, specializing in oils and watercolors of still life subjects and exhibited with the Northern Virginia Art Association. Influenced by our family's interest in the arts, my younger sister Marilyn Jane McCully became an art historian and authority on Picasso [6]. She now lives with her husband Michael Raeburn and their family in London, England.

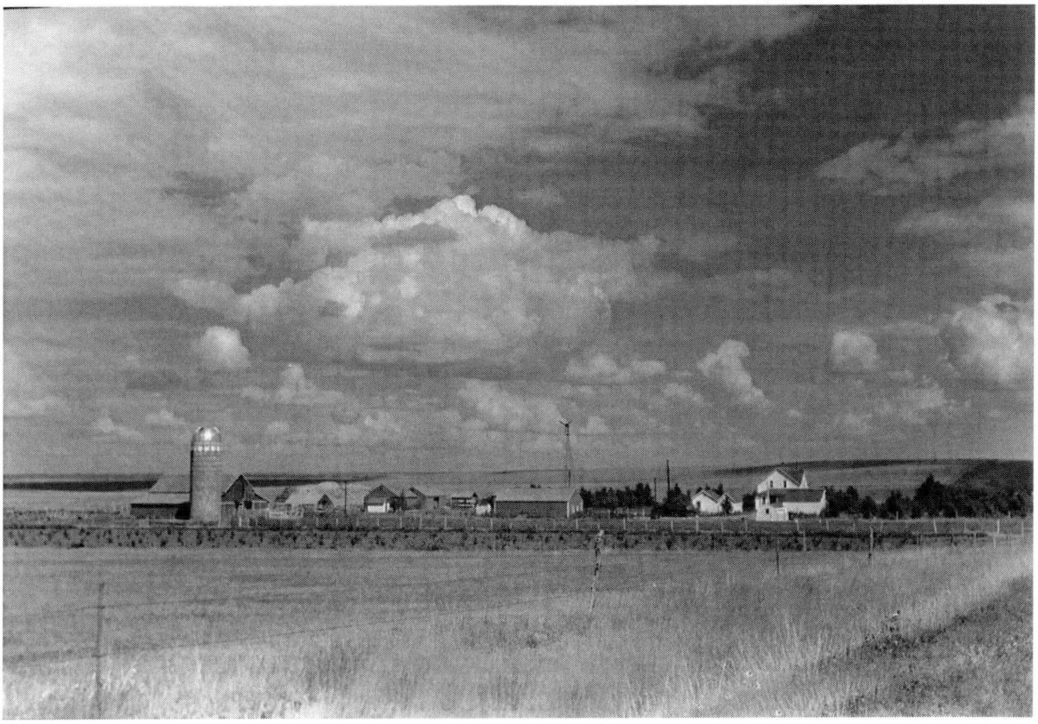

Personal collection of Kilmer McCully.

Figure 2. The 1890 homestead Spring Valley Farm of Juda and Maria Litwinenco is located near Herreid, South Dakota. The photo is from 1950 when it was owned by Glen and Elvina Tolstedt.

Harvard was recommended as a suitable college for me by a Harvard graduate friend of my father, since he knew of my record as valedictorian of the class of 1951 at George Washington High School in Alexandria, Virginia. When I was accepted at Harvard and awarded a scholarship by the Harvard Club of Washington DC, my college career was determined, even though I had never visited Harvard or Boston when I arrived there on the train from Washington in September 1951. President Conant had instituted a new policy of attracting students from a national pool of applicants after the Second World War, and I was a beneficiary of this new policy. I had previously been interested in attending Princeton University, but the co-ed status of Harvard, the strong musical traditions of Boston, and the generous scholarship helped me to decide on Harvard.

Harvard in 1951 was as intellectually lively as it had been in previous decades. The post-war group of student veterans had been graduated in 1947 and 1948. Many of my classmates, as I was, were attending college under a student deferment, and others were enrolled in Reserve Officers Training Corps. The Korean War had been raging for a year, and the Cold War with the Soviet Union had been increasing in intensity for five years, since the post-war confrontations between the USA under Truman, the UK under Churchill, and the USSR under Stalin. Yet in 1951 Harvard College had attained some semblance of its pre-war tranquility.

An increasing menace on the political horizon, however, was the publicity-seeking self aggrandizement of Senator Joseph McCarthy, who had begun his notorious campaign of hunting for communist sympathizers in Government, the film industry, and college campuses.

For my classmates and for me, the 17-year-old son of pioneer ranchers and farmers, these political conditions were a distant background noise in our excitement with life on the college campus. The rich cultural and intellectual environment of Harvard was much as it had been in previous generations of students [7]. In every aspect of campus life, stimulating opportunities presented themselves, and I was determined to make the most of them.

Because of an expressed interest in biochemistry, my assigned Freshman Advisor was Paul Zamecnik (Figure 3), a medical scientist who was in the midst of his prize-winning investigation of cellular protein biosynthesis in the Huntington Laboratory at Massachusetts General Hospital. Zamecnik encouraged me to take a broad selection of courses in science, the arts, and the humanities, even though I had expressed an interest in a career in medicine. He later became my advocate, mentor, and scientific collaborator, helping me to apply for admission to Harvard Medical School and later sponsoring my application for fellowships from the National Institutes of Health and the American Cancer Society. My course work for my first semester consisted of chemistry, mathematics, German and a humanities course under Conant's new curriculum, General Education in a Free Society, published by a Harvard faculty task force in 1948.

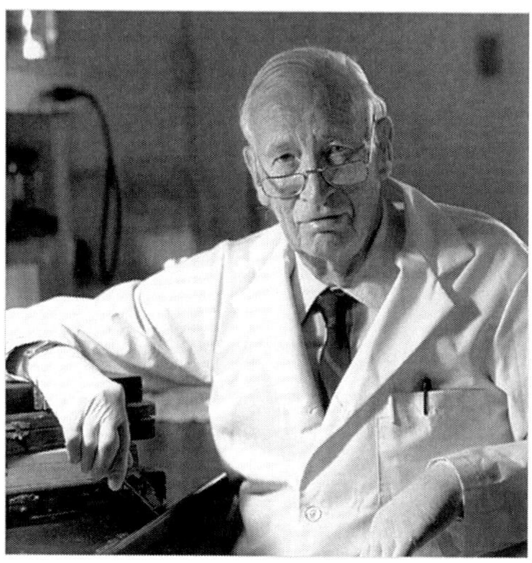

Courtesy of Mercer Photography/UMass Medical School.

Figure 3. Paul C. Zamecnik (1913-2009) was Professor of Oncologic Medicine at Harvard Medical School and Director of the Huntington Laboratories of Massachusetts General Hospital.

To combat a mild case of the Freshman Blues, I pursued my interest in music by auditioning as a violinist in the Harvard-Radcliffe Orchestra (Figure 4), conducted by an energetic free lance musician, Russell Stanger. In addition, I participated in chamber music and string quartet sessions coached by the beloved former conductor of the orchestra, Malcolm Holmes, who was, unknown to me, beginning to succumb to cancer. Making music in these two activities helped me to meet other students, overcome my home sickness, and adjust to college life. Later I was able to improve my proficiency of violin playing by studying with a fine teacher and violinist in the Boston Symphony Orchestra, Gaston Elcus, and, after graduation, by studying with Wolfe Wolfensohn, a fine violinist and pedagogue at the neighboring Longy School of Music in Cambridge. Wolfensohn once told me that I could make a career in music because of my talent for violin playing and possibly become a concertmaster of an orchestra. I had briefly considered music as a career for one day at the age of 15, but I was determined to keep music as an avocation, secondary to my interest in science and medicine.

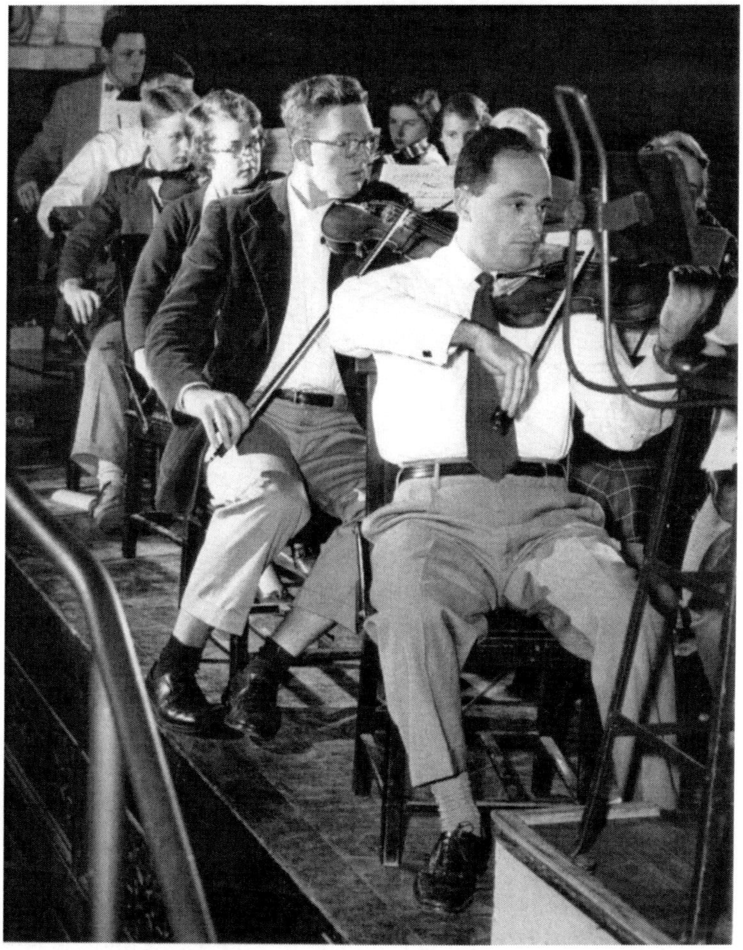

Personal collection of Kilmer McCully.

Figure 4. The Harvard-Radcliffe Orchestra is shown during rehearsal in 1952. From right to left the first three violinists are Sandor Shapiro, Kilmer McCully and Myrl Duncan.

During my three years with the Harvard-Radcliffe Orchestra, I became a member and Treasurer of the sponsoring organization, the Pierian Sodality of 1808, supposedly the oldest continuous musical organization in America. Two of the conductors of the orchestra were Richard Burgin, the concertmaster of the Boston Symphony Orchestra and Aaron Copland, who was a guest conductor in his incidental music to *Our Town*. In my senior year several of my classmates and I founded the Bach Society Orchestra, a chamber orchestra with a student conductor, which subsequently has had an illustrious following over the years.

During the spring term of our freshman year Larry Fane and I enrolled in a science course given by the brilliant young experimental psychologist, Burrhus Frederick Skinner [8]. In this course we were entranced by demonstrations of control of animal behavior by a system of rewards named "operant conditioning" by B.F. Skinner [9]. He showed how pigeons could be induced to play ping pong, among other demonstrations. Larry and I read his book *Walden Two* in which his psychological principles, including the "Skinner box" for child rearing, were applied to an imaginary utopian society [10].

Skinner was a frustrated writer and failed novelist, who turned to experimental psychology as a career at Harvard. He had a very clear understanding of the scientific method and used his insight to clarify the meaning of "mind" in behaviorist terms. To Skinner the mind was merely the description of the processes occurring in a "black box' which is the brain. The scientific method applied to behaviorist psychology consisted of creating conditions for an animal and observing the resulting effect on behavior.

Larry and I tried this approach on an unsuspecting room-mate, encouraging an unlikely interest in Georges Braque, an artist and cubist colleague of Pablo Picasso, by Skinner's "reinforcement techniques." Later I remember having a philosophical discussion about the meaning of causation in scientific experiments with Gerald Holton, a Harvard physicist and historian of science. Between Skinner's behaviorist concepts and Holton's understanding of causation in relating physical conditions one to another, I began to appreciate the power of the scientific method.

My father, Harold McCully, had turned in mid-life to study of educational psychology, receiving an EdD degree in Counseling Psychology from George Washington University while I was an undergraduate [11]. From this example and from Skinner's approach to behaviorist psychology, I decided to take more courses and switch my major to experimental psychology to pursue this interest. Coincidentally my course in biology was an introduction to biochemistry taught by George Wald, who later received the Nobel Prize for his studies on the biochemistry of vision. Biochemistry became so fascinating that I tried my hand at writing a multi-stanza poem regarding metabolism.

Discouraged with experimental psychology as a concentration major, I discussed a project that could combine my interests in science with my advisor, Paul Zamecnik. My first original concept for a scientific experiment was a proposal to study the effect of a brain metabolic poison, fluoroacetate, on animal behavior, using the operant conditioning techniques developed by Skinner. Zamecnik encouraged me to meet with Peter Dewes, a professor of pharmacology at Harvard Medical School, who was using Skinner's techniques to study the effect of drugs on animal behavior. This experiment was planned for my junior and senior years, but after some lengthy reflection, I decided to abandon this experiment and switch my major to chemistry so that I could undertake an intensive course in poetry analysis with the famous poet and playwright, Archibald MacLeish.

It was more than fifty years later that I met Phyllis Mullenix, a former toxicologist at the Forsythe Dental Research Institute in Boston, who had carried out the experiment that I had proposed in 1954. She was hired by Forsythe in 1984 to study the effects of various toxic materials used in dentistry, such as mercury and fluoride, on the behavior of animals, using the operant conditioning techniques of Skinner. Mullenix and her mentor Stata Norton of the University of Kansas Medical Center developed a computer-assisted method of quantifying changes in rat behavior by toxins by analysis of photographic images. Encouraged by Harold Hodge, a Consultant to Forsythe and the retired toxicologist from the Atomic Energy

Commission Laboratory of Toxicology at Rochester University, Mullenix used this powerful technique to demonstrate that moderate doses of fluoride had a profound effect on behavior, causing grossly abnormal reactions and preventing learning responses. As described in *The Fluoride Deception* by Christopher Bryson, the results of this experiment were met with derision and incredulity by the dental establishment, forcing Mullenix from her position at Forsythe and curtailing her scientific career [12].

While at Harvard, my own interest in poetry and writing were encouraged by contact with famous poets and writers. At Adams House where I was in residence, a poetry reading series was arranged by the house master and the senior tutor, Richard Wilbur, who later became Poet Laureate, and by President Conant, who was a friend of MacLeish. Visiting poets and scholars met with students, read from their works, and offered criticisms of student creations. At these sessions and at public lectures I was able to hear and meet many famous writers, including Robert Frost, Stephen Spender, Robert Lowell, and Dylan Thomas. When my own meager efforts at poetry were read by Wilbur and MacLeish, their advice was to pursue my interests in science and medicine. Years later, I met the writer John Updike, who had preceded me by one year at Harvard in the class of 1954. He confided to me that, while at Harvard, his application to MacLeish's creative writing course had been rejected, as mine was in my senior year.

Because of a long standing interest in history and biography, my junior year was partly occupied with a course in American history. The fall semester was devoted to study of the westward movement and settlement of western lands during the 18th and 19th centuries, affectionately dubbed "wagon wheels" by Harvard students and taught by Frederick Merk [13]. That course explained the context for my pioneer ancestry by the Kilmer family who arrived from London, England in Germantown, New York in 1709, the McCully family who arrived from Londonderry, Northern Ireland, in Truro, Nova Scotia in 1764, and the Litwinenco family who arrived from Odessa, Ukraine in Herreid, South Dakota in 1890. I later discovered that my great-great grand uncle, Jonathan McCully, a politician from Halifax, was a signatory of the Charlottetown Convention of 1864, a Father of Confederation and a founder of the country of Canada.

The Kilmer family is descended from German Protestant refugees who were driven from their homes in Kassel in Hesse, Germany in the late 17th century by the Catholic Sun-King, Louis XIV of France [4]. The Kilmer descendents settled around London and were sent by the British Navy to make turpentine from the forests of the New World. The Kilmer descendents became land grantees in New York near Rhinebeck after surviving the winter with the help of local natives, later migrating to New Brunswick, New Jersey, Philadelphia, Binghamton, and Ontario. My namesake great grandmother, Catherine Kilmer McCully, was a pioneer in Chatham, Ontario in the 19th century who married my great grandfather, Alfred McCully, the son of Cyrus McCully and Mary Tingley, a Mayflower descendent.

The Litwinenco family pioneered a farm in South Dakota, which remained in the family for 99 years, supporting three generations [5]. My grandfather Juda Litwinenco was a lay minister in the Adventist Church, and he was said to have befriended Chief Sitting Bull, who was killed on the Reservation in December, 1890. Partly from my experiences working on the farm as a teenager with my uncle Glen and aunt Elvina Tolstedt and my cousin Vern Tolstedt, I published an essay on Wheat in *Perspectives in Biology and Medicine,* describing the introduction of durum wheat in Dakota Territory from Ukraine by my grandfather and his friends [14].

The spring semester of my junior year at Harvard I studied the social history of America with Arthur Schlesinger Sr, and I learned about the social origins of the political movements of America in the 19th and 20th centuries. The next year in my senior year because of a need to earn some extra money to supplement my John Harvard Scholarship, I was offered a place as a "house boy" in the family home of the historian Arthur Schlesinger Jr. I worked with Marion Schlesinger during my senior year, helping with yard and house work, watching their children when the parents were away, and serving as a waiter at their many dinner parties at home [15].

At one of these dinner parties I helped to serve Reinhold Niebuhr, the elderly theologian. At another party I served Bernard DeVoto, the Harvard historian, a martini straight from SS Pierce, a Boston purveyor, rather than the 3.7:1 martini that he had specified in his column in *Harper's Magazine*. I did not have the opportunity to serve the junior senator from Massachusetts, John F. Kennedy, who had been a guest at the Schlesingers' dinner parties on other occasions.

Marion Schlesinger took an interest in my chemistry studies and my application to Harvard Medical School, because her father, Walter Bradford Cannon, was an illustrious physiologist and Dean at Harvard during the early 20th century. Arthur Schlesinger once commented to me about my professor of biochemistry, Konrad Bloch, that "the biochemists think that they can understand the secret of life."

My studies of chemistry were a consistent theme during my undergraduate years. In my freshman year I was treated to dramatic demonstrations of chemical reactions by Leonard Nash, using experiments taken from Black and Conant's book *Practical Chemistry* [2]. In my second year, the professor of organic chemistry, Louis Fieser, invited me and a dozen other students who were performing well in his course into his laboratory in the spring term. He said that he wanted his students to help him to verify a new method for purification of cholesterol that he had recently developed [16]. Fieser was a world class chemist specializing in polycyclic hydrocarbons and sterols, and he was noted for invention of the jellied gasoline weapon Napalm developed during the Second World War. Our task was to add bromine to cholesterol, re-crystallize the dibromo-cholesterol, and remove the bromine atoms with acetic acid, yielding pure cholesterol.

Some years later I met Bruce Taylor, a medical scientist at Albany Medical College, who had used Fieser's method to prove that highly purified cholesterol, protected from oxygen, had no effect on arteries of monkeys injected with or fed cholesterol. Taylor's group showed that oxidized derivatives of cholesterol, especially cholestane triol, hydroxycholesterol, and cholestanone, produced plaques in the arteries within 24 hours when administered to monkeys [17]. Fieser and one of his students, Allan Kliman, had begun similar experiments with rabbits, using cholesterol oxides to produce arterial plaques in the 1950s.

Because of my increasing interest in chemistry and biochemistry, I enrolled in an advanced organic chemistry course with Paul Bartlett in my junior year and in a course in advanced biochemistry with Konrad Bloch in my senior year. My other chemistry courses were analytical chemistry with JJ Lingane and physical chemistry with George Kistiakowsky and Paul Doty. Kistiakowsky, a friend and colleague of James Conant, was a White Russian explosives chemist who worked in Los Alamos on the Manhattan Project to produce the atomic bomb in the 1940s and later became Science Advisor to President Eisenhower.

As a result of these interests, my chemistry professors encouraged me to apply for a PhD program in chemistry at Harvard. However, in discussions with my advisor Paul Zamecnik, I decided to use my chemistry education in investigation of disease, after completing a medical degree. In my days as a boy scientist in Denver, I had read the fascinating book *Microbe Hunters* by Paul DeKruif and had been inspired to consider a career in medical science, emulating the great scientists, Koch, Pasteur, Ehrlich, Metchnikoff and others in their studies of the causation and treatment of disease [18]. To me these scientists and their discoveries represented accomplishments to which I could aspire in a medical research career. Paul Zamecnik, knowing of my interest in medical research, encouraged me to apply for admission to Harvard Medical School and said "it will not be necessary to apply to other medical schools."

During the summer of 1954 after my junior year, I decided to visit my girl-friend Annina Jacobs, who had transferred from Tufts University to UCLA two years previously and lived with her family in Camarillo, California. Paul Zamecnik helped me to find a position as a research assistant in the laboratory of James Bonner, a plant biochemist at the California Institute of Technology in Pasadena. My very first exposure to working in a basic research laboratory was to study the function of the plant growth hormone, indole acetic acid, in the growth of oats seedlings. The compound was labeled with carbon 14, and its uptake could be followed in the seedlings by using a Geiger counter. While at CalTech, I took the opportunity to attend seminars and lectures by some of their great faculty and visiting scientists. Linus Pauling discussed the amino acid replacement in the sickle cell hemoglobin molecule, Lazlo Zechmeister discussed polyterpenes and retinoids, and Melvin Calvin discussed carbon fixation in photosynthesis. After returning to Harvard in the fall, I heard Pauling give a lecture on the alpha helix structure of proteins. I was in awe of the accomplishments of these great scientists. I hoped that one day I would have the opportunity to use my knowledge and interest in chemistry and biochemistry to unravel the mystery of disease.

During my course in advanced biochemistry with Konrad Bloch, I learned of his pioneering experiments on cholesterol biosynthesis with Rudolf Schoenheimer. They used deuterated acetate to demonstrate that the cholesterol molecule is entirely constructed from acetate by a complex series of reactions in polyterpene synthesis [19]. These reactions include synthesis of mevalonate, isopentenyl and dimethylallyl pyrophosphate, geranyl pyrophosphate, farnesyl pyrophosphate, and squalene. Cyclization of squalene by oxidation produces a concerted reaction that yields the 4 rings of the cholesterol molecule.

I was so fascinated by the nature of this investigation that I approached Bloch about working as a student assistant in his laboratory during the summer of 1956 after my first year of medical school. My assignment was to purify the wool fat sterol lanosterol from pig liver by saponification with alkali, extraction of sterols by organic solvents, and purification by chromatography on activated alumina columns. I was permitted to use Professor Louis Fieser's special balance, mounted on a 60 foot column of granite, to weigh the miniscule amount of lanosterol that I had purified from kilograms of liver. Bloch was pleased when my repeat experiments were quantitative with 10% error [20].

During my four months in his laboratory, Bloch and I discussed other projects for me to design in the cholesterol field. Knowing of my interest in medicine, having completed my first year of medical school, Bloch told me that he had given up attending medical meetings on cholesterol because "the doctors do not understand how cholesterol participates in atherosclerosis." The work of Bloch's laboratory was supported by the Life Insurance Medical Research Fund that was predicated on the assumption that cholesterol causes heart disease and stroke. These experiences working in a world class research laboratory were exciting and fired my determination to pursue medical research when I completed medical school. Later I remember congratulating Konrad Bloch in his office after he had been awarded the Nobel Prize in Medicine in 1964 [19].

During my freshman year, one of my classmates, Paul Swartz, introduced me to Annina Elena Jacobs, a former classmate of his at Lynn English High School and now a freshman at Tufts University in nearby Medford. He said "you two should get along since your father is a psychologist and her father is a psychiatrist." On our first date, we indeed found an attraction for each other. Annina was a lively, attractive, vivacious girl, who finished near the top of her class at Lynn English High School. She was interested in drama, having participated in a state-wide drama festival and winning top honors in the state competition. At Tufts she was interested in French literature, music, and English. She later told me that, after our first date, she confided to her mother "that is the man I am going to marry!"

Annina's father, Salvador Jacobs, and her mother, Elisa Del Campo, were Italian immigrants who arrived in Boston as young children during the World War One period. Her father, who had little education and came from a poor family, attended Haverhill High School. He later attended college and medical school at Tufts University, supported by scholarships, graduating with the Tufts Medical School class of 1932. His name was changed from the Italian Jacobucci to an anglicized version Jacobs to ease his acceptance in New England society. Salvador Jacobs became a staff physician at the Danvers State Hospital in Danvers, Massachusetts in 1934, because his private patients could not afford to pay him during the height of the Great Depression. He later became a neuropathologist, studying as an apprentice with prominent neurologists and neuropathologists like Paul Yakovlev of Harvard, Houston Merritt, later of Columbia University, Raymond Adams of Harvard, and Muriel Canavan, later Commissioner of Health in Massachusetts. Later Salvador Jacobs studied psychiatry and became a founding Diplomate of the American Board of Psychiatry in the 1930s.

Annina's mother, Elisa Del Campo, came from a prosperous Italian immigrant family in Lynn, Massachusetts. Elisa's father, Jerome Del Campo, was a musician, music teacher, owner of a music store, and real estate investor, who became prosperous in the 1920s. Elisa attended Salem State Normal School in Salem, Massachusetts and became the first female teacher of Italian ancestry to teach in the public schools in Lynn. One of Elisa's brothers, Dante Del Campo, attended Boston University Medical School and later became a pediatrician in Texas. Dante was refused admission to Tufts Medical School, despite his precocious gifts as a student and musician, because, as he was told "the Italian quota is filled." Elisa's other brother Richard became a musician, her sister Ida married John Campello, an MIT graduate and engineer at Stone and Webster in Boston, and her other sister Elda married Charles Benedetti, a prominent psychiatrist who practiced in Lowell, Massachusetts for many years.

During the Second World War, Annina's family was affected because her father Salvador enlisted in the Army in 1943 at the age of 43. He was assigned to duty in Brownwood, Texas and Laughton, Oklahoma, eventually serving as a psychiatrist, living in a boxcar near the front lines in France in 1944 and 1945. My father Harold also enlisted in 1943 at the age of 37, serving as a director of the Navy Air Technical Training Center for navigators and bombardiers in Memphis in 1944 and 1945. Because of these war-time experiences, Annina and I shared vivid memories of living in the South and Southwest.

Our romance flourished because of our mutual attraction, the similarities of our family backgrounds, and our similar outlook on college life. Storm clouds appeared on the horizon, however, because of Annina's rearing as a Catholic and mine as a Protestant. My family hesitated to meet Annina, fearful that our relationship might jeopardize medical school attendance. Annina's mother and aunts, however, welcomed me during holiday events and supported our romance. Annina's father, meanwhile, had surprised his family by accepting a position as a psychiatrist in the State Hospital in Camarillo, California during Annina's freshman year at Tufts University. As a consequence, Annina transferred from Tufts to the University of California at Los Angeles for her final college years, while I was a student at Harvard College. For two years we corresponded by letters, and finally I decided to visit Annina and her family in California while I worked as a research assistant at CalTech during the summer of 1954. After Annina visited my family at Christmas, we decided to marry during the summer of 1955 after we had each completed college.

Annina was then as she is now a loving and steadfast wife, making a happy, stable and welcoming home during medical school, during my career vicissitudes, during my period of rejection by the medical establishment, and during the maturation of our two children, Michael Kilmer McCully and Martha Elizabeth McCully (Figure 5). By her energy, common sense, insight, and love of life, Annina helped me through my years of trial by establishing a happy, loving home life. My ultimate redemption and recognition by the medical establishment owe much to Annina's determination to provide a happy home life for me, our children and grandchildren.

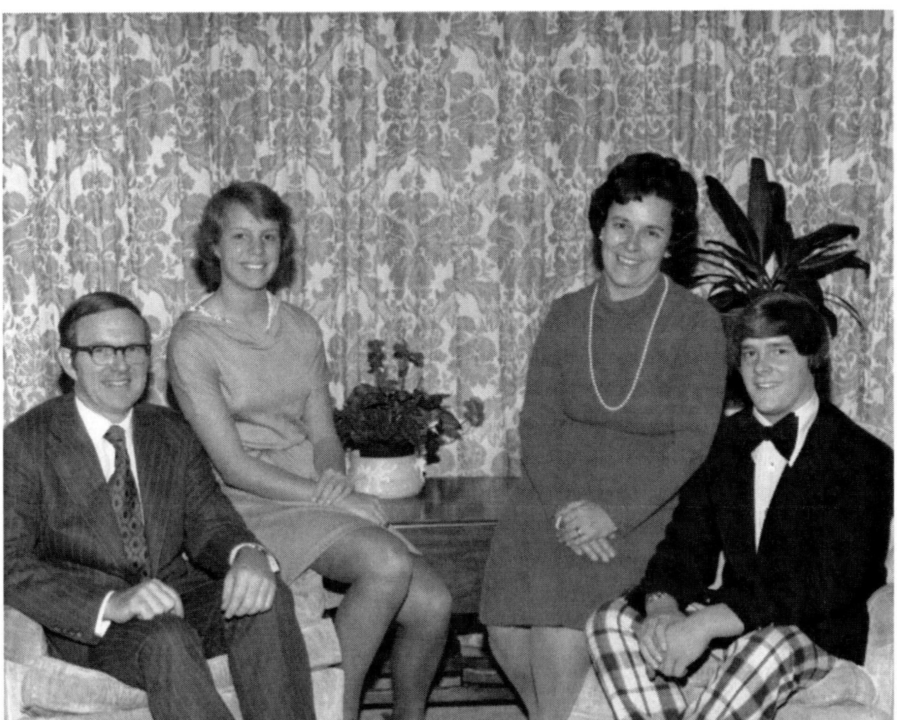

Personal collection of Kilmer McCully.

Figure 5. Kilmer and Annina McCully are shown in this 1973 photo with their children Michael Kilmer McCully and Martha Elizabeth McCully.

Our marriage was celebrated in the Appleton Chapel of the Harvard Memorial Church on August 14, 1955. The marriage service was performed by a Protestant Minister because negotiations with various Catholic Priests were unsuccessful. Part of the ceremony consisted of performances of an original organ prelude by a classmate of mine and a performance of a complete Bach Wedding Cantata by soloists, an orchestra of friends, and the Harvard Summer School Chorus. After a reception for friends and family, the newlyweds stayed in Cambridge to prepare for my attendance at Harvard Medical School and Annina's work in the personnel department of Gilchrist's Department Store in Boston.

Prior to our wedding, my summer employment took an unusual turn. Inquiring of the Civil Service Commission in Washington about summer jobs, the recruiter suggested that I could serve as a patent examiner in the US Patent Office. They gave me this opportunity because of my recently granted AB degree *magna cum laude* in chemistry from Harvard. At the Patent Office in the Department of Commerce in Washington, I participated in a three week training course which explained the history and laws governing patents, trademarks and copyrights. Thereafter, I was assigned to a senior patent examiner, who was my mentor in examining chemical patents covering chemical polymers such as Teflon and Rayon. When I left the position to prepare for my wedding and medical school matriculation, the Patent Office suggested that I should instead apply for admission to law school so that I could become a patent attorney. When I said that I was enrolled in medical school, they said that I could become a patent attorney after finishing medical school. I was kept on the rolls of the Patent Office as an unpaid employee for one year, in case I decided to change my career.

Harvard Medical School in 1955 was in a period of vigorous growth and adaptation to advances in basic fields of medical science under the leadership of the Dean, George Packer Berry, also a Professor of Bacteriology. Berry inspired students to combine an interest in basic science with applications to clinical medicine. It was apparent to me that my interest in chemistry and biochemistry could develop and flourish in the environment, as described in the book *Medicine at Harvard. The First Three Hundred Years* by Henry Beecher and Mark Altschule [21]. In subsequent years, Harvard Medical School has further developed into a world class colossus of medical education, medical research and clinical practice.

In contrast to some of my more clinically oriented classmates, I plunged into the first year basic science courses in anatomy, histology, physiology, and biochemistry with enthusiasm, learning the language and concepts of basic medical science. The second year courses of microbiology, pathology and pharmacology served to increase my enthusiasm, and I was thrilled to have John Enders, the Nobel Prize winner for polio virus cultivation, as one of my instructors. I also embarked on independent reading of recent developments in bioenergetics to continue my interest in basic biochemistry.

At one of the clinics for first year students, Frederick Stare described the experiments that he and his associates at the Harvard School of Public Health were conducting with monkeys concerning the origin of arteriosclerosis [22]. The monkeys were fed a synthetic diet of purified soy protein, vitamins, minerals, fiber, and sugar to which cholesterol was added. As part of their study they observed that the amino acid methionine caused a decrease in blood cholesterol levels and prevented plaque formation in the aortas of the animals. I was impressed by the emphasis on cholesterol in arterial diseases because of my study of cholesterol biosynthesis with Konrad Bloch during the previous year in college, and for that reason I applied for a position in his laboratory the following summer. It was 13 years later, as described in Chapter 3, that I returned to basic research on arteriosclerosis and its connection to homocysteine and methionine metabolism.

Partly because of my exciting experience in working in Bloch's laboratory during the summer of 1956, I approached Lewis Engel, a steroid biochemist at Massachusetts General Hospital about conducting an independent research project during my second and third years of medical school. The project involved analyzing the urinary metabolites of pregnenolone, a key steroid precursor of progesterone, by the newly developed method of countercurrent distribution analysis. Large volumes of urine from patients given pregnenolone were extracted and analyzed for evidence of conversion to the postulated intermediate, 17 alpha hydroxyl pregnenolone. Engel was enthusiastic about the project, but the results were not definitive, as described in a thesis that I submitted for honors with my medical degree. Engel suggested that I spend an extra year pursuing this study full time, but I declined because I was anxious to complete my degree and spend time later in full time post-doctoral fellowships. In addition, I found the area of steroid hormone research to be too narrow for my interests. My later research experience was influenced by learning basic concepts in this somewhat esoteric field.

An interesting requirement for the MD degree at Harvard in the 1950s was to complete a survey of the medical and public health resources and facilities of a community of the student's choosing. Through my wife's uncle, the psychiatrist Charles Benedetti, I was able to study and survey the medical facilities of Lowell, Massachusetts, where he had practiced for 15 years. My report was received enthusiastically by my mentor for the project, Dean Clarke, the Director of the Massachusetts General Hospital. Although the study was interesting, it reaffirmed that my interests were in basic medical research rather than in delivery of health care. The courses in Preventive Medicine with David Rutstein and in Legal Medicine with Michael Luongo, however, introduced me to statistical methods, epidemiology, and design of clinical studies, which helped me in my subsequent years in the field of atherosclerosis research.

During my third and fourth years of medical school, my studies of medicine, surgery, psychiatry and the subspecialties allowed my interest to expand more generally into clinical medicine. Partly because of my experience in cholesterol biosynthesis and steroid hormone research, I studied endocrinology for a month elective with John Crigler at Children's Hospital in Boston. Also I spent a fascinating month elective month as a sub-intern on the Neurology Service with Raymond Adams at Massachusetts General Hospital. I had another elective month on Hematology at Massachusetts General Hospital with William Beck, an expert on vitamin B12 metabolism. During my specialty rotations I was fortunate to study dermatology with Walter Lever at Massachusetts General Hospital, because I used this introduction in my later experiences in dermatopathology. During my surgery clerkship at Peter Bent Brigham Hospital, I was encouraged by Francis Moore, the Chief of Surgery, to consider an internship in surgery, but by my fourth year I had decided to apply for an internship in internal medicine. My experience in medicine and hematology was encouraged by learning about nutrition, vitamin B12 and pernicious anemia with William Castle, Charles Davidson, James Jandl, and Rudi Schmid of the Thorndike Laboratory at Boston City Hospital. Years later Charles Davidson told me that the Thorndike hematology group was cognizant of the significance of my discovery of the role of homocysteine in arteriosclerosis when it was published in 1969. By the end of eight years of education in college and medical school at Harvard, I was ready to enter internship and residency, rather than to attempt a PhD program in one of the fields of medical science.

In the spring of my fourth year of medical school I was delighted to learn that I was matched to my first choice of internship in medicine at Massachusetts General Hospital. My MD degree was awarded with honors, and I was admitted to Alpha Omega Alpha, the honorary medical fraternity. These qualifications and my interest in medical research helped me to secure this prized appointment. After graduation festivities were concluded in June, I began my internship on the Bulfinch medical ward at Massachusetts General Hospital on July 1, 1959. The medical resident with whom I shared my first two months of service was Robert Schimke, a brilliant clinician interested in basic medical research, as I was. Schimke later became a Professor of Biology at Stanford and won prestigious prizes and awards for his studies of protein catabolism.

In 1959 the medical internship at Massachusetts General Hospital consisted of 8 months of service on the medical wards, emergency ward, and private service, combined with one month each on Psychiatry, Neurology, Dermatology and Pediatrics. My 11 co-interns and I rotated among these services, meeting and working with the many outstanding physicians who attended and supervised resident responsibilities during the year. One of these physicians was John Stanbury, a thyroid specialist who pioneered the study of inherited diseases of the thyroid. He later co-authored the classic book on hereditary disease *The Metabolic Basis of Inherited Disease* and became a physician on the staff of Massachusetts Institute of Technology [23]. Other memorable physicians that I met during my internship were Paul Dudley White, the founder of American Cardiology, Edward Bland, Roman DeSanctis, Lloyd H (Holly) Smith, Jerome Gross, Alexander Leaf, and Kurt Isselbacher. The Chief of the Medical Service was Walter Bauer, a prominent rheumatologist who sponsored and mentored young physicians interested in combining basic medical science with academic medicine and medical practice.

During my year of medical internship I recall several medical triumphs of therapy, including a 65 year old man with acute bilateral pneumococcal pneumonia, a 5 year old child with hemophilus meningitis, and a 70 year old woman with pneumococcal meningitis, all of whom were saved by antibiotic therapy. Medical therapy was less impressive, however, for the many patients dying with metastatic cancer, for which little could be done beyond supportive measures and hospice care. During the year I was appalled at the many middle aged men and women admitted with acute heart attacks and stroke, frequently dying of complications of their underlying disease. My reaction to these experiences was a desire to find an area of medical research in which I could contribute to understanding the causes of cancer and arteriosclerosis.

My wife Annina and I had celebrated the birth of our first child, Michael Kilmer McCully in 1958 during my fourth year of medical school. During my internship year Annina again became pregnant and was due to deliver our second child, Martha Elizabeth McCully, in October 1960. Like many of my classmates, I had had a student deferment from the draft for 9 years and was now very likely to be drafted. The Korean War was over, the Cold War with the Soviet Union was heating up, but the Vietnam War had been postponed by President Eisenhower. Because of my interest in medical research and because of my draft status, I decided to leave my medical residency program and apply for active duty with the US Public Health Service, so that I could work in basic research full time at the National Institutes of Health in Bethesda, Maryland. I approached my former mentor, Konrad Bloch, who helped me to secure a position as Research Associate in the laboratory of Giulio Cantoni, one of his colleagues in biochemistry. Cantoni had recently been appointed as Chief of the Laboratory of Cellular Pharmacology in the National Institute of Mental Health. Cantoni was known for his discovery in 1953 of the important biochemical intermediate and co-enzyme, adenosyl methionine.

For all of these reasons and circumstances, I met with my Chief of Medicine, Walter Bauer, to discuss my plan. I explained to him that I had found the experience of medical internship to be stimulating and satisfying, but I wanted to take this opportunity to combine an experience in basic biomedical research with service in the US Public Health Service to satisfy my draft board, who was eager for me to enter a US military service. Bauer became upset that I would quit my internship immediately, but I re-assured him that I was quite interested in completing my year of training before leaving for the National Institutes of Health in July 1960.

REFERENCES

[1] Lawrence, Fane. *Machines of the Mind. Sculptures of Lawrence Fane.* Richmond: University of Richmond catalogue, 2002. Lawrence Fane was a private school graduate from Kansas City, the son of a prominent attorney. As room-mates, Larry and I became quite close because of our mutual interests in art, music, medicine and psychology. Larry was a pre-med student, but after acceptance to Washington University Medical School, he decided that he would become an artist and sculptor. He studied at the Boston Museum School and with George Demetrious of Rockport, Massachusetts before winning the Rome Prize and specializing in abstract sculpture. He was Professor of Fine Arts at Queens College in New York for many years and died in 2008 at the age of 75.

[2] Black, NH, Conant JB. *Practical Chemistry.* New York: Macmillan, 1934. This primer in high school chemistry was written by James Conant and Henry Black, Conant's teacher of chemistry at Roxbury Latin School in Boston, in order to interest students in the practical aspects of chemistry. Conant became an outstanding physical organic chemist at Harvard before he was appointed President of Harvard in 1933. One of Conant's faculty members, Leonard Nash, used some of the experiments from this book to excite Harvard freshmen about chemistry. One of the experiments was to inflate soap bubbles with hydrogen gas and ignite them with a spark to cause a loud explosion in the lecture hall. In repeating some of these experiments as a boy scientist in Denver and Memphis, my specialties were to ignite paper with sulfuric acid and potassium permanganate crystals, making firecrackers with black powder made from potassium nitrate, charcoal and sulfur, and igniting magnesium flares with burning black powder. I survived these experiments and an unsuccessful attempt to synthesize nitroglycerin from nitric acid and glycerin.

[3] Kuhn TS. *The Structure of Scientific Revolutions.* Chicago: University of Chicago Press, 1962.

[4] Kilmer CH. *The History of the Kilmer Family in America.* Elmira NY: Advertiser Association, 1897. The introduction of this genealogical book recounts the dramatic circumstances surrounding immigration of Johannes Kűhlmer and his family to the Hudson Valley in Germantown, New York in 1709. The name was anglicized to Kilmer in subsequent generations. The Kilmer family became land owners through a land grant from the King of England. Their descendants migrated widely throughout America, and many of them became ministers, doctors, and pharmacists. A prominent medicinal chemist, Frederick B. Kilmer, became Vice President and Director of Research at Johnson and Johnson Company in New Brunswick, New Jersey in the late 19th century. His son was Joyce Kilmer, a prominent journalist and poet in New York City, who was killed by a sniper's bullet on the last day of World War One in 1918.

[5] Tolstedt GL, Tolstedt V. *Seven Miles West of Herreid, South Dakota.* Rockford IL: Private publication, 1998. This book recounts the founding of the Spring Valley farm in 1890 by Juda and Maria Litwinenco near Herreid, South Dakota. The farm grew to 1000 acres and supported three generations of Litwinenco descendants until it was sold in 1989.

[6] Richardson J, McCully M. *Picasso. A Life. Volume 1 The early years.* New York: Random House, 1992. My sister Marilyn McCully is the art historian collaborator for this multi-volume biography of Picasso.

[7] Schlesinger A. *Veritas. Harvard College and the American Experience.* Chicago: Ivan R. Dee, 2005.

[8] Bjork DW. *B.F. Skinner, a life.* New York: HarperCollins, 1993.

[9] Skinner BF. *Schedules of Reinforcement.* New York: Appleton-Century-Crofts, 1957.

[10] Skinner BF. *Walden Two.* New York: MacMillan, 1948.

[11] McCully CH, Miller LL. *Challenge for Change in Counselor Education.* Minneapolis: Burgess, 1969. This collection of my father's essays and speeches, edited by Lyle Miller, describes his views of the philosophical basis for student counseling. He was Director of the Counseling Service for the Veterans Administration in the 1950s and later Specialist in the US Office of Education until his death in 1965.

[12] Bryson C. *The Fluoride Deception.* New York: Seven Stories Press, 2004. This book describes the important experiments of Phyllis Mullenix showing the neurotoxic effects of fluoride and the rejection of her discoveries by the dental and public health establishment.

[13] Merk F. *History of the Westward Movement.* New York: Knopf, 1978.

[14] McCully KS. The significance of wheat in the Dakota Territory, human evolution, civilization and degenerative diseases. *Perspectives in Biology and Medicine,* 2001;44:52-61. This article describes the settlement of Spring Valley farm near Herreid, South Dakota in 1890 by my grandparents, Judah and Maria Litwinenco and their three children, who had emigrated from Odessa, Ukraine. Durum wheat kernels were smuggled into New York in the pockets of my grandfather's overcoat, because his Ukrainian Russian friends told him that the climate of South Dakota is similar to that of Ukraine and would support growth of "macaroni wheat." The article also describes how milling of wheat leads to losses of micronutrients, including folic acid and pyridoxine, leading to nutritional deficiencies and degenerative diseases.

[15] McCully KS. Dinner with the Schlesingers. *The Culinary Times*, XVII, No. 2, fall 2007. This article describes my experiences as a "house boy" with Arthur and Marion Schlesinger during my senior year at Harvard.

[16] Fieser LF. Cholesterol and companions. VII Cholesterol dibromides. *Journal of the American Chemical Society*, 1953;75:5421-5422. This publication describes Fieser's important method for purification of cholesterol that was used by C. Bruce Taylor to demonstrate the inability of pure cholesterol to produce arterial plaques in animals.

[17] Peng S-K, Taylor CB. Cholesterol autoxidation, health and arteriosclerosis. *World Review Nutrition-Dieta,* 1984;44:117-154. This article describes the toxicity of cholesterol oxides in cells and tissues, the atherogenic effect of cholesterol oxides, and the inability of pure cholesterol to produce arterial plaques in animals.

[18] DeKruif P. *Microbe Hunters*. New York: Harcourt Brace, 1926.

[19] Bloch K. The Biological Synthesis of Cholesterol. *Nobel Lectures*, December 11, 1964.

[20] Gautschi F, Bloch K. On the structure of an intermediate in the biological demethylation of lanosterol. *Journal of the American Chemical Society*, 1957;79:684-689. A footnote to this article describes the quantitative isolation of lanosterol from pig liver by KS McCully.

[21] Beecher HK, Altschule MD. *Medicine at Harvard. The First Three Hundred Years.* Hanover, NH: University Press of New England, 1977. This book describes the rich intellectual environment of Harvard Medical School and the affiliated medical centers during the period when I was a student from 1955-1959.

[22] Mann GV, Andrus SB, McNally A, Stare FJ. Experimental atherosclerosis in Cebus monkeys. *Journal of Experimental Medicine*, 1953;98:195-218.

[23] Stanbury JB, Wyngaarden JB, Frederickson DS. *The Metabolic Basis of Inherited Disease.* 7th Ed. New York: McGraw-Hill, 1960. This classic text is now in its 7th Edition and describes the explosion of information about genomic medicine and disease. An important chapter on homocystinuria was written by S. Harvey Mudd in the 6th edition, describing the metabolic origin of this disease.

Chapter 3

DISCOVERY: THE AMINO ACID HOMOCYSTEINE IS IMPLICATED IN HEART DISEASE, CANCER AND AGING

Louis Pasteur's famous aphorism "Chance favors the prepared mind" is emblazoned on the vestibule wall of Vanderbilt Hall, the student residence at Harvard Medical School, located on Avenue Louis Pasteur in the Longwood section of Boston. Students and faculty alike are reminded when they read this aphorism that the key to discovery lies in the intellectual preparation of the mind of the discoverer. Chance, on the other hand, presents itself unexpectedly only to the discoverer. The scientist who has inadequate or inappropriate knowledge of a field will not be able to recognize a chance opportunity when presented and will not be able to make a discovery in medical science.

Scientific education and training for medical investigators typically follows a medical degree or a doctoral degree in medical science in the form of post doctoral fellowships. These research fellowships allow the young scientist to work with a senior scientist who acts as a mentor, introducing his younger colleague to his field of interest. Typically the senior scientist chooses a project or question to be answered by the research fellow. The advantage of this apprentice system is that the fellow becomes acquainted with the current state of knowledge in a particular field of medical research. The disadvantage is that the mentor expects the fellow to investigate some aspect of the conventional wisdom of a field, rather than to allow the fellow's creativity and curiosity to select the subject for study. In medical research the most difficult problem for the young scientist is selection of an appropriate question to answer.

Most problems and questions in a field of study have already been considered by thousands of other scientists. What is lacking is the creative insight to ask an important new question that can be answered by the available resources. The most apt description of the process of discovery was phrased by Albert Szent-Gyorgi, the discoverer of ascorbic acid, who said that "discovery is to see what everyone else has seen, but to think what no one else has thought [1]." This quote describes the creative imagination needed by the research fellow to ask a new question that is pertinent and can be answered by the resources at hand. When a chance observation is made by a scientist with a prepared mind, discovery is possible, but creative imagination is also necessary.

The scientific climate in 1960 was heavily influenced by the surprise launch of the sputnik satellite, the first artificial satellite in history, by the Soviet Union in 1957. Politicians and scientists were concerned that American science was falling behind Soviet science, potentially affecting the outcome of the Cold War. Accordingly, the 1960s were a period of expansion of basic science funding by the US Government. Those physicians and science graduates who were interested in opportunities for fellowships in basic medical science found it possible to seek research training by this means.

Working at the National Institutes of Health in the 1960s was an ideal opportunity for young physicians and scientists to gain experience and training in basic medical research, and many resident physicians at the Massachusetts General Hospital took advantage of this opportunity. In my case, this experience was a more attractive alternative than pursuing a PhD degree at a university, since active duty in the US Public Health Service, while working at the National Institutes of Health, would fulfill my draft board's requirement for two years of military service. In addition, the prospect of a modest salary was appealing, after nine years of education and internship experience. I contacted my previous mentor Konrad Bloch about securing one of these coveted positions at the National Institutes of Health, and he recommended working as a Research Associate in the laboratory of Giulio Cantoni at the National Institute of Mental Health.

My assignment for active duty with the US Public Health Service was to serve as a Research Associate in Biochemistry with Cantoni in his Laboratory of Cellular Pharmacology. During the 1950s Giulio Cantoni was recruited by the National Institutes of Health from Case Western Reserve University to direct a new program in basic medical research because of his discovery of the important co-enzyme of biological methylation, adenosyl methionine [2]. Cantoni was a medical graduate and refugee from Fascist Italy in 1939, who discovered this compound while working as a research fellow in the laboratory of Severo Ochoa at New York University.

When I reported for duty in Bethesda in July 1960, Cantoni was away on a sabbatical residence in Italy, and he had arranged for Maxine Singer, a biochemist in Leon Heppel's laboratory, to introduce me to methods of enzyme purification and assay of ribonuclease, an enzyme that hydrolyzes ribonucleic acid (RNA) to its constituent nucleotides. When Cantoni returned, my assigned project was to purify the T1 takadiastase ribonuclease from the fungus *Aspergillus oryzae*. This enzyme cleaves RNA adjacent to guanyl nucleotides of the molecule. Having worked with Singer on the structure of a newly discovered RNA molecule of importance in protein biosynthesis called soluble RNA, later called transfer RNA, Cantoni was interested in developing a method for determining the sequence of nucleotides in this molecule.

Transfer RNA was discovered by Robert Holley in 1956 while working as a research fellow in the laboratory of James Bonner at CalTech, the same laboratory in which I had worked as a student in 1954. Holley discovered that the process of activation of amino acids by ATP during protein biosynthesis was inhibited by ribonuclease [3]. During cellular protein synthesis, each transfer RNA molecule forms a complex with a different amino acid, which in turn is donated to the growing polypeptide chain of protein within ribosomal RNA. This process of protein biosynthesis was elucidated by Paul Zamecnik and his co-workers in his laboratory at Massachusetts General Hospital in the 1950s. Each transfer RNA molecule is considered to have a coding sequence of nucleotides that can recognize a specific amino acid that is bound to its activating enzyme. The amino acid transfer RNA complex is also considered to contain a separate coding sequence of nucleotides, the anti-codon, which can recognize the genetic code of messenger RNA. Messenger RNA is copied from the genetic code of DNA, directing the sequence of amino acids within the polypeptides of proteins. This whole process of translating the DNA genetic code into the amino acid sequences of proteins was dubbed the "central dogma" of molecular biology. By determining the nucleotide sequence of transfer RNA, Cantoni and many other investigators hoped to understand how its molecular structure dictates deciphering of the genetic code.

Using my preparation of purified takadiastase T1 ribonuclease, Cantoni and I treated transfer RNA from rabbit liver to determine whether all of the linkages adjacent to guanyl nucleotides had been cleaved. We discovered that the methylated bases of transfer RNA are resistant to this enzyme and published these results as my first published article in the scientific literature [4]. By combining T1 ribonuclease with pancreatic ribonuclease that cleaves RNA adjacent to uridine and cytosine nucleotides, we then separated the various resulting oligonucleotides by column chromatography, determined that the nucleotide sequence of transfer RNA is non-random, and assembled the data to produce a model sequence of the nucleotides of transfer RNA [5]. This model sequence employed a loop and Watson-Crick base pairing to form a rod shaped molecule containing a single loop.

Using the same approach, Robert Holley and his research group at Cornell determined the nucleotide sequence of highly purified alanine transfer RNA and proposed a clover leaf model of the molecule, as described in his Nobel lecture in 1968 [3].

On one memorable occasion I had the opportunity to demonstrate my sequence model of transfer RNA to Leo Szilard, the famous physicist who was visiting Cantoni's laboratory. Szilard was the inventor of the atomic bomb, having conceived of the idea of a nuclear chain reaction within a critical mass of purified uranium 235 in 1939. After the bomb had been exploded over Hiroshima and Nagasaki, Japan in 1945, Szilard became disillusioned with nuclear physics and turned to investigation of microbial physiology, inventing a feed-back process for growing bacteria. Szilard was interested in my model, and we discussed the theoretical change in entropy when transfer RNA molecules become oriented to the codons of messenger RNA.

While working at the National Institutes of Health, the intellectual atmosphere was stimulating because of the presence of many outstanding scientists, such as Earl Stadtman, Gordon Tompkins, Christian Anfinsen, Bruce Ames, Maxine Singer, Seymour Kety, Leon Heppel, Alan Mehler, Jules Axelrod, and Marshall Nirenberg. I attended many lectures and seminars by these scientists and other visiting scientists during my two years there. I also attended Earl Stadtman's legendary course in bacterial physiology and biochemistry. Once per week Cantoni and his associates, Harvey Mudd, Seymour Kaufman, Samuel Luborski, Werner Klee, and Kenji Tanaka held a journal club seminar at which a current article of interest was dissected and discussed. At these seminars there were many discussions concerning adenosyl methionine, methionine and homocysteine, the sulfur amino acids being investigated by Mudd and other members of Cantoni's laboratory. These discussions amounted to an intensive course on the biochemistry of sulfur amino acids.

Before leaving Cantoni's laboratory in 1962, I had arranged to work as a member of Paul Zamecnik's laboratory in Boston for one year as a post doctoral fellow. Zamecnik's team had developed a method for purification of a single transfer RNA molecule from yeast RNA. The plan was to use my method of ribonuclease cleavage and oligonucleotide analysis to determine the nucleotide sequence of their purified transfer RNA. However, when I arrived, I was disappointed to find that Zamecnik's method had failed to produce a significant quantity of highly purified transfer RNA for these experiments. Holley's team at Cornell used counter-current distribution to purify yeast alanine transfer RNA, and they were already using the takadiastase T1 ribonuclease method for determining its nucleotide sequence.

Paul Zamecnik acknowledged that my transfer RNA sequencing project was not a viable option for my fellowship and instead encouraged me to investigate site-specific chemical mutagenesis, a subject that he had studied with Lord Todd in England. Several experiments were completed with hemi-sulfur mustard gas, a highly reactive carcinogen. After studying some of the current literature in the carcinogenesis field, I had serious doubts whether this line of investigation would illuminate the idea that carcinogenesis and abnormal oxidative metabolism of cancer cells are causally related to DNA mutations. Therefore, instead of pursuing this field or the highly competitive field of transfer RNA structure, I decided to study the structure of polyribosomes using ultracentrifugation of purified liver extracts.

Another research fellow in the laboratory, Robert Allen, was also studying polyribosomes. When I suggested to Allen that ribonuclease cleavage would alter the pattern of polyribosome migration because of hydrolysis of messenger RNA, he performed the experiment and published the results with Zamecnik. My name was not included as co-author and there was no acknowledgement of my contribution. When I complained to Zamecnik about this oversight, he told me "that is the way scientific discoveries are published." I had also learned from Cantoni that "if results are not published, they are not research." The lesson I learned from this episode was that in the future I would publish my research results independently under my name before sharing them with colleagues.

Meanwhile, I had discussed with Zamecnik my desire to spend a year with Guido Pontecorvo, Professor of Genetics at Glasgow University, to expand my knowledge of genetics. Because of my Harvard connections, I secured a nomination to the Society of Fellows at Harvard University to support my year of fellowship in Zamecnik's laboratory and my trip to Scotland the next year. When I traveled to Cambridge from Bethesda in 1962 for interviews, I met with several prominent scientists, including Carol Williams, the experimental entomologist at Harvard, and Francis Crick, the discoverer of DNA structure with Watson and Wilkins. At the meeting Crick asked me to describe how I would design experiments to develop a theory of aging. One of the popular ideas about aging in the 1960s was that somatic mutations led to an accumulation of the wrong amino acids in proteins because of a mistaken reading of the genetic code. My work on the structure of transfer RNA seemed pertinent to this hypothesis, but I was disappointed with my lack of detailed knowledge of the process of aging.

Since I was not selected for the Junior Fellow program at Harvard, Paul Zamecnik encouraged me to apply for a five year Faculty Research Award from the American Cancer Society. After my year in Glasgow with Pontecorvo, I would be given the opportunity to work in James Watson's laboratory in the Biology Department at Harvard. This plan was appealing because of the general excitement in the scientific community about research in molecular biology following the dramatic solving of the molecular structure of DNA by Watson and Crick in 1953.

Arriving in Glasgow, Scotland in September 1963 with Annina and our two young children for my fellowship year in genetics was an exhilarating and stimulating experience. We had never traveled to Europe, we had to cope with learning the Glaswegian accent, the money was too large, the cars were too small and drove on the left hand side of the road, and our house was heated only by coal fireplaces. We rented a semi-detached house, surrounded by a lovely walled garden, overlooking the Clyde River in Old Kilpatrick, a suburb of Glasgow, from a professor on sabbatical in Africa. Our neighbors, my associates at the university, and the Scots in general were gracious, charming, friendly and interested in meeting our visiting American family.

Guido Pontecorvo (Figure 6) was an Italian scientist and refugee from Fascism, who arrived in Scotland in 1939 to study genetics at the University of Edinburgh. One of Ponte's brothers, Bruno Pontecorvo, was a nuclear physicist in Russia, another brother was an engineer in America, and the youngest brother became a film producer in Italy after the Second World War. Ponte, as everyone called him, was a brilliant microbial geneticist, who was selected to found a new Department of Genetics at Glasgow University in the 1940s. His research on the fine structure of the genes of the fungus *Aspergillus nidulans* was widely praised and described in his recent book *Trends in Genetic Analysis* [6]. I first heard Ponte lecture on his research findings when I was a Research Associate at the National Institutes of Health in 1962. Ponte was a charming and erudite biologist with a comprehensive knowledge of botany, classical and molecular genetics. His department was known for its advances in the field of molecular genetics and attracted a national and international collection of scientists and research fellows. Besides me, another American, Gordon Dorn, a Russian, Alexander Peckov, and several other Scottish and English scientists were working with Ponte on microbial and human genetics in his department.

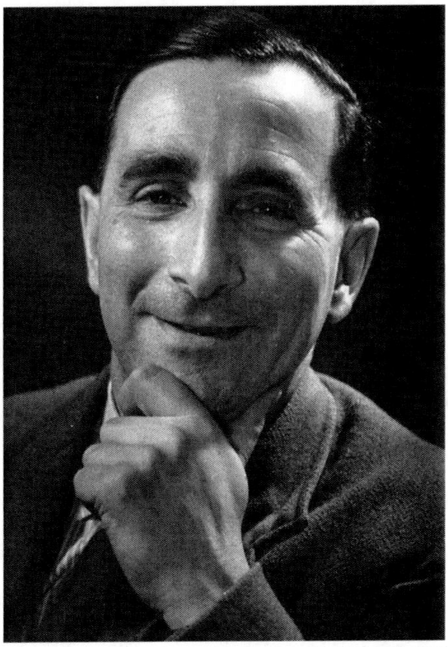

Courtesy of Glasgow University Archive Services, Ref. GB 0248 UPI-507-1.

Figure 6. Guido Pontecorvo (1907-1999) was Professor and founder of the Department of Genetics at Glasgow University from 1955 to 1968.

My project, as mutually agreed with Ponte, was to devise a way to select for mutants of transfer RNA and then to use the powerful methods of microbial genetics to study the detailed structure of the DNA genes that code for the transfer RNA molecule. First, however, I needed to learn the techniques of studying the genetics of *Aspergillus nidulans*. Ted Forbes, Ponte's chief assistant, had developed strains of *Aspergillus* that contained mutant markers on each of the eight chromosomes of the organism. My task was to combine these various strains into a single "master strain" that contained a mutant marker on each of its eight chromosomes. In this way, a new mutant could be assigned to a location on a particular chromosome by determining which of the known markers of the master strain did not segregate freely with the new mutant in haploidization of a created diploid strain. This method was perfected successfully and published in *Genetical Research* in 1965 to Ponte's and my pleasure [7].

The selection of mutants that are resistant to para-fluorophenylalanine, a toxic analogue of methionine, proved to be the wrong way to select for transfer RNA mutants, since all of the mutants that I studied proved to be resistant to the analogue because of impaired cellular transport of the analogue into the fungal cells. Some years later, Sydney Brenner, whom I met briefly during one of his visits to Glasgow, devised a successful way to select for transfer RNA mutants. By that time, however, Robert Holley had successfully completed his classic determination of the nucleotide sequence and structure of alanine transfer RNA by the T1 ribonuclease method, and genetic methods were not needed to determine its nucleotide sequence. In addition, later studies showed that many transfer RNA genes are located on mitochondrial DNA, further complicating the rationale for Ponte's and my approach to the problem.

One of the most delightful aspects of working with Ponte was the opportunity to discuss and question basic principles of genetics and molecular biology during our leisurely daily luncheons at the Glasgow University Faculty Club. My questions regarding fundamental genetics were patiently answered by Ponte, providing me with a year long course in the field. In addition, other faculty members in other science departments frequently joined Ponte, me and others for tea or coffee after lunch for wide-ranging discussions of science. Visiting scientists also gave seminars in the Genetics Department or at the Virology Research Department in the next door building in Glasgow University. The easy pace and style of academic life and scientific research in Glasgow contrasted with the intensive and frenetic style which characterized my experiences at the National Institutes of Health and Harvard.

Returning home to Boston in the fall of 1964 after my wonderful and stimulating year in Ponte's lab in Glasgow was a challenge and a shock to me and my family. We had become accustomed to the quiet, friendly and genteel world of Europe and Scotland with our beautiful view of ships on the Clyde River from our front window and my leisurely luncheons with Ponte discussing the latest advances in genetics and molecular biology. Because of its proximity to Cambridge and Watson's laboratory at Harvard University, we decided to live in Winchester, a suburb of Boston, so that our son could start elementary school in the fall and the family could re-adjust to the pace of American life. To this day we still reside in Winchester in an antique 1883 Victorian style house that we purchased in 1965.

Working with James Watson at Harvard in 1964 with one of the most famous scientists in the world was daunting. Much was expected of me, having published research articles on transfer RNA structure with Giulio Cantoni, sponsored by Paul Zamecnik, a leader in the field of protein biosynthesis, and having worked with Guido Pontecorvo, one of the leading geneticists of the world. Watson was most gracious and welcoming to me, taking me to lunch for a quiet discussion of my future plans for the year, and arranging for me to organize a seminar series for his Department.

Watson had been a precocious teenager and college student interested in ornithology. He told me that after he was rejected for his PhD studies at more prestigious universities, he settled at Indiana University where he became interested in studying genetics with Savatore Luria in their prominent biology department. After receiving his PhD in biology, Watson secured a post doctoral position in the Carlson Laboratories in Copenhagen. He angered the sponsors of his fellowship when he abruptly quit his studies and left Denmark for Cambridge University in England where he began his famous studies with Francis Crick and Maurice Wilkins on DNA structure [8,9].

Watson's experiences led to his rules for success in science [10]. His first rule is to study with superb scientists who are winners in the intense competition in the world of science. His second rule is to take risks by exploring a new unrecognized approach to a significant problem. In taking this risk, a scientist has to be prepared to "get into deep trouble." because colleagues and rivals will tell you that you are "very likely to be unqualified to succeed." This risk taking often leads to criticism because "your very willingness to take on a very big goal will offend some people who will think that you are…crazy." Watson's third rule is to have scientific allies "who will save you when you find yourself in deep [trouble]." Max Perutz and John Kendrew of Cambridge University saved Watson when his American fellowship was cut off for tackling the DNA structure problem. Watson's fourth rule is "never do anything that bores you." You must persist with a scientific problem that is exciting and appealing to you. As Louis Pasteur once said, "the scientist's most precious possession is his enthusiasm" for investigating a problem that interests him. Because the scientist who takes risks is likely to encounter criticism and ridicule, it is necessary to turn to experts who have knowledge in other fields for advice and to "constantly expose your ideas to informed criticism."

My situation in Watson's Department was tenuous. My strategy for selecting transfer RNA mutants of *Aspergillus* was unsuccessful, and Robert Holley was successfully using methods for transfer RNA nucleotide sequence analysis that I had studied with Cantoni. The other members of Watson's group, Walter Gilbert, Mark Ptashne, and Mario Capecchi, among others, were interested in applying the latest techniques of molecular biology to understanding genetic expression in micro-organisms. I began to feel that I had lost sight of my original goal for medical science as a career, using my knowledge of science to study the cause of human diseases. With my prospects for using Ponte's *Aspergillus* system to analyze transfer RNA at a standstill, I had reached a scientific impasse.

With the advice of Charles Benedetti, Annina's psychiatrist uncle, I decided to pursue my long range goal in medical science by re-entering the medical world. My choice was between continuing my residency in medicine, where I was welcomed by the Chief of Infectious Diseases, Morton Swartz, at the Massachusetts General Hospital, or to enter another specialty field of medicine. I finally decided on a residency in pathology, after interviewing a pathologist colleague of Benedetti's who was practicing pathology at a hospital in Lowell, Massachusetts. After reviewing my previous experience and interest in pathology in medical school, I determined that I had scored one of my highest grades in pathology when I had taken the first part of the National Board of Medical Examiners test while in medical school.

After conferring with Watson about my decision to enter a residency in pathology, I contacted Benjamin Castleman (Figure 7), Chief of Pathology at Massachusetts General Hospital, whose lectures and teaching of pathology I had admired during medical school. During my interview in the late fall, we determined that I could enter his residency program in anatomic and clinical pathology as a Clinical and Research Fellow in Pathology, while maintaining my Faculty Research Award from the American Cancer Society. This support assured me that I could continue my research program while learning the specialty of pathology for three years. In addition, my years of research experience in biochemistry and microbiology earned one year of residency credit for me from the American Board of Pathology. Castleman was eager for me to enter his residency program "tomorrow," but we settled on January 1, 1965 as my starting date.

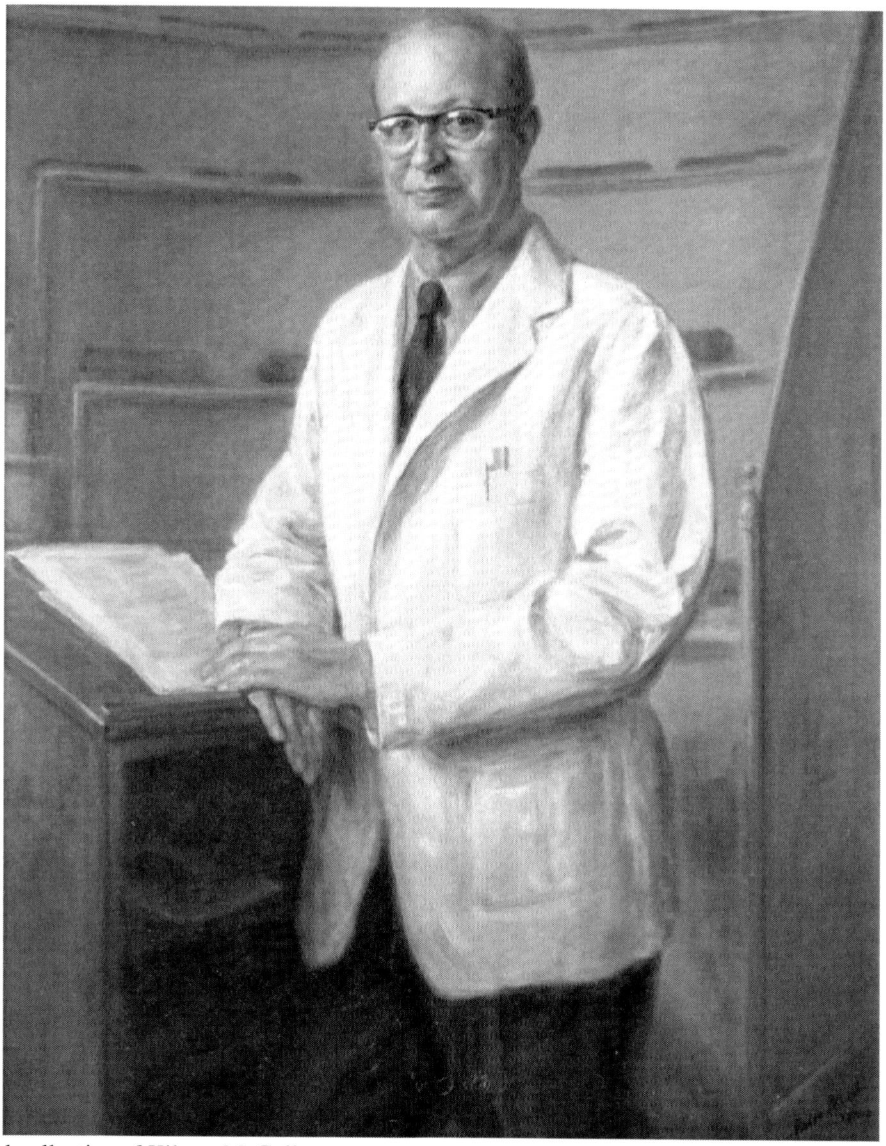

Personal collection of Kilmer McCully.

Figure 7. Benjamin Castleman (1906-1982) was Professor of Pathology at Harvard Medical School and Chairman of Pathology at Massachusetts General Hospital. This portrait shows Castleman in the Ether Dome, where he directed the Clinical-Pathological Case Conferences for many years.

After four and one half years of intensive experience in biochemistry, molecular biology and microbial genetics, entering pathology residency training seemed like re-learning the lost language of medicine. Nevertheless, my enthusiasm for learning pathology and investigating medical science was re-kindled by the experience. I soon became proficient in anatomic pathology, performing 165 autopsies, studying thousands of surgical pathology, neuropathology and cytopathology cases, and learning the fundamentals of immunohematology, clinical chemistry, hematology, immunology, and microbiology with my fellow residents. The experience and atmosphere in pathology training suited my interests in studying disease more than the basic science approach that I had undertaken in the four and one half years since completing my medical internship.

My Chief, Benjamin Castleman, was known for his clinical expertise in pathology, his teaching at Harvard Medical School, and his publication of the Cabot cases of clinical-pathological conferences in the *New England Journal of Medicine*. On one of his trips he had met Etienne Wolf, an experimental pathologist from Paris, who had developed a method for growing human tumors on chick embryo cultures. Knowing of my interest in cancer research, Castleman suggested that I should try to repeat Wolf's experiments, a project worthy of my support from the American Cancer Society. In this study my technician and I succeeded in maintaining viable fragments of human tumors on chick embryo cultures for periods of two to three weeks, demonstrating that the cancer cells incorporated radioactive amino acids into proteins [11]. I was disappointed, however, that the malignant cells failed to multiply and invade the tissues of the chick embryo in these experiments, as Wolf had claimed. Because of this work, an energetic and brilliant resident in surgery, Judah Folkman, approached me about collaborating with him in investigating his concept of tumor angiogenesis. By that time, however, I had become interested in the pathology of human genetics and declined his offer.

My three years of pathology residency and my support from the American Cancer Society were completed during 1968, and Castleman offered me a position in the Pathology Department after I completed my training and passed the American Board of Pathology examinations. To support my research program, he encouraged me to apply for a National Institutes of Health research grant. Because the organ culture method for human tumors seemed laborious and unproductive, I decided to renew my interest in *Aspergillus* genetics and base my grant application on study of transfer RNA mutants in this organism. After intensive study of anatomic pathology and clinical pathology, I passed my Board examinations in 1968. I was also appointed Instructor in Pathology at Harvard Medical School and Assistant Pathologist at Massachusetts General Hospital.

Having completed my residency training and Board examinations in pathology, I became discouraged with my current research projects on organ cultures of tumors and transfer RNA mutants in *Aspergillus*. To broaden the outlook of my research program I decided to meet with John Littlefield to discuss participating in the activities of the Human Genetics Unit, to which he had recently been appointed as Chief. Littlefield was a member of Paul Zamecnik's research group at the Huntington Laboratories, and we had become acquainted while I worked there as a student and research fellow. My new idea was to specialize in the pathology of inherited diseases in children in order to find a new field of investigation that suited my background and interests. Littlefield had experience in growing human cells in culture, and he offered to help me set up a cell culture operation in my laboratory. In the meanwhile, I became a member of the Genetics Unit, visiting patients with inherited diseases in the Pediatrics and Medical wards of the hospital. Some other members of the Human Genetics group were Lewis Holmes, Richard Erbe, Harvey Levy and Vivian Shih.

In the summer of 1968 Harvey Levy and Vivian Shih presented a case of the recently discovered disease homocystinuria at one of the Human Genetics Clinical Conferences. The patient was a 9-year-old girl with mental retardation, dislocated ocular lenses, accelerated growth with tall stature and flushing of the skin of her face, arms and legs [12]. Mary Efron, a pediatrician who had studied inherited diseases with Charles Dent in England, and Vivian Shih recognized that this patient had symptoms of homocystinuria. Having recently founded an Amino Acid Laboratory in the Department of Pediatrics, Efron and Shih demonstrated excessive amounts of the amino acid homocystine in the plasma and urine of the child by paper and column chromatography.

Having extensive experience in transfer RNA structure and function, protein biosynthesis, and methionine and homocysteine metabolism, I became intensely interested in this new disease and decided to read the available medical literature on the subject. My interest was further heightened when Levy and Shih stated that, according to the child's mother, an uncle of the child had died of a similar disease in the 1930s which was the subject of a published case report in the medical literature. Mary Efron and Vivian Shih traced the uncle's case to a clinical-pathological conference report published in the *New England Journal of Medicine* in 1933 [13].

The amino acid homocysteine was discovered by the American biochemist Vincent DuVigneaud in 1932. He and other scientists established homocysteine as a key intermediate in methionine and sulfur amino acid metabolism [14]. Homocysteine is converted to cystathionine and cysteine by an enzymatic pathway that requires the co-enzyme pyridoxal phosphate. Homocysteine is also converted to methionine by transfer of methyl groups from folic acid or choline, a process termed transmethylation.

Although the biochemistry of homocysteine was extensively studied by DuVigneaud and other scientists from 1932 to the 1950s, little was known of its significance in human disease until 1962, when cases of the disease homocystinuria were described almost simultaneously from clinics and research institutions in Belfast, Northern Ireland, Milwaukee, and Philadelphia. The most complete clinical description of the new disease was published by Carson and Neill from Belfast in 1962 [15]. In their survey of urine samples from children with mental retardation, they discovered several children who excreted large amounts of the amino acid homocystine, as demonstrated by paper chromatography. The children also had dislocated ocular lenses, accelerated growth in childhood with long fingers, arms and legs, skeletal abnormalities, and severe osteoporosis. Some of the children had died of thrombosis of arteries and veins to vital organs, and a description of the pathological changes in the organs was published by Gibson, Carson and Neill in 1964 [16]. Because the clinical abnormalities resembled some features of Marfan's Syndrome, several cases of homocystinuria, previously diagnosed with Marfan's Syndrome, were reported in a study from the Johns Hopkins Human Genetics Unit [17]. Several other cases of homocystinuria were described by the research group from Belfast and their team [18].

In the case report from 1933 the clinical and pathological description of the uncle's disease indicated that he had almost certainly died of homocystinuria [13]. He had mental retardation, dislocated optic lenses, and genu valgum, a congenital deformity of the knee and hip joints. Some of these features were found in his niece in 1965 [12]. The uncle had died suddenly three days after developing vomiting, coma, nystagmus and facial weakness, symptoms of an acute stroke. In his description of the pathological findings Tracey Mallory found a thrombus occluding the carotid artery and a large infarct of the brain which had killed the child. Mallory described the changes in the wall of the carotid artery as narrowing by "a very marked intimal thickening which could be the end result of an inflammatory endarteritis or of a simple sclerotic process such as one sees in elderly people." His pathological diagnosis was cerebral infarct secondary to carotid thrombosis and arteriosclerosis of the carotid artery.

My former colleague Harvey Mudd and his group at the National Institutes of Health had discovered in 1964 that inherited deficiency of the enzyme cystathionine synthase was responsible for the new disease homocystinuria [19]. My medical school classmate, George Spaeth, an ophthalmologist at the Wills Eye Institute in Philadelphia, and his co-investigator, Winton Barber, had independently discovered homocystinuria in a child with dislocated ocular lenses in 1962 and had referred the family to Harvey Mudd for study [20]. The enzyme cystathionine synthase and the co-enzyme pyridoxal phosphate catalyze the reaction of homocysteine with serine to form cystathionine, an intermediate discovered by DuVigneaud in the 1930s [14]. Because this reaction is blocked in children with homocystinuria, the amino acid homocysteine and its precursor methionine increase in the plasma, causing excretion of homocystine in the urine.

I was intrigued by the possibility that the increase in plasma homocysteine or methionine might have been responsible in some way for the arteriosclerosis, carotid thrombosis and death from cerebral infarct in the archival 1933 case of homocystinuria. Since the case had been completed in the Pathology Department where I was working, I was able to find the original autopsy protocol, six original glass slides of tissue sections, and a lump of paraffin containing tissues from the case. When I studied these slides and new slides made from the tissues in paraffin, I confirmed what Tracey Mallory had described in 1933. To me the fibrous arteriosclerotic plaques of the carotid artery and other smaller plaques scattered through the arteries had many of the same characteristics as the fibrous arterial plaques in the many patients with arteriosclerosis that I had studied in my pathology residency.

It was noteworthy that the arterial plaques in the 1933 case had no cholesterol crystals or fat deposits, such as commonly found in plaques from patients with atherosclerosis dying with stroke or myocardial infarct. I was surprised that none of the previous publications on the pathology of homocystinuria had compared the arterial abnormalities to arteriosclerosis, since their illustrations closely resembled the fibrous arteriosclerotic plaques that I had found in the 1933 case. Instead the arterial changes were compared with the changes in the aorta produced by the experimental disease lathyrism, resulting from feeding chicks with beta propionitrile, a toxic component of *Lathyrus odoratus*, found in sweet pea seeds.

The important question concerning whether the arteriosclerotic plaques that Tracey Mallory had observed in the 1933 case of homocystinuria and confirmed by my own study of this case were caused by homocysteine could not be answered easily. Indeed two other scientists, Charles Butterworth, a professor of nutrition, and the pediatrician Gerald Gaull had previously discussed this question independently without resolution. One possibility was that elevation of plasma methionine or deficiency of plasma cystathionine could be responsible for the thrombosis and arterial abnormalities. In my discussions with Pontecorvo I had clarified my understanding of the distinctions between genotypic and phenotypic expressions of genetic abnormalities in *Aspergillus* mutants. These discussions helped me to understand that limitations of knowledge of the characteristics of pathological changes and metabolic abnormalities in homocystinuria precluded a definitive conclusion about causation of arterial plaques by homocysteine.

The impasse in my understanding of the origin of arterial plaques in homocystinuria was broken several months later in the fall of 1968 when another case of homocystinuria was discussed at another Human Genetics Conference. This case was quite different from the 1933 case that I had studied, since it occurred in a 2-month-old baby boy. This desperately ill child was referred to the Pediatrics Service of Massachusetts General Hospital because of failure to gain weight and aspiration pneumonia. The urine and plasma of this child were found to contain homocystine, cystathionine and methyl malonic acid, and the methionine level in the plasma was abnormally low. Intensive studies by Harvey Levy and Vivian Shih at Massachusetts General Hospital, Harvey Mudd at National Institutes of Health and Robert Abeles at Brandeis University revealed that the child suffered from a rare, previously unknown disease of cobalamin (vitamin B12) metabolism subsequently called cobalamin C disease [21]. In this disease an abnormality of intracellular cobalamin transport results in failure of methylation of homocysteine to produce methionine. As a result, methionine levels are low in plasma, and homocysteine and cystathionine levels are elevated. In addition increased amounts of methyl malonic acid are excreted in the urine because of the cobalamin abnormality. Despite therapy with vitamin B12, vitamin B6, folic acid, choline and other methyl donors, the baby died at the age of two months.

When I learned that this child with the new disease of homocysteine metabolism had an autopsy, I became intensely excited by the possibility that the arteries of this child may exhibit arteriosclerotic plaques similar to those that I had found in the 1933 archival case of homocystinuria. If the autopsy demonstrated arteriosclerotic plaques in this child, it would mean that the amino acid homocysteine would be implicated in their genesis. The reason was that the methionine and cystathionine concentrations were dramatically different in these two inherited diseases of metabolism caused by different enzymatic abnormalities. If no arteriosclerotic plaques were found in the autopsy, it would mean that plasma homocysteine and cystathionine could become highly elevated without affecting the arteries.

When the Conference was concluded, I remember rushing back to the Pathology Department with excitement and anticipation to find the results of the autopsy. The case had been completed and filed in the archives by one of our most talented residents, Bernard Forget, who later became a professor of hematology at Yale Medical School. In the autopsy protocol there was a detailed and fascinating discussion of the biochemical abnormalities of this index case of cobalamin C disease in the medical literature. In reading the protocol further, I was crestfallen to find that there was no description of any pathological abnormalities in the aorta, arteries or arterioles in the major organs. There was moderate fat deposition in the liver cells, a peculiar squamous metaplasia of gastric glands in the stomach, and the severe aspiration pneumonia that killed the baby. There was no indication that either the resident or the staff pathologist who reviewed the findings in this case was aware of the arteriosclerosis and thrombosis found in earlier cases of homocystinuria in the medical literature.

Discouraged but undaunted because of my prior study of the archival case of homocystinuria, I found the original slides for the cobalamin C case and a large jar of formalin containing all of the organs from the baby boy. When I studied the arteries from this case in the original slides and the many new slides made from the saved tissues, I was astounded to find widespread arteriosclerotic plaques scattered through the arteries of this baby! My fellow resident had not found this abnormality because he had either not recognized or searched for plaques in the arteries, as I did. I immediately realized that the origin of arteriosclerotic plaques could be traced to elevated plasma levels of homocysteine, since the methionine and cystathionine levels were very different in the two types of homocystinuria (Figure 8). This discovery meant that, at least in the case of human inherited diseases, plaque formation could be attributed to a direct effect of the amino acid on the cells and tissues of the arteries. In neither case was there evidence of cholesterol or fat deposition in the arterial plaques, so the process leading to arteriosclerosis in these cases was independent of the conventional view of the genesis of atherosclerosis.

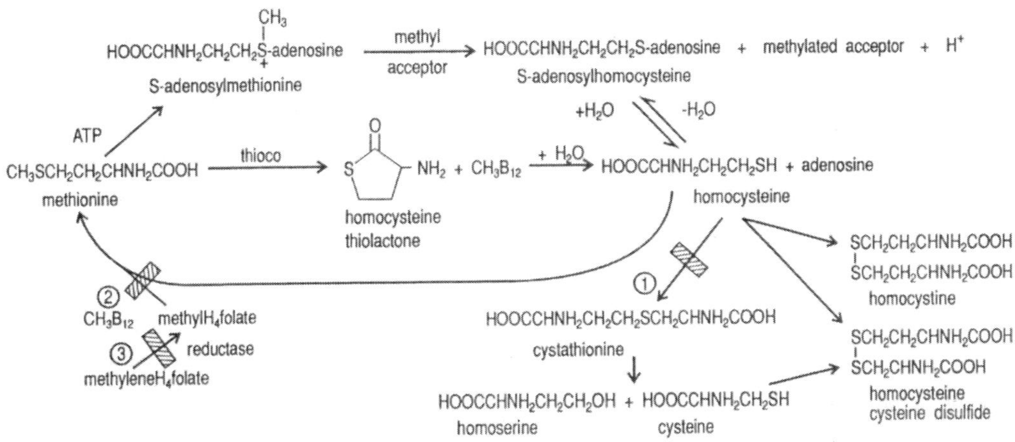

Reprinted from Annals of Clinical and Laboratory Science, 1993, Volume 23, page 483 by permission of the Institute for Clinical Science, Inc.

Figure 8. Enzymatic disorders of homocysteine metabolism. Biochemical pathways of synthesis of homocysteine thiolactone, adenosyl methionine, and homocysteine from methionine are indicated. Inherited deficiencies of cystathionine synthase (1), methionine synthase (2), and methylenetetrahydrofolate reductase (3) cause accumulation of homocystine and homocysteine cysteine disulfide in tissues and body fluids.

To say the least, I was greatly stimulated and extremely excited with the realization that I had made a significant observation concerning the most important cause of disease and death in America. With my background of knowledge and experience in the field of amino acid function in transfer RNA and cellular protein biosynthesis, I knew that I had the resources to address the many questions raised by my discovery about the importance of homocysteine in disease. Many of the abnormalities in children with homocystinuria –accelerated growth, thrombosis, dislocated lenses, arteriosclerosis, developmental abnormalities of skeleton, osteoporosis – might be explained by investigation of the biochemical and physiological effects of homocysteine. So many possibilities for investigation crowded my mind that I had difficulty sleeping through the night for over two weeks. I woke up early in the morning with ideas for experiments racing through my mind. My wife told me that I began to spout chemical formulas in my sleep.

From my previous years of fellowship I had learned that Mother Nature guards her secrets very closely. It was human nature to leap to conclusions that may not be justified when all of the facts are known. In addition, I kept the excitement of my discovery to myself, not discussing my findings explicitly with my colleagues. Instead I determined that I must verify the validity of my discovery by reviewing my observations with other sources of information. I asked Benjamin Castleman for assistance in reviewing the pathological findings in cases of homocystinuria that had been published from Belfast, Northern Ireland, and from Johns Hopkins Medical School. Through a pathology colleague at Johns Hopkins, Castleman was able to borrow tissue slides from a number of published authentic cases of homocystinuria. Indeed I verified that the plaques in my two cases closely resembled the features of those in the published cases.

Another way of verifying the significance of my discovery was to show that the plaques in the arteries of my cases are similar to plaques occurring in patients without homocystinuria. My colleague James Caulfield studied the arterial plaques from my cases of homocystinuria by electron microscopy and demonstrated that these plaques have the ultrastructural features of fibrous plaques from control cases of arteriosclerosis without homocystinuria. In addition I reviewed the peculiar squamous metaplasia of gastric glands of the child with cobalamin C disease with another colleague Robert Scully, who told me that similar changes are found in the stomach of patients with multiple vitamin deficiencies, including vitamin A. Indeed I had read Honor Fell's articles from Cambridge University in England, about her experiments with organ cultures demonstrating squamous metaplasia in experimental retinoid (vitamin A) deficiency.

The child with cobalamin C disease had marked elevation of cystathionine in plasma and urine and also excreted large quantities of methyl malonic acid in the urine. To exclude the possibility that these metabolites could be responsible for the arterial plaques, I reviewed previous studies of cases with cystathioninuria or methyl malonic aciduria caused by inherited diseases of metabolism. None of the reports in the literature contained descriptions of arterial plaques. In addition, cases of elevation of methionine levels without elevation of homocysteine, caused by inherited enzyme abnormalities or liver disease, revealed no evidence of arterial plaques.

In a discussion of my findings with John Littlefield of the Genetics Unit I recalled a comment in my notes from medical school that experimental dietary deficiency of vitamin B6 (pyridoxine) causes arteriosclerotic plaques in monkeys [22]. We remembered that these studies were reported by James Rinehart, working at Boston City Hospital and later at the University of California Medical School in San Francisco. My interpretation that homocysteine causes arteriosclerotic plaques explained Rinehart's findings, since pyridoxine is the co-enzyme of cystathionine synthase, the enzyme that is deficient in the classic type of homocystinuria, and deficient intake of this vitamin would lead to elevated levels of plasma homocysteine. Indeed later studies with animals confirmed this interpretation.

Another experimental study from Toronto showed that dietary deficiency of choline, a methyl group donor responsible for converting homocysteine to methionine, also causes arteriosclerotic plaques in coronary arteries of rats. This result could be explained by assuming that choline deficiency causes elevation of plasma homocysteine because of impaired methylation of homocysteine to methionine, leading to arterial plaques because of the effect of homocysteine on the cells and tissues of the arteries. Indeed later studies with choline-deficient animals demonstrated elevation of plasma homocysteine.

The experimental production of atherosclerosis by dietary cholesterol was related to methionine metabolism, as I recalled from my first year medical school presentation by Frederick Stare. The monkeys were fed autoclaved soy bean meal that was known to be deficient in methionine, as well as added cholesterol. Dietary methionine caused a decrease in plasma cholesterol levels and prevented arterial plaques in the monkeys. Later studies showed that deficient production of adenosyl methionine from dietary methionine deficiency causes elevation of plasma homocysteine in animals and humans. Finally the Stare group found that hypothyroidism, induced in animals by thiouracil, exacerbates experimental atherosclerosis in rats, an effect explained by the subsequent finding that plasma homocysteine is elevated in both human and experimental hypothyroidism.

Armed with demonstration of arteriosclerotic plaques in the two types of homocystinuria and supported by these new interpretations of experimental arteriosclerosis, I wrote my first article on homocysteine and sent it to the *American Journal of Pathology* [23]. When I mailed the completed manuscript, I remember thinking that this discovery might prove to be highly significant for understanding the cause of heart disease and stroke in the population. To my astonishment the manuscript was accepted for publication without revision in three weeks. Within the next two months I received reprint requests by post card, in the days before the internet and xerography, from more than 400 scientists world-wide. Evidently, other scientists understood the significance of my discovery of a field for future research on the causes of arteriosclerosis. In my discussion of the implications of this discovery, I suggested that elevated plasma homocysteine levels from dietary, toxic, metabolic, hormonal, hereditary, environmental or other predisposing factors might prove to be important in causation of arteriosclerosis in the general population. As examples, I cited diabetes, hypothyroidism, hypertension, radiation injury and smoking as factors leading to elevation of plasma homocysteine and arteriosclerosis. All of these factors have now been confirmed to cause elevation of plasma homocysteine by subsequent studies. Finally I discussed the possibility that deposition of plasma lipids in atherosclerotic plaques is secondary to the arterial damage caused by homocysteine. I was careful about discussing involvement of cholesterol and lipoproteins, because there was no evidence of deposition of these substances in the arterial plaques in my two cases of homocystinuria.

In my view, this discovery of the role of homocysteine in arteriosclerosis illustrates the validity of Pasteur's aphorism. My mind had been prepared to make this discovery by my fellowships and experiences with transfer RNA, protein biosynthesis, and microbial genetics. The chance to review the pathological findings in the world literature's first case of cobalamin C disease gave me the opportunity to make this discovery. Moreover, many other previous investigators had studied the metabolic and pathological findings in cases of homocystinuria, but my new thoughts about the significance of these findings led to this advance in medical science, illustrating Szent-Gyorgi's description of the process of discovery.

References

[1] Moss RW. *Free Radical. Albert Szent-Gyorgi and the battle over vitamin C.* New York: Paragon House, 1988.

[2] Cantoni GL. S-adenosyl methionine: present status and future perspectives. In F Salvatore, E Borek, V Zappia, HG Williams-Ashman, F Schlenk, editors. *The Biochemistry of Adenosylmethionine*. New York: Columbia University Press, 1977.

[3] Holley RW. Alanine transfer RNA. *Nobel lectures*, December 11, 1968.

[4] McCully KS, Cantoni GL. On the specificity of takadiastase T1 ribonuclease. *Biochimica et Biophysica Acta*, 1961;51:190-192.

[5] McCully KS, Cantoni GL. Studies on soluble ribonucleic acid (S-RNA) of rabbit liver. A base sequence model of S-RNA. *Journal of Molecular Biology*, 1962;5:497-505.

[6] Pontecorvo G. *Trends in Genetic Analysis*. New York: Columbia University Press, 1958.

[7] Forbes T, McCully KS. The use of p-fluorophenylalanine with "master strains" of Aspergillus nidulans for assigning genes to linkage groups. *Genetical Research (Cambridge)*, 1965;6:352-359.

[8] Watson JD. *The Double Helix: A personal account of the discovery of the structure of DNA*. New York: Norton, 1980.

[9] Watson JD. The involvement of RNA in the synthesis of proteins. *Nobel Lectures*, December 11, 1962.

[10] Watson JD. Succeeding in science: some rules of thumb. *Science*, 1993;261:1812-1813.

[11] McCully KS. Protein synthesizing activity of human neoplastic and normal thyroid tissue in chick embryo mesonephros organ cultures. *International Journal of Cancer*, 1968;3:142-149.

[12] Shih V, Efron M. Pyridoxine unresponsive homocystinuria. Final diagnosis of case 19471 from 1933. *New England Journal of Medicine*, 1970;283:1206-1208.

[13] Case Records of the Massachusetts General Hospital. Marked cerebral symptoms following a limp of three week's duration. *New England Journal of Medicine*, 1933;209:1063-1066.

[14] DuVigneaud V. *A Trail of Research in Sulfur Chemistry and Metabolism*. Ithaca NY: Cornell University Press, 1952.

[15] Carson NAJ, Neill DW. Metabolic abnormalities detected in a survey of mentally backward individuals in Northern Ireland. *Archive of Diseases of Childhood*, 1962;37:505-513.

[16] Gibson JB, Carson NAJ, Neill DW. Pathological findings in homocystinuria. *Journal of Clinical Pathology*, 1964;17:427-437.

[17] Schimke RN, McKusick VA, Huang T, Pollack AD. Homocystinuria. Studies of 20 families with 38 affected members. *Journal of the American Medical Association*, 1965;193:711-719.

[18] Carson NAJ, Dent CE, Field CMB, Gaull GE. Homocystinuria. Clinical and pathological review of ten cases. *Journal of Pediatrics*, 1965;66:565-583.

[19] Mudd SH, Finkelstein JD, Irreverre F, Laster L. Homocystinuria: an enzymatic defect. *Science*, 1964;143:1443-1445.

[20] Spaeth GL, Barber GW. Homocystinuria in a mentally retarded child and her normal cousin. *Transactions of the American Academy of Ophthmology and Otolaryngology*, 1965;69:912-930.

[21] Mudd SH, Levy HL, Abeles RH. A derangement in the metabolism of vitamin B12 leading to homocystinuria, cystathioninuria and methylmalonic aciduria. *Biochemical and Biophysical Research Communications*, 1968;35:121-126.

[22] Rinehart JF, Greenberg LD. Arteriosclerotic lesions in pyridoxine-deficient monkeys. *American Journal of Pathology*, 1949;25:481-491.

[23] McCully KS. Vascular pathology of homocysteinemia: implications for the pathogenesis of arteriosclerosis. *American Journal of Pathology*, 1969;56:111-128.

Chapter 4

EXPLORATION: HOMOCYSTEINE RESEARCH AND THE MOLECULAR BASIS OF DISEASE

In his book on scientific exploration, *The Way of an Investigator*, Walter Bradford Cannon describes the intensity and dedication with which the scientific investigator approaches a new field of discovery [1]. Cannon was the illustrious professor of physiology at Harvard Medical School in the early 20th century, who later became an influential Dean of the school. He was interested in explaining physiological functions of the human body by utilizing new discoveries in basic medical science. He was the first physiologist to use the newly discovered X-rays by Wilhelm Rőntgen in 1897 for studying the physiology of swallowing and gastric motility by use of fluoroscopy following a meal of barium sulfate. He later described the "fight or flight" response of the sympathetic nervous system and adrenal hormones, explaining how stress affects the physiological activation of the heart, blood circulation, nervous system, and gastro-intestinal system.

In his book Cannon describes the situation confronting the investigator when addressing an important new concept or discovery by laboratory experimentation. The investigator must devise experiments and gather data to verify or disprove the new concept. The intellectual process of investigation is exacting on the abilities of the investigator, requiring hours of diligent study and performance of experiments with intense concentration and commitment.

Cannon also introduced the case study method of teaching medicine in which discussion of clinical and pathological findings in a case is used to illustrate the disease process as it occurs in an individual. The case conference known as clinical-pathological conference was utilized by Richard Cabot at Massachusetts General Hospital for publication in the *New England Journal of Medicine*. The archival case of homocystinuria that I had studied, first suggesting a connection between homocysteine metabolism and arteriosclerosis, was presented in one of these conferences and published in the *New England Journal of Medicine* in 1933. After his retirement in 1945, Cannon died as a martyr to scientific discovery because he developed the malignant skin disease, mycosis fungoides. This disease is related to leukemia, and it was caused by his exposure to X-rays during fluoroscopy. He was the father of Marion Schlesinger, whose family I served as "house boy" during my fourth year of college in 1954.

My discovery of the role of the amino acid homocysteine in causing arteriosclerosis in children with homocystinuria, as described in Chapter 3, confronted me with many challenges for exploration of this new concept. In order to explain the suggested causation of arteriosclerosis in the human population without these rare inherited diseases, the biochemical, physiological and pathological effects of homocysteine on cells and tissues would have to be understood. The connections with the current hypothesis that dietary cholesterol and fats were involved in the pathogenesis of arteriosclerosis would have to be explained. Indeed the new concept of the causative effect of homocysteine in producing arterial plaques would have to be supported by studies in experimental animals and later in human subjects. It was a tall order! In order to tackle such a broad approach to understanding the causes of the most important disease affecting 20th century Americans, evidence would have to be gathered concerning many aspects of this fundamental question.

Fortunately for me, my grant application to the National Institutes of Health for study of protein synthesis in *Aspergillus nidulans* transfer RNA mutants had just been funded in 1969 after I had finished my residency training. This grant provided me with three years of research funds to study my discovery about homocysteine, and my American Cancer Society Faculty Research Award was scheduled to conclude in 1968. To resolve my dilemma about investigating an area of study that was not specifically described in my grant application, I met with Paul Zamecnik for his guidance. He told me that study sections recommending funding for grant proposals were sympathetic to changes in objectives, provided that the new direction of research efforts was productive. He said that if I was convinced of the importance of my new discovery, I should devote all my efforts to experimentation to support this concept, and when the grant was up for renewal after the first three years, I should explain to the study section my rationale for changing the focus of the research program and provide evidence in the form of published research articles supporting the change in direction. This situation was risky for my future as a scientist, but Zamecnik's advice was excellent, and I was fortunate to be able to show evidence of progress when my grant came up for renewal. After all, my new research program was to be devoted to investigation of the amino acid homocysteine in human disease, rather than protein synthesis in *Aspergillus* mutants.

My initial strategy in tackling this daunting research challenge was to utilize as best I could my knowledge of experimental methods in basic science that I had been studying during my student and fellowship years. My experiences in studying cholesterol chemistry and biosynthesis with Louis Fieser and Konrad Bloch, steroid hormone metabolism with Lewis Engel, transfer RNA structure and function with Giulio Cantoni, protein biosynthesis and molecular biology with Paul Zamecnik and James Watson, and microbial genetics with Guido Pontecorvo gave me a broad repertory of techniques and concepts of basic science with which I could investigate my discovery. On the other hand, I had little experience with clinical studies of patients, clinical chemistry for analysis of blood specimens, or epidemiology of disease in populations. Finally I decided to use the manifestations of physiological, biochemical, and pathological changes in human subjects with homocystinuria as a guide to my approach. Understanding how the cellular and tissue changes produced by homocysteine lead to arterial plaques would be my highest priority. In addition, the acceleration of normal growth and the connective tissue abnormalities of artery, cartilage, and bone in children with homocystinuria were certainly worthy of study. My most pressing question was where to begin.

After publication of my article in 1969 describing my discovery about the connection between homocysteine and arteriosclerosis, I was in a position to subject my ideas to informed criticism and advice by other medical scientists with knowledge in related fields. In order to develop an assay for analyzing homocysteine in plasma and tissues, I turned to Vivian Shih and Harvey Levy, who were experts in analysis of amino acids in plasma and urine by the column chromatography methods developed by Stein and Moore at Rockefeller University in the 1950s [2]. Shih and Levy helped me to devise a column chromatography system in my own laboratory to construct a make-shift amino acid analyzer. After my grant was renewed three years later, I was able to purchase a state-of-the-art Beckman Amino Acid Analyzer to study amino acid composition of research specimens. I turned to John Littlefield for help with setting up a human cell culture laboratory, and he helped me to secure a cell line of skin fibroblasts from a child with homocystinuria. These cultured cells contained the defective enzyme cystathionine synthase, the same abnormality found in the liver of these children, as demonstrated by Harvey Mudd's research group at the National Institutes of Health.

Periodically my Chief, Benjamin Castleman, asked each staff pathologist in his Department to discuss the pathological findings in selected interesting cases presented in the Ether Dome Conference Room, where the clinical-pathological conferences were held. At one of these conferences I discussed the pathological findings in a 38 year old woman with diabetes who had died of coronary occlusion and myocardial infarct. After the conference I was approached by a member of the audience, Moses Suzman, a prominent cardiologist from South Africa, who wanted to discuss my recently published article on homocysteine and arteriosclerosis. Suzman, the husband of the famous South African political leader, Helen Suzman, told me that he had some experience with vitamin B6 (pyridoxine) and arteriosclerosis. Suzman had been a Rockefeller Fellow in Nutrition at Harvard and Massachusetts General Hospital in the 1940s and was a friend and colleague of James Rinehart, another Rockefeller Fellow in Nutrition at Harvard and Boston City Hospital.

Suzman told me about the day when he was having lunch with James Rinehart at Boston City Hospital when Rinehart told him of the results of his initial experiments with monkeys and nutritional deficiencies. Rinehart had been trying to produce cirrhosis of the liver by various vitamin deficiencies. He announced to Suzman that "my experiments failed to produce cirrhosis of the liver, but the monkeys with deficiency of vitamin B6 developed arteriosclerosis!" Rinehart later became Chairman of Pathology at the University of California Medical School at San Francisco and published a series of articles describing atherosclerotic plaques, cirrhosis of the liver, dental caries, and abnormal bone development in monkeys with severe, chronic, intermittent dietary deficiency of vitamin B6 [3-5].

During the next several months Suzman visited me on a regular basis in my laboratory in the Pathology Department to discuss my progress in investigating homocysteine and arteriosclerosis. On these occasions he would come to my office carrying a thick stack of 3x5 cards containing references to literature articles and descriptions of significant publications in the history of arteriosclerosis research. I had already read the reports of the pioneering studies of Wladimir Sergius Ignatowsky from 1908, showing that feeding of meat, eggs and milk to rabbits, a vegetarian species, produced atherosclerotic plaques in the arteries. I had also read the account of Nicolai Anitschkow's experiments from 1914 in which feeding cholesterol to rabbits produced cholesterol deposition in the tissues of the animals, including atherosclerotic plaques filled with lipids.

Suzman introduced me to the fascinating experiments by the early American medical scientist, Harry Newburgh, who repeated Ignatowsky's experiments while serving as Professor of Clinical Medicine at University of Michigan Medical School in the 1920s. Newburgh repeated Ignatowsky's experiments utilizing meat powder from which all cholesterol and fats had been removed by extraction with organic solvents. Newburgh found that feeding the meat powder to rabbits produced arterial plaques, effectively disproving Anitschkow's suggestion that cholesterol was responsible for the arterial plaques in Ignatowsky's animals. Newburgh then infused individual amino acids into rabbits and dogs, discovering that several amino acids produced kidney failure, reproducing Ignatowsky's original observations. None of Newburgh's animals contained arterial plaques because he did not use methionine or homocysteine, which had not yet been discovered in the early 1920s. If Newburgh had used these amino acids, he would have discovered their potential for producing arterial plaques in the 1920s [6].

It was not long after my publication of my discovery concerning homocysteine and arteriosclerosis that Benjamin Castleman invited me and several other staff members of his Pathology Department to present their research findings to the Scientific Advisory Committee of the Massachusetts General Hospital. Several of the members, including Lewis Thomas of Yale Medical School, George Klein of Karolinska Hospital in Sweden, and Edward Tatum of Rockefeller Institute in New York, were world leaders in basic medical research. In their report in 1970, the Committee praised my findings as "an almost ideal example of experimental pathology, profiting from the application to a problem of a variety of techniques and concepts of basic science."

Later in 1972 I called Konrad Bloch to tell him about my discovery and to ask for his criticism and advice about my plans for future investigations. By this time I had published several research reports describing my initial findings in cell cultures, metabolism of homocysteine in liver, and production of arterial plaques in rabbits by homocysteine. Bloch invited me to present my findings to his research group in the Department of Chemistry at Harvard University. After my presentation, Bloch contacted me and invited me to lunch at the Harvard Faculty Club to discuss my progress in investigating homocysteine. After lunch we spent about two hours discussing what I had discovered and what my prospects were for advancing the field of research. Bloch told me that my discovery was significant, I needed a full time biochemist to help follow all of the leads, and that "other laboratories would in the future make independent observations to validate your findings." After that meeting, I felt that key scientists at Harvard would be examining the significance of my research discoveries.

In studying the cell cultures taken from the skin of children with homocystinuria, I found that the cells synthesize a flocculent, granular matrix rather than the fibrillar matrix produced by normal control cells [7]. Examining the cultures with polarized light revealed loss of birefringence by the homocystinuric cells, and this abnormality correlated with the appearance of the granular matrix, as demonstrated in stained cell preparations. Growing normal cells in culture medium containing homocysteine converted some of the fibrillar matrix to the granular form. Analysis of the amino acids of proteins of the cell cultures showed that the matrix substance had the composition of extracellular proteoglycan rather than collagen. Adding homocysteine to the culture medium of the homocystinuric cells resulted in a dramatic decrease in growth, demonstrating a toxic effect on growth in culture. Labeling studies with radioactive sulfate showed that the homocystinuric cells bound more sulfate to the granular matrix than the normal cells. In addition, I found that homocysteine thiolactone, the reactive anhydride of homocysteine, produced a shift in color of toluidine blue dye to a red-violet color, called metachromasia. This effect is known to be caused by interaction of the dye molecule with charge-transfer complexes. I later hypothesized that the change from the helical configuration of normal fibrillar matrix to the random coil configuration of homocysteine-induced aggregated matrix was induced by charge transfer complex formation between homocysteine thiolactone and the acidic carboxyl groups of proteoglycan molecules, increasing the binding of sulfate to alter their charge distribution and conformation [8].

In experiments with cultured homocystinuric cells we studied the effect of homocysteine thiolactone labeled with radioactive sulfur in the culture medium [7]. We found that the homocystinuric cells converted the sulfur atom to sulfate as effectively as normal cells. This finding demonstrated a new pathway for sulfate synthesis from homocysteine, because the deficiency of cystathionine synthase in the homocystinuric cells blocked the only known pathway for conversion of homocysteine to cystathionine, cysteine and sulfate. This pathway had been established by DuVigneaud's research group in the 1940s. Previous reports in the literature indicated that vitamin A is needed for sulfation of extracellular matrix, and I later suggested a scheme for participation of thioretinamide, the retinoic acid amide of homocysteine, in this new pathway for sulfation. These findings helped to explain the deposition of extracellular matrix in the arterial plaques of children with homocystinuria. Other studies from the literature showed that developing arteriosclerotic plaques in animals and humans actively bind sulfate to the matrix deposited in the plaques. The binding of sulfate to cartilage matrix during normal growth is mediated by "sulfation factor" now know as insulin-like growth factor, which is under the control of growth hormone.

In order to gather evidence supporting the causative function of homocysteine in production of arteriosclerotic plaques, rabbits were given the pure amino acid in the thiolactone form by injection and by feeding experiments. Subcutaneous injection of the amino acid in moderate doses, similar to the normal human daily dietary intake of methionine, produced fibrous plaques in coronary arteries, aorta, and arteries to the major organs within 3-5 weeks [9]. Addition of cholesterol to the diet of the animals injected with homocysteine produced lipid deposits within the fibrous plaques. Animals given five fold higher doses of homocysteine or methionine developed more prominent plaques in the aorta and major arteries. While these experiments were in progress, I remember receiving a call from my assistant on the weekend, telling me that two of the rabbits had died. When I examined the vena cava and iliac veins of these animals, I found large blood clots that had migrated to the veins of the lungs to produce pulmonary infarction, a process known as pulmonary embolism. In animals also injected with vitamin B6, there was no evidence of thrombosis or embolism. Another interesting finding was that the animals given these large doses of homocysteine or methionine gained much more weight than the controls, showing a dramatic stimulation of growth within one month. Other members of our Department visited the animal lab out of curiosity to see "McCully's giant rabbits."

When we studied tissue sections of the arterial plaques in these animals, we found prominent changes in connective tissue of aorta and arteries [10]. We found fibrosis, deposition of sulfated matrix, destruction of elastic fibers, hyperplasia of smooth muscle cells, and areas of calcium deposition. However, no lipids or cholesterol were observed in these fibrous arteriosclerotic plaques. In later experiments, we found that feeding butter with the synthetic diet containing homocysteine produced fibrolipid plaques containing abundant fat deposits in the arteries of the rabbits.

While these experiments were in progress, I received a call from Gerald Gaull, a pediatrician at a hospital for mentally retarded children in New York, inviting me to visit his laboratory and give a seminar describing our production of arteriosclerotic plaques in rabbits. Gaull had studied patients with homocystinuria in collaboration with Charles Dent's research group in England and Northern Ireland. After my seminar, he offered to repeat our rabbit experiments in his lab and send me the slides of the arteries for interpretation. They chose to use baby weanling rabbits, but we had used older yearling rabbits in our experiments. In their report published in the *American Journal of Pathology*, Gaull's group reported some thickening of the aorta, but they published a photomicrograph of a normal artery and claimed that their experiment failed to support our original observations. He did not allow me to add my description of the plaques produced by his experiments and did not acknowledge my participation in the experiments, claiming that the abnormalities he found were "spontaneous" rather than secondary to the effects of homocysteine. My own examination revealed in 5 of 14 animals injected with homocysteine that the aortas contained "marked multiple focal plaques with deposition of matrix and focal destruction of elastic lamellae [7]." I later learned that this episode was related to difficulty that Gaull's research group had encountered from their Institutional Review Board because of my publication of production of arteriosclerotic plaques in rabbit arteries. Because of my publication, Gaull's Institutional Review Board was reluctant to approve his experiments, involving giving homocysteine to human subjects with mental retardation.

Several years after the results of my experiments had been published in 1975, Fumio Kuzuya, a Professor of Geriatrics in Japan, sent me several articles describing his experiments with vitamin B6 and homocysteine in monkeys and rabbits. Kuzuya had studied with Rinehart and Greenberg in San Francisco in the 1950s and had continued to work with this animal model after returning to Japan. He confirmed Rinehart's findings of arteriosclerotic plaques in monkeys fed a diet deficient in vitamin B6, and he later showed that the arterial plaques induced by vitamin B6 deficiency regressed when the monkeys were subsequently treated with vitamin B6. He also published an article showing that he could produce arteriosclerosis and pulmonary embolism in rabbits by injecting homocysteine and prevention by vitamin B6, confirming our previously published results [10,11]. I did not know about this publication because it was published in Japanese, and the citation was not available in Index Medicus, the main citation service available before PubMed or other internet citation services were introduced years later.

As studied in the early 20th century, many investigators found that feeding a diet containing no ascorbic acid produces a disease in guinea pigs that has many features of the human disease scurvy. S. Bert Wolbach, the Professor of Pathology at Peter Bent Brigham Hospital and Harvard Medical School, described the pathological changes observed in guinea pigs with experimental scurvy. He found that the extracellular matrix of connective tissues becomes attenuated and diminished, the capillaries become thinned and susceptible to spontaneous hemorrhage, and the cartilage of growing epiphyses in long bones becomes abnormal, causing a profound inhibition of growth in young animals.

Later investigators demonstrated a failure of collagen synthesis in connective tissues and inhibition of hydroxylation of proline to hydroxyproline, leading to a failure to heal wounds in animals with experimental scurvy. Many of these abnormalities are observed in the human disease. Scurvy devastated sailors and explorers in the 16th and 17th centuries, because the long sea voyages led to many deaths from a lack of fresh fruits and vegetables in their diet. When the British Navy introduced the use of citrus fruits and limes to prevent scurvy in sailors in the 19th century, the disease was prevented and the sailors became known as "limeys." Ascorbic acid was identified as the substance in fresh fruits and vegetables that prevents scurvy by Albert Szent-Gyorgi, the Hungarian biochemist, in 1932.

Because of our observations on binding of sulfate to proteoglycans and the newly discovered pathway for sulfate synthesis from homocysteine thiolactone in cultured homocystinuric cells, I suspected that ascorbic acid might have a function in sulfation of the matrix of connective tissues. Other investigators had found decreased synthesis of chondroitin sulfate in the cartilage cells of guinea pigs with experimental scurvy. Because of this finding, I surmised that the profound inhibition of growth in scurvy might result from abnormal homocysteine metabolism. In addition, children with homocystinuria have accelerated growth in childhood, pointing to a role for homocysteine in the normal process of growth. For these reasons I suspected that homocysteine metabolism is involved in the sulfation of connective tissue matrix during normal growth. I also conjectured that homocysteine or homocysteic acid, the fully oxidized form of homocysteine, might alleviate the profound inhibition of growth in young guinea pigs with experimental scurvy.

In our studies of homocysteine metabolism in experimental scurvy, we found that the metabolism of radioactive homocysteine thiolactone, labeled either with C14 or S35, was indeed abnormal in guinea pig liver. Extracts of liver showed a profound inhibition of conversion of homocysteine thiolactone to homocysteic acid and oxidized forms of homocysteine. Instead, free homocysteine accumulated in the liver and in microsome preparations of liver from scorbutic animals. In these experiments, we also studied the conversion of synthetic homocysteic acid, labeled with S35, to phosphoadenosine phosphosulfate, the co-enzyme for sulfation of connective tissue matrix, discovered by Philip Robbins of MIT and Fritz Lipmann, the famous biochemist working at the Massachusetts General Hospital in the 1950s. By column chromatography, we demonstrated conversion of the sulfur atom of synthetic homocysteic acid, labeled with S35 to radioactive phosphor-adenosine phosphosulfate. These results provided an explanation for sulfate synthesis that occurs in cultured homocystinuric cells lacking cystathionine synthase (Figure 9). I was thrilled when my report describing these experiments was published in the prestigious journal *Nature* in 1971 [12].

To test my idea about growth inhibition in experimental scurvy from failure of conversion of homocysteine to sulfate, I decided to inject homocysteic acid, the precursor of sulfate, into young scorbutic guinea pigs to study the effect on growth. The homocysteic acid injections failed to restore growth and failed to prevent death from experimental scurvy. However, we found that the normal animals injected with homocysteic acid grew faster than normal uninjected animals. In this experiment I had failed to cure scurvy, but I had discovered a role for homocysteic acid in normal growth. This result agreed with our finding that rabbits given large doses of homocysteine, homocysteic acid, or methionine also had accelerated growth. In experiments with cell cultures of normal fibroblasts, we found that addition of homocysteic acid to the culture medium increased the binding of radioactive sulfate to the matrix of these cells. This effect was similar to the effect of homocysteine on sulfate binding to cartilage fragments found by other investigators, an effect attributed to "sulfation factor." The action of growth hormone on cartilage cells was discovered by other investigators to be mediated by a substance produced in the liver known as "sulfation factor" later termed "somatomedin" and now known to be identical with insulin-like growth factor of plasma.

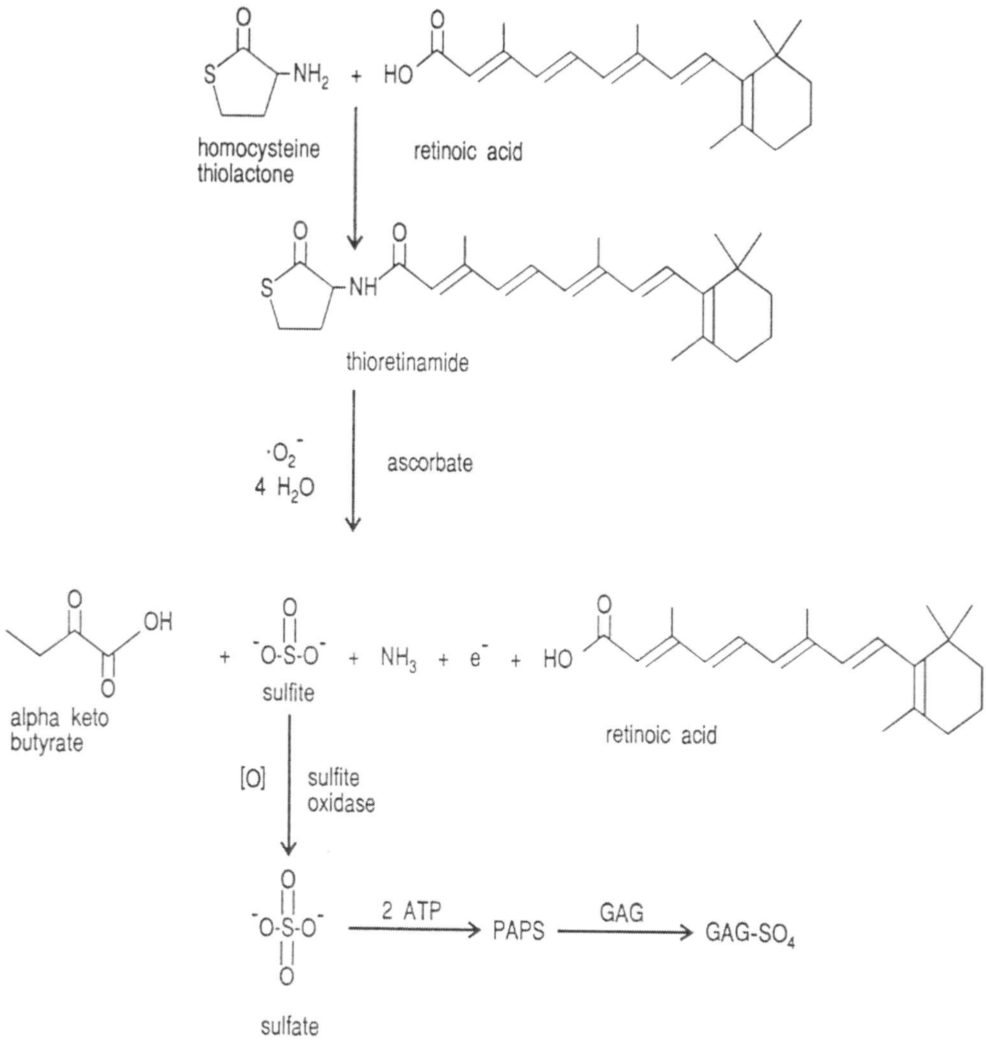

Reprinted from Annals of Clinical and Laboratory Science, 1994, Volume 24, page 47 by permission of the Institute for Clinical Science, Inc.

Figure 9. Pathway for synthesis of thioretinamide from homocysteine thiolactone and retinoic acid, oxidation to sulfite and sulfate, and activation of sulfate to phosphoadenosine phosphosulfate (PAPS) by ATP, explains sulfation of glycosaminoglycans (GAG) to form sulfate esters.

To investigate how homocysteine produces accelerated growth of children with homocystinuria and to explain how homocysteic acid stimulates growth of normal rabbits and guinea pigs, we decided to study the effect of homocysteic acid on growth of rats from which the anterior pituitary gland had been removed. The pituitary gland normally secretes growth hormone, which in turn causes the liver to produce "somatomedin." This factor stimulates growth of epiphyseal cartilage and increases sulfate binding to the matrix of growing cartilage cells in bone. With Virginia Smith and Peter Clopath we used a standard assay for growth hormone, involving measuring the width of the epiphyseal cartilage of bones of rats from which the pituitary gland had been removed. We found that these hypophysectomized rats without a source of growth hormone showed a positive growth response to homocysteic acid if the animals were treated with the thyroid hormone, thyroxine. Thyroxine corrects the deficiency of thyroid hormone in hypophysectomized animals resulting from their lack of thyrotropic hormone. Using another assay for growth hormone, we also found that homocysteic acid and thyroxine stimulated tail growth in young hypophysectomized rats. Using a standard assay for "somatomedin," we found that the serum of hypophysectomized rats treated with homocysteic acid and thyroxine contains normal amounts of the factor that increases sulfate binding to cartilage fragments. We were delighted when our report of these findings was published in the prestigious journal *Science* in 1976 [13].

In order to explore the significance of our findings in normal growth and sulfation of cartilage matrix, Roberta Ricci, a visiting research fellow from Rome, grew chick embryo chondrocytes in culture to study sulfation of their extracellular matrix. Ricci had studied the effect of para-fluorophenylalanine on *Aspergillus* in Pontecorvo's lab in Glasgow after I had completed my fellowship year there in 1964. Using her culture system, Ricci found that chondrocytes exposed to human plasma from a hypopituitary patient bind fewer sulfates than chondrocytes exposed to normal human plasma. She also found that decreased sulfate binding to cultured chondrocytes in the presence of plasma from a hypopituitary patient is restored to normal levels by addition of homocysteic acid to the culture medium. Homocysteic acid had a similar effect on sulfate binding to chondrocytes as the effect of plasma from a hypopituitary patient treated with growth hormone. Use of this assay for purification and identification of insulin-like growth factor in chromatography of plasma showed increased sulfate binding to chondrocytes in fractions of plasma containing homocysteic acid. The results of these experiments supported our previous findings of growth stimulation of hypophysectomized animals by homocysteic acid [14].

Because of these interesting results with young animals, we decided to study the influence of aging on metabolism of homocysteine thiolactone in the liver of rats and guinea pigs. We found that young animals convert a larger fraction of injected homocysteine thiolactone labeled with C14 to homocysteic acid and homocysteine sulfinic acid than older fully grown animals. This conversion in hypophysectomized young rats resembles that observed in older rats. Free homocysteine accumulated in rat liver, compared with only traces of the compound in guinea pig liver, showing a species difference. These experiments show that young growing animals form the oxidized homocysteine derivative homocysteic acid with somatomedin activity and homocysteine sulfinic acid more than older fully grown animals, correlating with their age and growth status [15].

In 1934 Harry Baernstein of the University of Wisconsin discovered homocysteine thiolactone, a new compound formed by reaction of hydriodic acid with methionine. This compound is the cyclic anhydride of homocysteine, the amino acid discovered by DuVigneaud in 1932. Working with homocysteine thiolactone, DuVigneaud found that hydrolysis with strong alkali produces homocysteine, but hydrolysis with dilute alkali produced an insoluble polymeric substance composed of the dimerized homocysteine thiolactone, homocysteine diketopiperazine. Homocysteine is re-converted to homocysteine thiolactone by the action of strong acid, such as sulfuric acid. Since homocysteine thiolactone was not found in the urine of children with homocystinuria, it was assumed that this compound is rapidly hydrolyzed to homocysteine by non-specific esterases in plasma, cells, and tissues. In the 1950s investigators at Columbia University discovered that homocysteine thiolactone reacts with free amino groups of proteins to form peptide-bound homocysteine containing a free sulfhydryl group, a process termed thiolation of proteins.

In experiments with Eliot Spindel in our lab we looked for evidence that methionine is converted to homocysteine thiolactone during normal metabolism. When we injected guinea pigs with methionine labeled either with C14 or S35, we demonstrated conversion to homocysteine thiolactone. The radioactivity from labeled methionine was demonstrated in the homocysteine thiolactone peak separated from liver extracts by the amino acid chromategraphic technique of Stein and Moore. In other experiments we synthesized the perchlorate salt of homocysteine thiolactone by treating the hydrochloride salt of the compound with perchloric acid, followed by crystallization from chloroform-methanol solvent. Using a total lipid extract of liver from a guinea pig injected with labeled methionine, we demonstrated labeled homocysteine thiolactone by co-crystallization with synthetic homocysteine thiolactone perchlorate [16].

Some years later Heironim Jakubowski discovered that homocysteine thiolactone is synthesized from methionine by methionyl amino acyl synthase, the enzyme that activates methionine transfer RNA with methionine [17]. Jakubowski and his research team also discovered that paraoxanase, an extracellular enzyme associated with high-density lipoprotein HDL and bleomycin hydrolase, an intracellular enzyme that inactivates the antineoplastic compound bleomycin, both hydrolyze homocysteine thiolactone to homocysteine.

When cancer cells are grown in culture, they exhibit a loss of contact inhibition of growth, causing the cells to pile up and form multiple layers on the surface of the culture dish. Unlike normal cells, cancer cells can be grown as independent colonies in soft agar gel. These features are not found in normal cells, suggesting that the growth of cancer cells in tissues and organs is related to these abnormal growth properties. Our experiments with cultured skin cells from homocystinuric children showed a loss of contact inhibition of growth, resembling the growth of cultured cancer cells, associated with production of highly sulfated, aggregated extracellular matrix. In the 19th century Rudolf Virchow and other pathologists had compared the proliferating smooth muscle cells of atherosclerotic plaques to benign neoplasms of artery wall, and in the 1960s Earl Benditt had demonstrated clonal growth of these cells in human arteriosclerotic plaques. The proliferating cells of arterial plaques in children with homocystinuria and in experimental animals treated with homocysteine also exhibit smooth muscle cell proliferation. These observations suggested a possible role for homocysteine metabolism in the abnormal growth properties of malignant cells.

My colleague, Paul Black, whom I had met in Glasgow while he was a research fellow at the Virology Research Institute at Glasgow University, offered to give me several cell culture lines of fibroblasts resulting from SV40 polyoma infection, so-called transformed cells. He also gave me cell lines cultured from malignant tumors induced in animals by SV40 polyoma virus. Two other malignant cell lines, cultured from rat bladder cancers induced by chemical carcinogens were given to me by James Daly, a pathologist also in training when I was a resident. In studying sulfation of the matrix of these various cell lines by radioactive sulfate and homocysteine thiolactone, we found a peculiar phenomenon only in the cancer cells but not in normal or viral transformed cells grown with homocysteine thiolactone. When extracts of these cells were placed on chromatography columns, the pressure in the column rose rapidly causing the column to burst. We surmised that the reaction of homocysteine thiolactone with cellular constituents formed aggregates that occluded solvent flow in the columns.

The answer to this phenomenon became apparent when the extracts of the cancer cell cultures were dialyzed to remove free homocysteine thiolactone, followed by acid hydrolysis and chromatography of the free amino acids. To my surprise we discovered that the dialyzed proteins contained radioactive homocysteine that had become linked to protein by a peptide bond. The nature of the peptide bond was established by showing that the radioactive homocysteine was displaced from protein by pronase, an enzyme that hydrolyzes peptide bonds, or by alkaline hydrolysis. The radioactive homocysteine was precipitated by trichloroacetic acid, and it was resistant to displacement by mercaptoethanol, a reagent that disrupts disulfide bonds. In contrast, normal cultured skin cells or fibroblasts transformed by SV40 polyoma virus incorporated no radioactivity from homocysteine thiolactone into peptide-bound homocysteine. Instead these cells converted most of the radioactivity from homocysteine thiolactone into sulfate.

I interpreted this discovery to indicate that normal cells contain a regulatory compound that catalyzes conversion of homocysteine thiolactone to sulfate, whereas malignant cells lack this substance, causing them to accumulated peptide-bound homocysteine within cellular proteins. This finding is similar to the discovery by Rudolf Benesche and Ruth Benesche from Columbia University in 1953 that homocysteine thiolactone reacts with free amino groups of proteins to form peptide-bound homocysteine. Our observation was the first to show that this process occurs in cultured malignant cells, but not in cultured normal cells [18].

Several investigators had found that, unlike normal cells, cancer cells are unable to grow in culture without methionine in a medium containing homocysteine, cobalamin and folic acid. Because of our discovery of failure of conversion of homocysteine thiolactone to sulfate in malignant cells, I hypothesized that an unknown derivative of homocysteine thiolactone was depleted from cancer cells. In normal cells this unknown compound presumably catalyzes conversion of homocysteine thiolactone to sulfate and allows the cells to grow in culture without methionine. This hypothesis implies that homocysteine thiolactone accumulates in malignant cells, resulting in thiolation of proteins by homocysteine and causing the widespread abnormalities of cell membranes in malignant cells. In addition, other macromolecules containing free amino groups, such as DNA, RNA and glycosaminoglycans are also presumed to react with accumulated homocysteine thiolactone to form peptide-bound homocysteinyl groups. Some evidence for this hypothesis was reported by Jakubowski and Goldman in 1993, demonstrating accumulation of homocysteine thiolactone in cultures of malignant cells [19].

Because of this important hypothesis, Peter Clopath, a visiting research fellow and chemist from Switzerland, and I set out to determine the molecular nature of this unknown derivative of homocysteine thiolactone that is presumed to prevent accumulation of homocysteine thiolactone in normal cells. From our previous results with normal liver cells, showing release of homocysteine thiolactone by hydrolysis, we reasoned that the substituent of the unknown compound must be on the nitrogen atom of homocysteine thiolactone. Therefore, we set out to synthesize about 35 new derivatives of homocysteine thiolactone by organic synthesis and to test these new compounds for their ability to inhibit growth of transplanted malignant tumors in mice.

We were encouraged to find that the amide synthesized from arachidonic acid and homocysteine thiolactone significantly decreased the growth of transplanted breast cancer in mice [20]. The amide from oleic acid and homocysteine thiolactone increased tumor growth, but there was no effect of the amides made from butyric acid, linoleic acid, linolenic acid, or succinic acid on tumor growth. This result indicated that the unknown N-substituted homocysteine thiolactone compound in normal cells most probably contains a system of conjugated double bonds, similar to those of arachidonic acid, adjacent to the carbonyl group of homocysteine thiolactone amide. Earlier experiments showed that the perchlorate salt of homocysteine thiolactone increases growth and the amount of necrosis within transplanted breast tumors. Another compound, pyridoxal homocysteine thiolactone enamine, synthesized from vitamin B6 and homocysteine thiolactone, significantly decreased tumor growth if given for 2 weeks before tumor transplantation and continued for another 2 weeks of tumor growth. In unpublished results we found significant inhibition of tumor growth by the amide formed from retinoic acid (vitamin A acid) and homocysteine thiolactone.

During the years when my research group was studying these biochemical, physiological, and pathological process of homocysteine metabolism in normal and abnormal growth, I was recruited by Harvard Medical School, where I had an appointment as Assistant Professor of Pathology, to be one of the three founding faculty members of a new course in General Pathology for students in the newly formed Harvard-MIT Program in Health Sciences and Technology. Alan Natapoff, a mathematician from MIT, Harvey Goldman, a pathologist from Beth Israel Hospital, and I organized this new course in 1971. In this course I introduced the first year medical and technology students to some basic observations about homocysteine in health and disease. To this day graduates of this course approach me to describe how my introduction to homocysteine research had influenced their careers. This teaching assignment was taxing and time consuming, but I met a talented group of younger physicians and investigators through this course. Today 40 years later a modified version of this course is still taught in the Harvard-MIT combined medical curriculum.

After my American Cancer Society Faculty Research Award concluded in 1968, grants from other agencies, including the American Heart Association, the American Cancer Society, and the Massachusetts Heart Association, and the National Institutes of Health grant supported my research activities. Because of my progress in investigating homocysteine, my Chief, Benjamin Castleman, recommended me for a prestigious NIH Career Development Award that supported my research activities for five years from 1971 through 1976. During this period I gave many lectures and seminars at Harvard, MIT, Massachusetts General Hospital and other local and national research institutes. I was visited by a senior member of the NIH study section that sponsored my NIH grant to discuss my progress. And I was visited by Professor Fernand Chatagner, a French biochemist specializing in sulfur amino acid chemistry and biochemistry to discuss my research results.

On a memorable occasion in 1973 Bridget Wilcken, an Australian pediatrician, visited my laboratory while traveling from England to Australia, where she was to join her husband, the cardiologist, David Wilcken. Wilcken's lab in Australia became interested in homocysteine research and had found that patients with kidney failure accumulate homocysteine in the plasma. The Wilckens were interested in studying homocysteine metabolism in patients with coronary heart disease. Bridget Wilcken and I spent several hours discussing how to detect abnormal homocysteine metabolism in these patients. We agreed that giving a moderate oral dose of the amino acid methionine, the only precursor of homocysteine in metabolism, would stress the pathway for homocysteine accumulation, leading to elevated levels of homocysteine and methionine in the plasma. David Wilcken's research team had developed a system of amino acid analysis of plasma that could detect small quantities of homocystine, the disulfide of homocysteine, as well as the mixed disulfide formed from cysteine and homocysteine, in patients with homocystinuria and in patients with kidney failure. In 1976 the Wilcken group reported that human subjects with coronary heart disease accumulated more homocystine and cysteine homocysteine mixed disulfide in plasma than normal controls, following an oral dose of methionine [21]. This successful study was the first demonstration of abnormal homocysteine metabolism in human subjects with arteriosclerosis, confirming the prediction in my original article published in 1969.

On another occasion I was invited to attend a seminar devoted to the effects of contraceptive hormones, sponsored by the National Institutes of Health in Mobile, Alabama. One of the prominent investigators to attend this conference was Victor Herbert, a hematologist from New York. Herbert was an expert on folic acid, cobalamin and anemia, who had conducted a famous study in which he subjected himself to a diet depleted of folic acid. He developed anemia after several months, and the anemia was cured by taking pure synthetic folic acid. At this symposium I discussed recent findings from the Armed Forces Institute of Pathology showing that users of oral contraceptive hormones developed arteriosclerotic plaques and an increased risk of thrombosis in young women, suggesting that abnormal homocysteine metabolism might be involved [22]. I was aided by my experience in studying pregnenolone metabolism with Lewis Engel during medical school. The subject has proven to be complex, with no clear answer about the effect of these hormones on homocysteine metabolism. There is a slight increase in plasma homocysteine during the estrogenic phase, compared with the progestational phase of the normal menstrual cycle. Homocysteine metabolism changes after menopause, however, and plasma homocysteine levels in post-menopausal women increase to the levels observed in men of the same age, correlating with increasing risk of arteriosclerosis.

An independent experimental study with baboons, carried out by Leonard Harker and Russell Ross of Seattle, showed that intravenous homocysteine thiolactone causes arterial plaques and thrombosis of arteries within 2-3 weeks, in agreement with our findings in rabbits [23]. Their report published in 1976 supported the homocysteine theory of arteriosclerosis that I had proposed in my previous articles. Another important publication in 1976 showed that a child who died with methylenetetrahydrofolate reductase deficiency and homocystinuria had arteriosclerotic plaques in the arteries that were almost identical with the plaques that I had found in my two original cases of homocystinuria published in 1969 [24]. This third major type of enzymatic deficiency causes elevation of plasma homocysteine, similar to that found in the two other types, cystathionine synthase deficiency and methionine synthase deficiency (Figure 8). The finding of arterial plaques in this patient was independent confirmation of my conclusion that arteriosclerotic plaques are caused by a direct effect of homocysteine on the cells and tissues of the arteries.

In the 7 years since publication of my discovery of arteriosclerosis in children with homocystinuria, my exploration of the homocysteine field produced new insights into the biochemical, physiological, cellular and pathological processes in normal growth, arteriosclerosis, cancer and aging. We had succeeded in producing the essential pathological abnormalities of blood vessels in homocystinuria, produced by three different inherited enzymatic abnormalities, by administration of homocysteine to rabbits, reproducing the disease in an animal model. We had discovered a new biochemical pathway for conversion of homocysteine thiolactone to sulfate, correlating with production of abnormal matrix in cultured cells from a child with homocystinuria. We had discovered a fundamental abnormality of sulfate metabolism in cancer cells, by demonstrating the inability of cancer cells to metabolize homocysteine thiolactone to sulfate. We had demonstrated abnormalities of homocysteine metabolism in experimental scurvy and in aging animals.

Because of these new studies, there were many new hypotheses to investigate, and independent investigators had confirmed and extended some of our basic findings. Because of my previous experiences and disappointments as a research fellow, I was very encouraged that my findings were productive and moving forward successfully. It was an altogether exciting and exhilarating experience in medical science that I had dreamed of accomplishing as a boy scientist in Denver, reading about Paul DeKruif's *Microbe Hunters* working in the 19th century. I was so convinced of the validity and importance of my discoveries that I explored the idea of writing a book or monograph to explain to a wider scientific audience what I had discovered [7].

I was not prepared for the disastrous reaction of the medical establishment to my publications on my career as a medical scientist during the next two years in 1977 and 1978.

REFERENCES

[1] Cannon WB. *The Way of an Investigator. A scientist's experiences in medical research.* New York: Norton Press, 1945.

[2] Moore S, Spackman DH, Stein WH. Chromatography of amino acids on sulfonated polystyrene resins. *Analytical Chemistry*, 1958;30:1185-1190.

[3] Rinehart JF, Greenberg LD. Arteriosclerotic lesions in pyridoxine-deficient monkeys. *American Journal of Pathology*, 1949;25:481-491.

[4] Rinehart JF, Greenberg LD. Pathogenesis of experimental arteriosclerosis in pyridoxine deficiency. With notes on similarities to human arteriosclerosis. *Archives of Pathology*, 1951;51:12-18.

[5] Rinehart JF, Greenberg LD. Vitamin B6 deficiency in the rhesus monkey. With particular reference to the occurrence of atherosclerosis, dental caries and hepatic cirrhosis. *American Journal of Clinical Nutrition*, 1956;4:318-328.

[6] McCully KS. Hyperhomocysteinemia and arteriosclerosis: historical aspects. *Clinical Chemistry and Laboratory Medicine*, 2005;43:980-986.

[7] McCully KS. The homocysteine theory of arteriosclerosis: development and current status. In: Gotto AMJr, Paoletti R, editors. *Atherosclerosis Reviews*, Volume 11. New York: Raven Press, 1983, pp 157-246.

[8] McCully KS. Homocysteine and vascular disease: role of folate, choline and lipoproteins in homocysteine metabolism. In: Szuhaj BH, Zeisel SH, editors. *Proceedings of the 7th International Symposium on Phospholipids*, Champaign IL: ACOS Press, 1998, pp 117-130.

[9] McCully KS, Ragsdale BD. Production of arteriosclerosis by homocysteinemia. *American Journal of Pathology,* 1970;61:1-11.

[10] McCully KS, Wilson RB. Homocysteine theory of arteriosclerosis. *Atherosclerosis,* 1975;22:215-227.

[11] Kuzuya F, Yoshimine N. [Homocysteine theory of arteriosclerosis.] *Domyakukoka (Journal of the Japan Atherosclerosis Society*), 1978;6:135-139.

[12] McCully KS. Homocysteine metabolism in scurvy, growth and arteriosclerosis. Nature 1971;231:391-392.

[13] Clopath P, Smith VC, McCully KS. Growth promotion by homocysteic acid. *Science*, 1976;192:372-374.

[14] Ricci R, McCully KS. [Effect of homocysteic acid on chondrocytes *in vitro*.] *Atti Assozione Genetica Italia*, 1972;17:25-28.

[15] McCully KS. Growth disorders and homocysteine metabolism. *Annals of Clinical and Laboratory Science*, 1975;5:147-152.

[16] Spindel E, McCully KS. Conversion of methionine to homocysteine thiolactone in liver. *Biochimica et Biophysica Acta*, 1974;343:687-691.

[17] Jakubowski H. Proofreading *in vivo*: editing of homocysteine by methionyl t-RNA synthetase in Escherichia coli. *Proceedings of the National Academy of Sciences USA*, 1990;87:4504-4508.

[18] McCully KS. Homocysteine thiolactone metabolism in malignant cells. *Cancer Research*, 1976;36:3198-3202.

[19] Jakubowski H, Goldman E. Synthesis of homocysteine thiolactone by methionyl tRNA synthetase in cultured mammalian cells. *Federation of European Biochemical Sciences*, 1993;3:237-240.

[20] McCully KS, Clopath P. Homocysteine compounds which influence growth of a malignant neoplasm. *Chemotherapy*, 1977;23:44-49.

[21] Wilcken DEL, Wilcken B. The pathogenesis of coronary artery disease. A possible role for methionine metabolism. *Journal of Clinical Investigation*, 1976;57:1079-1982.

[22] McCully KS. Homocysteine, atherosclerosis and thrombosis: implications for oral contraceptive users. *American Journal of Clinical Nutrition*, 1975;28:542-549.

[23] Harker LA, Ross R, Slichter SJ, Scott CR. Homocystine-induced arteriosclerosis. Role of endothelial cell injury and platelet response to its genesis. *Journal of Clinical Investigation*, 1976;58:731-741.

[24] Kanwar YS, Manaligod JR, Wong WK. Morphologic studies in a patient with homocystinuria due to 5,10-methylenetetrahydrofolate reductase deficiency. *Pediatric Research*, 1976;10:598-609.

Chapter 5

REJECTION: THE MEDICAL ESTABLISHMENT REJECTS HOMOCYSTEINE RESEARCH

From the vantage point of more than 30 elapsed years, the context of the disastrous events for my medical research career during the 4 years between 1977 and 1981 seems clearer to me now than it did at the time. Although I did not realize it at the beginning of this period, I was due for an intense experience in scientific, medical and academic politics. All of the senior faculty and medical staff at Massachusetts General Hospital and Harvard Medical School who were involved with decisions about my career during this period are long since retired or, in many cases, now deceased. At the time, I had little appreciation of the maneuvering, rivalry and competition surrounding my current position in an elite scientific academic environment and my impending transition to an outside institution. There is an old saying that "academic politics are so fierce because so little is at stake." In my case, finding a position that would allow me to follow up on my very promising discoveries about homocysteine and disease was at stake.

While I was in the midst of my exploration of homocysteine research, my Chief, Benjamin Castleman, announced his plans for retirement in 1972. After one year of service as Acting Director of the Massachusetts General Hospital, Castleman retired in 1974. During the previous ten years he had supported my residency training in pathology, encouraged my research interests, provided an excellent laboratory facility for my research on homocysteine, appointed me as Associate Pathologist in his Department, and helped me to secure an academic position as Assistant Professor of Pathology at Harvard Medical School.

Before his retirement Castleman encouraged me to become interested in developing a computer based system for printing and storage of pathology reports. However, existing computer memory capacity was inadequate for this project in the early 1970s, and I had little background or interest in such a career. He also offered me the opportunity of developing a Division of Laboratory Medicine within the Pathology Department. To support my research activities, he discussed establishing a research laboratory in the kitchen area in the basement of an old clinical building that was later demolished. After careful consideration, I decided that the administrative task of consolidating the scattered laboratories conducting clinical testing in the Department of Medicine into a Division of Laboratory Medicine would discourage my research program.

While I thought that I might be considered as a successor to Castleman as Chief of Pathology, there was no inquiry or interest in my candidacy for this position from senior hospital or Harvard officials. Several national candidates were interviewed for Castleman's position, and I met with several of them to explain my research program. After a prolonged search, Robert McCluskey, an immunologist and pathologist associate of Baruj Benacerraf, the Chairman of Pathology at Harvard Medical School, was ultimately chosen for the position in 1976.

Before the arrival of Robert McCluskey, Castleman explained to me that my research laboratory was scheduled to be moved out of the Pathology Department into a large laboratory in the Jackson Tower building at the hospital. This lab space was formerly occupied by the prominent biochemist, Herman Kalckar, who had recently retired from his research program. This was indeed a palatial research laboratory that offered my research team wonderful facilities and space for continuing my exploration of homocysteine. For several months I was encouraged to believe that I could use this opportunity to increase the productivity of my research program.

It was not to be, because after one year, my laboratory space was unceremoniously claimed by the Chief of Cardiology, Edgar Haber, for his research program on immune aspects of coronary heart disease. When I complained about this discouraging situation to Robert McCluskey, he told me that he had no control over lab space in the Research Building or in the Department of Medicine. He then informed me that my research program was to be moved to a windowless, tiny, ancient space in the Department of Medicine, located in the basement of the Bulfinch Building, the original historic location of the Massachusetts General Hospital built in 1821. By this time, most members of my research team had "seen the handwriting on the wall" and had left for other opportunities, leaving me with my equipment and one research technician, totally isolated from the Pathology Department and cut off from the other research activities in the hospital.

During this period in 1975 I had the opportunity to become acquainted with Baruj Benacerraf, the Chairman of Pathology and Harvard Medical School. Benacerraf was appointed to this position in 1970, following a research career in immunology at New York University and National Institutes of Health. For his studies on the genetic control of responsiveness to antigens by the Ir gene, he was awarded the Nobel Prize in Medicine in 1980. On several occasions Benacerraf invited me to his apartment for rehearsals of music with his wife, who played the harpsichord, a cellist and an oboist. At a following musical event at the medical school, our ensemble performed the Bach concerto for oboe and violin. There was a strange tinge to this experience, because the tempo of the concerto during the performance was considerably more brisk than our rehearsal tempo. Benacerraf never mentioned my research program, but he did make a few obscure comments about the future of the Pathology Department at the Massachusetts General Hospital. His intentions were obscure then and were never made clear during several subsequent meetings at his office.

Meanwhile Castleman's retirement and the removal of my research lab to inferior facilities totally isolated me from the intellectual atmosphere of the other scientists in the hospital and made my position in the Pathology Department very tenuous. My National Institutes of Health Career Development Award had expired in 1976, and the salary support for my research program was now taken from my research grant expense funds. This arrangement put the support for my position partially on "soft money" from my research grant. The remainder of my salary was paid by my teaching activities in the Harvard-MIT

Program in Health Sciences and Technology and by the hospital for my clinical work as Associate Pathologist.

When I met with my new Chief, Robert McCluskey, about my future in his Department, he delivered an ultimatum about renewal of my National Institutes of Health research grant. If my salary could not be supported by renewal of this grant, I could not be continued as a member of his Department or recommended for continuation of my academic position at Harvard. Under the conditions of my isolation from the Department, the inferior conditions of my research facilities, and the loss of my key collaborators and technical staff, I could not in conscience ask for renewal of this grant. This situation was an academic "catch 22" asking me to accomplish an impossible task merely to continue my association with the hospital. In addition, he made it clear that there would be no recommendation for promotion or tenure at Harvard.

From his ultimatum, it became clear that I must leave the hospital and seek a position elsewhere to continue my research on homocysteine and disease. My opportunity as a promising investigator in medical science at Harvard had come to an end after an affiliation of 27 years, comprising college and medical school education, internship in Medicine, residency in Pathology, and 11 years of service as Associate Pathologist.

In previous discussions with my former Chief, Castleman had complained that I "had not convinced" the senior faculty of the significance of my findings and that I "needed to show the efficacy of your theories in diagnosis and treatment" of patients with arteriosclerosis. When I met with Charles Sanders, the cardiologist recently installed as Director of the Massachusetts General Hospital, to complain about my treatment and ask for the reasons for the decision about my career at the hospital and Harvard, he told me that the senior faculty had determined that I "had not proven [my] theories." Negotiation with Sanders had determined that December 31, 1978 was to be my last day of affiliation with Massachusetts General Hospital. My position as Assistant Professor of Pathology at Harvard Medical School was scheduled to expire on July 1, 1979.

In an earlier attempt to relate my discoveries about homocysteine to current opinions of followers of the popular cholesterol/lipid hypothesis, I attended a series of seminars and informal research meetings held by Robert Lees, a medical school classmate of mine and Director of the Arteriosclerosis Research Center at Massachusetts Institute of Technology. Lees had developed a convenient method of determining lipoprotein fractions from plasma of patients with atherosclerosis. He had spent several years at the National Heart Institute, where he collaborated with Donald Frederickson, Robert Levy and other members of the lipid research group. After completing further fellowship training at Massachusetts General Hospital, Lees secured a position at MIT and won a prestigious grant to establish a Specialized Center in Arteriosclerosis Research. After attending these meetings for several months, I decided that the focus of this group was not helpful to my concepts about homocysteine and vascular disease. It was difficult for me at the time to relate my discoveries to the conventional approach of the cholesterol/lipid investigators. Lees and I did make one attempt to determine homocysteic acid in plasma samples from patients with atherosclerosis, but our efforts to determine homocysteine levels by conventional amino acid chromatography were unsuccessful.

During the mid 1970s two young neuroscientists at MIT, Stephen Raymond and Edward Gruberg, became interested in my homocysteine theory of arteriosclerosis. They were recent MIT doctoral graduates in neuroscience who had secured junior faculty positions at MIT.

They became interested in homocysteine research through discussions with Moses Suzman, the South African cardiologist who had given me an informal course on the history of atherosclerosis research. In seminars at MIT Suzman described his success in preventing coronary heart disease with vitamin B6 and other therapeutic vitamins [1]. He related my discovery about homocysteine and arteriosclerosis to the success he had achieved in his therapeutic program. Suzman traveled widely in the US and Europe, giving seminars about his success and the explanation of his results by the homocysteine theory of arteriosclerosis. Suzman told me that when he gave these seminars to groups of cardiologists, his explanations were greeted by "stony silence."

Despite their training in neuroscience and lack of medical qualifications, Gruberg and Raymond became so enthusiastic about the homocysteine theory that they wrote the first book for the general reader on the subject entitled *Beyond Cholesterol. Vitamin B6, arteriosclerosis and Your Heart* [2]. Prior to publication of this book in 1981, they published an article entitled "Beyond Cholesterol" in *Atlantic Monthly* in 1979, introducing the general reader to the homocysteine theory of arteriosclerosis for the first time [3]. During the writing of this book and article, both Suzman and I regularly met with Gruberg and Raymond to assist them and check for accuracy of their approach.

When the *Atlantic Monthly* article "Beyond Cholesterol" was published in 1979, there was a flurry of attention paid to the striking conclusions of the article in the conventional media, especially the *Boston Globe* and *Time Magazine*, but also in the tabloid press, including *The National Enquirer*. When Robert Lees was questioned by a reporter from the *Boston Globe* about the article, he labeled the approach as "errant nonsense," and "a hoax perpetrated on the public." When the *Boston Globe* reporter called me for my comments, I said that supporters of the conventional wisdom about heart disease became upset when new findings and discoveries appeared to undermine their life work in the field.

After *Beyond Cholesterol* was published in *Atlantic Monthly*, I was contacted by a reporter and photographer from *Time Magazine*, which had become interested in this brewing controversy in Boston medical circles. *Time Magazine* published an unflattering photograph of me and briefly described my theory of heart disease [4]. They quoted William Castelli, the Director of the Framingham Heart Study, as saying that the approach of giving vitamins to prevent heart disease is "crazy." The *Time Magazine* article also described recent findings by Catherine Fabricant of Cornell demonstrating that a type of herpes virus could induce arteriosclerosis in chickens. If the chickens were free of virus, they were resistant to the effects of cholesterol in inducing arterial plaques, suggesting a role for virus infection in the disease.

Some contacts of mine told me that Frederick Stare, the Chairman of Nutrition at Harvard School of Public Health was heard to say that "no one on the Harvard faculty would ever say that vitamins had anything to do with heart disease." George Mann, an investigator in Stare's group, had repeated the experiments of Rinehart and Greenberg by feeding a diet deficient in vitamin B6 to young monkeys [5]. The monkeys had become so deficient in vitamin B6 that they became emaciated and anemic. Several of the animals died, and the survivors had no arterial plaques containing fats. Rinehart had subjected his monkeys to intermittent deficiency of vitamin B6, allowing them to survive more than one year up to 18 months. The arteries in Rinehart's animals developed fibrous plaques without fat deposition, and no fat was observed in the plaques unless the animals survived more than one year, explaining why Mann's experiments were unsuccessful.

During the period of my intensive exploration of the homocysteine theory, I was invited by David Korn, the Chairman of Pathology at Stanford Medical School and my former classmate at medical school, to present a seminar on my findings to his Department in 1973. After my presentation, Korn asked me whether I would be interested in organizing a Division of Laboratory Medicine in his Department. My reaction to this offer was similar to what I had told Castleman about a similar opportunity at Massachusetts General Hospital. I felt unqualified for the responsibility and believed that the administrative demands of the position would discourage further productive research on homocysteine and disease. Later, unknown to me Baruj Benacerraf and Robert McCluskey recommended that I interview for a position as Chairman of Pathology at St. Louis University Medical School. They did not discuss the proposal or inform me of their recommendation, and I declined the offer because I felt that the administrative responsibilities of such a position would spell the end of my research career.

When the reality of my situation became totally clear in 1977, my reaction to this stressful and disastrous conclusion of my research career was that of bewilderment and incomprehension. I was deeply disappointed that I had failed to convince the scientific and medical establishment and leaders of Boston medicine that my findings were important and worthy of further study. In my many lectures and seminars to the medical science community in Boston and elsewhere, there had been no credible refutation of the validity of my findings. Instead the principal reaction to my discoveries and theories was disbelief, lack of interest, and in Suzman's words "stony silence." There was no confidence that my findings were sufficiently significant or documented to modify any aspect of the conventional views about cholesterol, lipoproteins, and dietary fats as the underlying cause of atherosclerosis. Of course, I took these failings as a reflection on my abilities as a scientist, not suspecting the extent to which political motives and conditions affected my situation.

On New Year's Eve 1978, after an affiliation of more than 27 years with Harvard and Massachusetts General Hospital, I left my lab for home in Winchester to an uncertain future. I left under a cloud, dismissed by the new Chief of Pathology, the Director of the hospital, and the Chairman of Pathology at Harvard Medical School. There were no parties, no good-byes, and little acknowledgement that I had ever been a part of Harvard medicine. I had no laboratory, no research funding, no hospital or academic position, and no prospects for finding a position that would allow continuation of my medical science career. I felt that my efforts, publications, discoveries, and personal affiliations with Boston medicine had been totally and utterly rejected. To say the least, I felt that my treatment and ostracism had been unusually cruel and cold-hearted.

Naturally I scrutinized my conscience and my research results over the previous decade for any statements that could be construed as misleading or inaccurate. In my publications I had always based each conclusion on my own solid experimental observations. I had tried to refer appropriately to published research results by other investigators in the field. Whenever I discussed the possible relation of my homocysteine theory of arteriosclerosis to the conventional opinions about cholesterol, lipoproteins and dietary fats, I was careful to offer possible connections between the two theories in my articles and lectures. In my original article about the children with homocystinuria, I suggested that deposition of fats and cholesterol in arterial plaques was a secondary event following arterial damage by homocysteine. I could find no credible evidence that the motivation for my treatment by the medical science establishment was a reaction to any ethical or personal shortcomings as a medical scientist. I always had confidence in the validity of my findings and was certain that future investigators would corroborate my theories by independent scientific studies. For all of these reasons, I was determined to find a position in another institution that would permit continuation of my scientific research career. I was confident that my discoveries would ultimately prove to be important in diagnosis, treatment and prevention of arteriosclerosis and other important human diseases.

When I discussed my predicament with Robert McCluskey, my former Chief, he advised me to "quit research and enter clinical practice." He referred me to several openings in local hospitals that were looking for staff pathologists. I felt that I was over-qualified for these practice opportunities and knew that they would not permit continuation of my research career. When I discussed my treatment with Paul Zamecnik, he referred me to Alan Rabson, Director of the National Cancer Institute. His answer was that there are "no openings." In a later attempt to meet with Robert Levy, Director of the National Heart Institute, to discuss my findings and theories, he refused to see me and sent a letter of "no interest." Benjamin Castleman suggested that I might return temporarily to the Pathology Department on a Without Compensation basis, but this arrangement was vetoed by Charles Sanders, the hospital Director.

In 1979 after I left the Massachusetts General Hospital, the article "Beyond Cholesterol" by Gruberg and Raymond was published in *Atlantic Monthly*. Publication of this article was followed by the attack on my theories by Robert Lees in the *Boston Globe* and by William Castelli in *Time Magazine*. I was then approached by Canadian Television, and they broadcast an interview in which I explained my theory of heart disease. Following these episodes, Martin Bander, the Director of Public Relations of the Massachusetts General Hospital, called me at home and told me to "shut up!" He said that he "did not want the name McCully associated with Harvard or Massachusetts General Hospital at any time in the future." Prior to this episode, my former mentor, Paul Zamecnik, had retired as Director of the Huntington Laboratories, and I was not invited to the luncheon or other festivities. All of these circumstances and events emphasized that I had been ostracized and put in the position as a pariah to the Boston medical science establishment.

After my forceful removal from Boston medicine and science, my professional situation and reputation were precarious. Although I did not know it at the time, I had fulfilled several of James Watson's four rules for success in science, as described in Chapter 3 [3]. In my research program, following my serendipitous discovery of the relation of homocysteine to arteriosclerosis, I had tackled the two most important diseases causing mortality in the US, arteriosclerosis and cancer. My totally new theoretical approach to understanding these diseases was very ambitious and a very large risk to my career. Although I had a strong and broad background of knowledge and experience in basic medical science, my lack of direct experience in the lipoprotein field might have been criticized by some scientists as a disqualification for my investigation in this field. Because of the risk that I had taken in investigating these new concepts, I now found myself totally adrift with no prospects for securing a position that would allow me to continue my scientific studies. I desperately needed a scientific ally, as Watson had found when he was adrift investigating DNA structure, who could help me to escape from my critics and to resume my career in medical research. I needed to find someone outside of the Harvard orbit who was sympathetic to my predicament and ambitions. Although I was discouraged at my arrival at a scientific dead end, I was optimistic that somehow I could find some opportunity to re-kindle my enthusiasm for investigating homocysteine and disease. In Pasteur's phrase, I had not lost my "most precious asset" of confidence and enthusiasm for my ideas and discoveries. In fulfilling Watson's last rule for success, I had subjected my ideas to informed criticism by experts in related fields and had asked for their advice. Although my discoveries had been ridiculed by some experts in the arteriosclerosis field, I felt that no qualified scientist had found a weakness or fatal flaw in my scientific arguments.

Although my scientific career situation was desperate, there was a glimmer of hope that my previous service in Castleman's Department could help me from my unemployment predicament. Since 1971 I had served as Pathology Consultant and co-founder of the Clinical Laboratory at Massachusetts Rehabilitation Hospital, an affiliate of Massachusetts General Hospital. The Laboratory Manager, Terry Valdez, and I had started this new clinical laboratory and built it into a successful operation. The laboratory continues to this day as a support service at Spaulding Rehabilitation Hospital, named for its founder Cyrus Spaulding. My role as Consultant in Pathology continued with responsibility for directing the laboratory and serving on several hospital committees. Because the compensation for this service was so meager, I was only able to devote a few hours per month to these duties.

Another opportunity arose through my violin playing interest. While I was working in Cantoni's laboratory at the National Institutes of Health, I became acquainted with William Sunderman Jr (Figure 10), a young physician and pathologist, who sometimes played the viola in our evening string quartet sessions. Sunderman's father, William Sunderman Sr, was a violinist and a prominent clinical pathologist and clinical chemist in Philadelphia. The older Sunderman was a founder of clinical pathology in the US, who introduced the concept of proficiency testing in clinical chemistry laboratories.

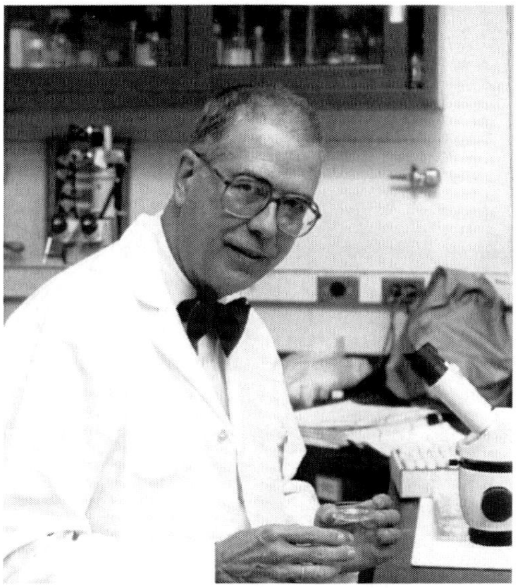

Personal collection of Kilmer McCully.

Figure 10. F. William Sunderman, Jr. (1931-2011) was Professor of Laboratory Medicine at the University of Connecticut and Secretary of the Association of Clinical Scientists. His father, F. William Sunderman, Sr. (1898-2003), was a founder of Clinical Pathology in America and founder of the Association of Clinical Scientists.

The younger Sunderman had a successful research career investigating nickel toxicity and had recently been appointed Chairman of the Department of Laboratory Medicine at the University of Connecticut at the new Medical School and Health Center in Farmington. Hearing of my predicament and unemployment, he offered me a part time position to support his investigation of the pathological effects of nickel toxicity in experimental animals. Several of the nickel compounds with which he was working are carcinogenic in man and animals, and I became interested in assisting in his research studies because of my discovery of abnormal homocysteine thiolactone metabolism in malignant cells. While conducting this research collaboration, Sunderman arranged for my appointment as Visiting Professor of Laboratory Medicine at the University of Connecticut Medical School. My friend and colleague Sunderman had stepped into my situation as a scientific ally in much the same way that Max Perutz and John Kendrew had helped James Watson, when he encountered difficulty for tackling the DNA structure problem with Francis Crick.

Leaving a full time position at a critical juncture in my medical career proved to be financially distressing for my family. The part time positions at Massachusetts Rehabilitation Hospital and the University of Connecticut, although helpful, did not substitute for full time employment and compensation. Both of our children had entered college, and their tuition bills were partially paid by financial aid programs at Cornell and Princeton because of my inability to pay these bills. The children had been interested in a possible career in medicine when they entered college, but they both lost interest in pre-med studies when they observed my treatment by the medical establishment. Because of our precarious financial circumstances, my wife Annina decided to give up her volunteer role as "Empress of Suburbia" and re-enter the workplace after an hiatus of 18 years, initially as a temporary office worker and eventually as Personnel Manager of a high tech company, Atex, located in nearby Bedford. Under these strenuous financial conditions, it was necessary to refinance our home in Winchester and use some of the equity in the house to pay college expenses and to maintain our residence.

My search for a position that would allow me to resume my medical and research career proved to be arduous and fraught with difficulty. My first promising opportunity was a vacancy for Chief of Pathology at Memorial Hospital in Pawtucket, Rhode Island. Through Harvey Goldman, pathologist at Beth Israel Hospital in Boston and the leader of our course in General Pathology for the Harvard-MIT Program in Health Sciences and Technology, I learned of this vacancy and contacted Frank Dietz, the President of the hospital. When I met with the pathology staff at Memorial Hospital, there was some interest in my candidacy and a verbal offer was given, promising a permanent position with appropriate compensation. I also met with Sumner Zacks, a neuropathologist at Miriam Hospital in Providence, who was the current Professor and Chairman of Pathology at Brown Medical School and a former resident at the Massachusetts General Hospital where I had just departed. After a delay of several months, the salary offer from Memorial Hospital was reduced considerably. Later I received a letter stating that another candidate had been selected. Frank Dietz of Memorial Hospital told me on the phone that I had "political problems" at Harvard and Massachusetts General Hospital.

Another promising opportunity was arranged through a surgeon colleague, Reuben Gittes, who later became Professor of Urology at Brigham and Womens' Hospital in Boston. A philanthropist, Leo Roon, and another philanthropist, Conrad Taff, had given a substantial endowment to establish a cardiovascular research center to the Scripps Clinic and Research

Foundation in La Jolla, California. After visiting Scripps and presenting a lecture on my homocysteine theory of arteriosclerosis, I met with Charles Edwards, the President of Scripps, to discuss a position there. Although I was interested in this opportunity, no offer was forthcoming. Later I was told by non-medical friends that key staff at Scripps had received negative phone calls from the Chairman of Pathology at Harvard Medical School about my candidacy. The position was finally given to Lawrence Harker, the investigator and colleague of Russell Ross in Seattle, who had demonstrated arteriosclerotic plaques in baboons treated with homocysteine in 1976.

Through a long standing friend and pathologist colleague in Philadelphia, George Hermann, I learned of a vacancy for Chief of Pathology at Fox Chase Cancer Institute in Philadelphia. After traveling to Fox Chase for interviews, I was informed that they wanted a surgical pathologist to be Chief of Pathology at the affiliated Jeannes Hospital, not a research scientist. Benjamin Castleman and Robert McCluskey supported my candidacy in letters to the President of the Institute, but when I spoke to his secretary she told me that she was having "ringing in the ears" after hearing a telephone conversation about me. Castleman told me that the Chairman of Pathology at University of Pennsylvania had recommended against my appointment to this position. I was disappointed not to be selected because of the fine reputation of the Fox Chase Cancer Institute in cancer research.

During my search for a position, I visited Cantoni's laboratory at National Institutes of Health to explore renewal of his previous offer of a position in his Department. In addition, I interviewed with several other scientists and administrators to inform them of my interest in a position there. Harvey Mudd told me of his new study of family members with homocystinuria. He later published his findings, claiming no increased risk of coronary heart disease in subjects that are heterozygous for the cystathionine synthase gene. Later studies from Ireland, however, concluded that this genetic marker increases the risk of coronary heart disease, contradicting Mudd's findings. In general, there were many critical questions regarding my experiments on homocysteine metabolism and growth stimulation by homocysteic acid, and the overall reaction to my ideas was frigid. Certainly no offer of a position was forthcoming, following interviews in the National Institute of Mental Health, the National Cancer Institute, the National Heart Institute, and the National Institute of Metabolic Diseases.

Through another contact at Harvard, Bette Uzman, former Professor of Pathology at Children's Hospital in Boston, I was recommended to interview for the position of Chief of Pathology and Laboratory Medicine at the Veterans Administration Medical Center in Dallas. After interviews with the Director of the hospital, the Chief of Staff, and the Search Committee, there was no interest in my candidacy. I later found that the position was given to another candidate rather than to me because of my lack of experience as a laboratory director. Through William Sunderman, I learned of a vacancy as a Staff Pathologist at the VA Medical Center in Providence. After interviews there, I was selected for the position, but the offer was later delayed in February 1981 because of a question about renewal of my medical license to practice medicine in Massachusetts.

During the period of 26 months in my quest for a permanent position from January 1979 to March 1981, I pursued a total of 51 opportunities nationwide through letters, phone calls and interviews. All of these inquiries met with rejection. When I met with McCluskey about my inability to find a position, he told me that I was "irresponsible" not to have found a position earlier. When I met with Castleman, he told me that I was not contacting the right individuals or the appropriate opportunities for my training and interests. When I met with the Dean of Harvard Medical School, Daniel Tosteson, to complain about my difficulties, he assured me that "nobody at the medical school is giving you a bad reference." I became suspicious when the records of my Continuing Medical Education at Massachusetts General Hospital were not available and did not reflect the extent of my education credits. These credits were necessary for renewal of my license to practice medicine in Massachusetts. In spite of rumors of "poison phone calls" and "negative emanations" I was never able to establish exactly who was preventing my success in finding a position.

It was clear that some sort of harassment campaign was in place and that I was being thwarted at every turn. In trying to understand the motivation for this campaign against me and my research discoveries, I concluded that nobody in the Harvard orbit would care about my fate if there was no validity to my discoveries and theories. The only conceivable reason for my treatment was a policy decision on the part of senior officials to discourage further investigation of my discoveries. Of course, this political decision had the effect of discouraging other scientists from entering the homocysteine field. The motto on the Harvard emblem is "Veritas" which means truth in Latin. Through my scientific research I had tried to find the truth, and now I was being coerced into abandoning my search for the truth. I could never find evidence that commercial interests were a part of the campaign against my theories, and the cholesterol cartel was never interested in my research discoveries or theories, except to ignore and ridicule my conclusions.

As I told Zamecnik, Bloch, Castleman and McCluskey, who had acted as mentors for my research career, I was certainly ready to leave the environment where my discoveries and theories were unwelcome for another institution more sympathetic to my research program. Yet during the four years from 1977 to 1981, I was unable to find such an opportunity. The harassment campaign had not only succeeded in closing the doors to all promising opportunities, but it had also succeeded in questioning my ability to continue the profession of medicine. As the victim of a campaign of harassment, I was blamed for my own predicament. Because of my failure to secure a suitable position, there were insinuations about my mental and emotional stability. Remarkably, however, throughout this ordeal I was able to maintain my composure and optimism, confident that some new opportunity would materialize.

The latest of my opportunities was beginning to succumb to a cloud of suspicion and doubt. My selection for the Staff Pathologist position at the Providence VA Medical Center was placed on hold because of my failure to renew my license to practice medicine in Massachusetts over the Continuing Medical Education issue. Since my situation had become totally intolerable, I discussed the possibility of legal action to stop the harassment campaign with my personal attorney. He assured me that a legal action to stop the harassment campaign would certainly destroy my meager financial assets and might permanently compromise my professional standing as a medical scientist, even if I were to receive some sort of settlement for my complaints. Instead he recommended that I explain my case to the important Boston civil rights attorney, William Homans, and ask for his recommendation.

As a descendant of several prominent Massachusetts families, Homans was, to quote his February 13, 1997 obituary in the New York Times, "a Boston civil rights lawyer who championed the downtrodden and the out-and-out villainous with such verve that he became a legend in Massachusetts legal circles." Some of his triumphs were his arguments in the State Supreme Court leading to abolishment of the death penalty in 1975, a landmark decision on appeal overturning conviction of a Boston obstetrician for performing a legal abortion, and his defense of defendants convicted of draft evasion in the Vietnam War era, leading to their acquittal. In a tribute to Homans after his death, the *Massachusetts Lawyers Weekly* quoted Superior Court Judge Julian T. Houston that Homans was "a hero to every lawyer in this Commonwealth who knows him, not only because of his extraordinary career, but because he has never succumbed to bitterness or turned his back on his responsibilities to his clients."

For my appointment with this legendary attorney, I prepared a detailed memorandum describing my unemployment problems, my education and professional experience, my dismissal from Massachusetts General Hospital and Harvard Medical School, my 51 unsuccessful documented attempts to secure a position elsewhere, and the threat to my license to practice medicine in Massachusetts. My interview with Homans took place at 4:00 pm on March 4, 1981 at his office in Boston. He sent his staff home, and the two of us discussed my situation for more than two hours, interrupted only by several enigmatic phone calls. We determined that it was in my best interest to settle my problem amicably without resort to law suits or administrative hearings. He recommended writing a letter to the Massachusetts Board of Registration in Medicine requesting re-instatement of my medical license in preparation for my new position at the VA Medical Center in Providence. He then told me that he knew several members of the Board of Trustees of the Massachusetts General Hospital and that he would "make a few phone calls on your behalf" to resolve the problem.

After my meeting with Homans, the clouds began to lift and rays of sunshine appeared. The Board of Registration in Medicine renewed my medical license to practice in Massachusetts promptly, and I sent a copy of my license to the Providence VA Medical Center. When Eleanor Travers, the chief of Pathology and Laboratory Medicine at the Providence VA called and asked me to report for duty on March 13, 1981, I knew that my ordeal was over. The nightmare of systematic harassment was over after 26 months of unemployment and uncertainty and after four years of medical politics that forced me to leave Boston medicine and medical science. My future career was to unfold at the Providence VA Medical Center. I was extremely grateful to Homans for his advice and assistance, and except for one phone call advising me to write to the Board of Registration in Medicine, I never heard from him again. Despite my offer, Homans never sent me a bill for his invaluable service and rescue of my career.

The position of Staff Pathologist at the Providence VA Medical Center qualified me for appointment on the faculty of Brown Medical School, and interviews with Sumner Zacks, the Chairman of Pathology at Brown with whom I had interviewed two years before, resulted in my appointment as Associate Professor of Pathology. My friend and colleague, William Sunderman, was instrumental in persuading Eleanor Travers of the VA and Sumner Zacks of Brown Medical School to accept my application for this position. The senior staff at the VA Medical Center and at Brown University was interested in my pursuing a research program, teaching students and residents from Brown Medical School, and practicing anatomic pathology and clinical pathology to serve veterans of the US armed forces.

References

[1] Suzman MM. Effect of pyridoxine and low animal protein diet in coronary artery disease. *Circulation*, 1973;48:Supplement IV-254. This abstract describes Suzman's experience with 17 patients with coronary artery disease given a low animal protein diet and 100 mg/day of vitamin B6 plus a B complex supplement for 13 months. All patients experienced increased exercise tolerance with complete or partial relief of angina, regression of electrocardiographic abnormalities, and improvement of the glucose tolerance test in 2 diabetic patients. Controlled prospective trials of this approach were recommended.

[2] Gruberg ER, Raymond SA. *Beyond Cholesterol. Vitamin B6, arteriosclerosis and your heart.* New York: St. Martin's Press, 1981. This 1981 book contains the first description of the homocysteine theory of arteriosclerosis published for the general reader. The book describes the status of the theory in the late 1970s and provides detailed information and references to the scientific literature to support the previous article in *Atlantic Monthly* in 1979. Moses Suzman and I consulted with and advised the authors while they were compiling the information and writing the manuscript for this book.

[3] Gruberg ER, Raymond SA. Beyond Cholesterol. A new theory on arteriosclerosis. *Atlantic Monthly*, May 1979, pp 59-65. This article for the general reader excited controversy and media interest when published in 1979. This is the first presentation of the homocysteine theory of arteriosclerosis published by the non-scientific press.

[4] Diet Debate. Is cholesterol the culprit? *Time Magazine*, August 6, 1979.

[5] Mann GV. Blood changes in experimental primates fed purified diets: Pyridoxine and riboflavin deficiency. *Vitamins and Hormones*, 1968;26:465-485. This article describes the effect of profound deficiency of vitamin B6 in the diet of monkeys. The animals became anemic, emaciated, several died, and the aortas contained no lipid deposits by fat staining. This apparent contradiction of the earlier results of Rinehart and Greenberg is attributed to the severity of the experimental deficiency of vitamin B6 in Mann's monkeys, explaining why he did not observe arteriosclerotic plaques. Rinehart and Greenberg's monkeys experienced intermittent deficiency of vitamin B6 and survived up to 18 months without severe anemia and emaciation.

[6] Watson JD. Succeeding in science: some rules of thumb. *Science*, 1993;261:1812-1813.

[7] Sunderman FWJr, Hopfer SM, Knight JA, McCully KS, Cecutti AG, Thornhill PG, Conway K, Miller C, Patierno SR, Costa M. Physicochemical characteristics and biological effects of nickel oxides. *Carcinogenesis*, 1987;8:305-313. This article summarizes the experiments with nickel toxicity that were completed while I collaborated with William Sunderman's research group in 1980. During 1980 my faculty appointment was Visiting Professor of Laboratory Medicine at the University of Connecticut.

[8] William P. Homans, Jr. Obituary. *New York Times*, February 13, 1997.

[9] Bellefontaine EJ. Appreciation of William P. Homans, Jr. "Enigmatic giant" was a hero to attorneys. *Massachusetts Lawyers Weekly*, 25MLW2141 June 16, 1997. In this tribute Bellefontaine describes Homans as "a criminal lawyer of great genius, a civil libertarian, a hero and role model for a generation of lawyers, and an advocate committed to his clients and their causes. During his legal career he defended the civil liberties of clients both rich and poor whose causes were both popular and unpopular."

Chapter 6

EXILE: AFTER BLACK-BALLING, A NEW OPPORTUNITY OPENS IN MEDICAL SCIENCE

Arriving in Providence on March 13, 1981, I passed the Capitol of Rhode Island located near the VA Medical Center in the Smith Hill district of the city. Atop the imposing marble dome of the Capitol building is an impressive statue of The Independent Man, dedicated to the memory of Roger Williams, founder of the Colony of Rhode Island and Providence Plantations in the 17th century. Williams had been expelled from the Colony of Massachusetts by the Puritan leaders of Boston because of his independent religious convictions. He founded the new Colony as a haven for seekers of a refuge from religious and political persecution and intolerance. My situation seemed similar to that of Roger Williams, as I was escaping from a political campaign of harassment against me. I had been expelled from Boston medicine because the medical establishment found my discoveries, ideas, and theories to be intolerable to the *status quo.*

A system of Veterans benefits and soldier's homes was first established by President Abraham Lincoln in 1865 "to care for him who shall have borne the battle, his widow and his orphan." The first veterans' hospital was established in Togus, Maine, adjacent to Augusta, the Capitol of Maine in 1866. In 1930 President Herbert Hoover founded the Veterans Administration to provide benefits, medical care, and memorials to the veterans of the Great War of 1914-1918 and earlier wars. The Veterans Administration expanded in scope and responsibility after World War Two and became the second largest government agency after the Department of Defense. It was established as a Cabinet Department as the Department of Veterans Affairs in 1989 by President Ronald Reagan. As the son and son-in-law of veterans of the Second World War and a veteran myself of the US Public Health Service, I felt that my service to veterans of the US Armed Forces was a worthy endeavor to which I could dedicate the remainder of my medical career. The Veterans Affairs Medical Center of Providence was constructed in 1949 in Davis Park, a beautiful arboretum and estate in the Smith Hill district of Providence, to care for the large numbers of veterans returning to Rhode Island and Southeastern Massachusetts after the Second World War.

The Pathology and Laboratory Medicine Service of the Providence VA Medical Center is located in a clinical addition built in 1979 to house outpatient facilities and the clinical laboratory, serving the needs of hospital in-patients and the out-patient clinics. After my arrival, my colleague and sponsor, William Sunderman of the University of Connecticut

Health Center in Farmington, paid a visit to the VA facility in Providence and approved of my new situation. He pointed out that the Laboratory Service offered a wide range of clinical services, comprising clinical chemistry, microbiology, hematology, blood bank, surgical pathology, autopsy pathology, and cytopathology. My training and experience qualified me for my duties as Staff Pathologist for these clinical services. The Chief of Service, Eleanor Travers, welcomed me to the Service along with Edward Avila, a young pathologist from Rochester, New York, who also became a Staff Pathologist in our Service. However, after 3 months Eleanor Travers departed the Service to become Director of Pathology and Laboratory Medicine for all VA laboratories in the nation in the VA Central Office in Washington DC. The Acting Chief of Pathology was Jesus Rodil, a long term VA physician originally from Galicia in Northern Spain, who had trained at McGill Medical School in Montreal and at a large teaching hospital in Winnipeg.

Our Service was affiliated with the Brown Medical School Residency Program in Pathology, and one senior resident joined our Service for 6 months to study clinical chemistry in preparation for his Board Examination in Anatomic and Clinical Pathology. With the departure of Eleanor Travers, however, our Service failed to attract other residents, and our residency program was maintained only on the periphery of the Brown program. Sumner Zacks, Chairman of Pathology at Brown University, recommended my appointment as Associate Professor of Pathology at Brown, and the President of Brown University awarded me an honorary MA ad eundum degree in 1983. For the next 20 years I participated in teaching residents and fellows in Surgery, Medicine, Dermatology and other Services from the Brown Medical School residency programs. I participated in teaching conferences in dermatopathology, gastrointestinal pathology, mortality and morbidity conferences, and tumor board conferences. These duties renewed my enthusiasm for clinical practice and teaching of pathology and laboratory medicine. I was especially pleased to devote my career to the medical care of veterans of the US Armed Forces.

After the departure of the former Chief of Pathology at the VA, a new Chairman of Pathology, Nelson Fausto, was appointed at Brown University. A political disturbance occurred between Brown Medical School and the Providence VA concerning appointment of a successor to the departed Chief at the VA. Nelson Fausto proposed appointing a faculty member at Brown to be titular Chief at the VA but maintain their principal operation at Brown University, effectively converting the Chief position at the VA to a part time appointment. The Chief of Staff at the VA and the Director of the VA Medical Center objected to this arrangement, and, as a consequence, none of the outside candidates for the position was selected. After a hiatus of more than 2 years, my colleague Jesus Rodil was finally selected to be Chief of Pathology at the Providence VA Medical Center. The impact of this political dispute was to remove our Service from active participation in the Brown Residency Program in Pathology. Rodil served as Chief of Pathology until his retirement in 1995. He was a generous and genuine person who encouraged my service to veterans in clinical practice, teaching and research.

Nelson Fausto, the new Chairman of Pathology at Brown Medical School, had spent a post-doctoral fellowship in the Huntington Laboratories at Massachusetts General Hospital, working with Nancy Bucher on the molecular pathology of regenerating liver. Fausto had studied the methylation of DNA during the active proliferation of liver cells during liver regeneration after experimental resection of liver in animals. Nancy Bucher had devised a biochemical system for the study of cholesterol biosynthesis in liver that had been used extensively by my former mentor, Konrad Bloch. I had become acquainted with Nancy Bucher during my study of steroid hormone metabolism with Lewis Engel and later as a post-doctoral fellow working with Paul Zamecnik on polyribosomes and protein biosynthesis at the Huntington Laboratories. Fausto was not interested in my research on homocysteine, even though some aspects intersected with his own studies of methylation of DNA by Cantoni's compound, adenosyl methionine. Fausto never encouraged my participation in teaching of Brown medical students, and he eventually discontinued the participation of the Providence VA Pathology Service in the Brown Residency Program in Pathology. Because of his antipathy to my research interests and because of the discontinuation of the VA in the Brown residency program, he terminated my appointment as Associate Professor of Pathology at Brown in 1988.

Because of my position as Staff Pathologist at the Providence VA Medical Center, I was no longer able to continue my consultation duties at the Massachusetts Rehabilitation Hospital in Boston. My experimental collaboration with William Sunderman at the University of Connecticut had concluded with publication of 9 interesting articles on the carcinogenic effects of nickel subsulfide and the related effects on erythropoiesis and arteriosclerosis in these experimental animals. Through these studies of nickel subsulfide, we established a relationship between the ability of this carcinogen to produce cancer and arteriosclerosis by effects on oxidative metabolism.

Several years after relocating to the Providence medical sphere, I was approached by my former colleagues at Harvard Medical School to conduct a discussion about the conflict between the traditional cholesterol hypothesis of heart disease and my work on homocysteine and arteriosclerosis. There was to be a confrontation between my classmate Robert Lees and me before the Harvard Medical School class in pathophysiology. I declined this opportunity for several reasons, among them a desire to maintain my distance from Boston medicine, an incomplete understanding of how homocysteine interacts with lipoproteins in producing arterial plaques, and a reluctance to confront a spokesman for the cholesterol cartel. For all of these reasons, I felt that my scientific medical research career should make a new departure from my previous ostracism from the Harvard and Boston medical sphere of influence.

When I began my second medical career at the Providence VA Medical Center, I was uncertain whether I could resume my studies of homocysteine and disease. The Medical Center sponsored a modest program of medical research, and VA faculty in different services of surgery, medicine and psychiatry had research grants for their research programs at the VA. Some of these research programs were conducted in collaboration with faculty at Brown Medical School. I approached the Associate Chief for Research and Development at the VA, Walter Brown, about my interest in resuming my research career. Brown offered me a position on the Research and Development Committee and suggested that I share some laboratory space in the old research building on the VA campus. Several years later I served as Chairman of the Research and Development Committee at the Providence VA Medical Center.

One of the effects of my ostracism from Harvard Medical School and Massachusetts General Hospital was that few investigators were interested in following the lead of my discoveries, theories and ideas about homocysteine and disease developed during the previous decade of exploration of the homocysteine field. Except for David and Bridget Wilcken in Australia and Lawrence Harker and Russell Ross in Seattle, there were few investigators publishing studies in the homocysteine field. In reading Index Medicus about homocysteine, there were few citations other than my own and those of the Wilckens in the early 1980s. It was not until 1984 when Lars Brattstrom of Sweden published a study demonstrating elevated plasma homocysteine levels in stroke patients that other investigators became interested in the field [1].

My first priority was to complete the lengthy monograph that I had begun in my last year at Massachusetts General Hospital in 1978. This monograph "Homocysteine theory of arteriosclerosis: development and current status" is the first publication in the medical literature to summarize my contributions to the discovery and exploration of homocysteine in human disease. I was pleased when my monograph was accepted for publication by Raven Press as part of their series of monographs, *Atherosclerosis Reviews*, in 1983 [2]. The administration of the Providence VA Medical Center supported this publication by a modest grant to defray publication costs. *Atherosclerosis Reviews* was edited by Antonio Gotto, a distinguished lipoprotein investigator from Baylor College of Medicine, and by Rodolfo Paoletti, a distinguished scientist from the Institute of Pharmacy in Milan, Italy.

In my monograph I discussed the experimental production of arteriosclerosis by feeding meat, milk and eggs to rabbits by Ignatowsky and by feeding of cholesterol to rabbits by Anitschkow. These results seemed to point to a nutritional origin of the disease. Furthermore, the experiments of Harry Newburgh, as described in Chapter 4, supported the concept of arteriosclerosis as a disease of protein intoxication. The later experiments of Rinehart and Greenberg, demonstrating arteriosclerotic plaques in monkeys with dietary vitamin B6 deficiency, also supported the concept of arteriosclerosis as a nutritionally induced disease. My monograph recounts the discovery of the homocysteine theory of arteriosclerosis through study of pathological findings in children with homocystinuria caused by different inherited enzymatic deficiencies, as described in Chapter 3. My monograph summarizes and describes our experimental production of arteriosclerotic plaques and thrombosis in rabbits, the growth stimulation of normal rabbits and guinea pigs and hypophysectomized rats treated with thyroxine, the production of aggregated sulfated matrix by cultured homocystinuric cells, the discovery of a new biochemical pathway for conversion of homocysteine thiolactone to sulfate, and the disturbances in homocysteine thiolactone metabolism in scorbutic guinea pigs and in aging animals, as described in Chapter 4.

My monograph describes the status of the homocysteine theory of arteriosclerosis in 1980 and attempted to explain the origin of the disease in the human population. The important study by David and Bridget Wilcken in 1976 was the first demonstration of abnormal homocysteine metabolism in human subjects with coronary heart disease. The early evidence for deficiency of vitamin B6 in human arteriosclerosis was published from Russia, showing that the plasma pyridoxine coenzymes, pyridoxal phosphate and pyridoxamine phosphate, were 23 nanograms per milliliter in the normal controls and 5 nanograms per milliliter in the diseased group. Declining plasma levels of pyridoxine coenzymes are correlated with aging and with increased susceptibility to arteriosclerosis. Experimental deficiency of vitamin B6 in human volunteers produces excretion of cystathionine and homocystine in the urine, further supporting the importance of dietary deficiency of this vitamin in human arteriosclerosis. Human populations have sub-optimal dietary intake of vitamin B6, because traditional methods of food processing, such as milling of grains, canning, extraction of sugars and oils, destroys 80-90% of this sensitive vitamin. By comparing the daily intake of methionine in vegetarians and non-vegetarians with the daily intake of vitamin B6, it was determined that dietary consumption of more than 2 micrograms of pyridoxine per milligram of methionine is associated with protection against arteriosclerosis in the population.

Several early examples of successful control of arteriosclerosis in human populations by utilizing the principles of the homocysteine theory are the Kempner rice diet for control of hypertension, the Pritikin program of exercise, stress reduction and vegetarian diet, and religious or other groups consuming a predominantly vegetarian diet. In all of these examples, the quantity of dietary methionine is decreased because plant foods contain approximately one half as much methionine as animal foods, and the dietary consumption of vitamin B6, folic acid and other micronutrients is increased by elimination of highly processed foods. These vegetarian groups and populations have lower blood pressure, lower body weight, and lower plasma cholesterol levels than groups eating a mixed diet, correlating with decreased susceptibility to vascular disease.

The small clinical trial by Suzman, as described in Chapter 5, was a specific application of principles of the homocysteine theory of arteriosclerosis [3]. In a group of 17 patients with coronary heart disease and angina pectoris, reduced dietary intake of animal protein combined with 100 milligrams of vitamin B6 and vitamin B complex supplements for 3 to 18 months produced improved exercise tolerance, decreased angina, and improvement in electrocardiographic abnormalities. Two patients with diabetes mellitus experienced improved glucose tolerance. This preliminary study was intended to stimulate larger, prospective studies in the future with more detailed clinical and laboratory documentation of improvement in morbidity and mortality outcomes. Suzman traveled widely in the US, Africa and Europe where his presentation of these findings was met by "stony silence" on the part of medical and cardiology audiences.

Epidemiological evidence shows that mortality from coronary heart disease increased steadily in the US during the 20th century, until a decline began in the mid 1960s. A conference sponsored by the National Institutes of Health in 1978 examined the known risk factors for the disease, including coronary care, smoking cessation, diet, blood cholesterol, exercise and hypertension in an attempt to explain the reasons for the decline [4]. The conference found encouraging trends in several known risk factors, but there was uncertainty whether the observed changes were sufficient to explain the magnitude of the decline in coronary heart disease mortality. The conclusion of the conference was that "although…the decline in coronary heart disease is real, the probably cause or causes could not be precisely identified."

My monograph presented an analysis of consumption of synthetic pyridoxine in the US food supply from 1944 until 1979. About 95% of synthetic pyridoxine is used for human consumption in the form of vitamin supplements and voluntary fortification of breakfast cereals. The per capita consumption of pyridoxine was quite small until 1961, when 0.53 milligrams per day, or approximately 25% of the Recommended Dietary Allowance, was consumed. During the 1960s importation of pyridoxine steadily increased, and during the 1970s, imported pyridoxine supplied larger quantities during the second half of the decade. Consumption of synthetic pyridoxine supplied 2 to 3 milligrams per day, exceeding the Recommended Dietary Allowance of this vitamin in 1974, 1977, 1978 and 1979. The conclusion from this analysis is that the decline in coronary heart disease mortality in the US was related to increased consumption of synthetic pyridoxine in the 1960s and 1970s.

In addition to pyridoxine, folic acid was also added to the US food supply beginning in the 1960s. Like pyridoxine, folic acid is susceptible to destruction by food processing.

Because of studies showing reduction in birth defects of the neural tube type following supplementation by folic acid, the National Research Council and the Food and Drug Administration mandated addition of folic acid to refined grain foods in 1998. Addition of folic acid to fortified grain foods caused a doubling of the average plasma levels of folate and a 15% decrease in homocysteine levels, as shown by the Framingham Heart Study [5]. The continued decline in coronary heart disease mortality in the past four decades is attributed to lowering of plasma homocysteine levels in the population by fortification of enriched grain foods and dietary supplements with pyridoxine and folic acid. A recent 2007 meta-analysis of stroke mortality concluded that significant lowering of plasma homocysteine over periods of 3 or more years led to the continuing decline in mortality from stroke since 1998 [6]. A study from the Centers for Disease Control and Prevention concluded that the decline in stroke mortality accelerated after folic acid fortification of the food supply in the US and Canada in 1998, but there was no effect on the decline in the UK where folic acid fortification is not mandated [7].

At about the same time that my monograph was accepted for publication in 1982, a new Staff Surgeon, Michael Vezeridis, was recruited by the Providence VA Medical Center. Vezeridis had trained in surgical research as a Research Fellow in Surgery at the Massachusetts General Hospital during the 1970s. He became interested in the factors controlling metastasis of malignant tumors and spent several years as an oncologic surgeon at the Roswell-Park Cancer Institute in Buffalo. After his arrival in Providence, we discovered our mutual interests in cancer research and decided to collaborate on studying cell cultures and mouse models of metastasis of malignant tumors. When the former Chief of Medicine at the Providence VA Medical Center departed for private practice, his VA research grant was given to Michael Vezeridis. This research grant supported a modest program of collaboration between Vezeridis and my research team for the next 9 years. I had tried to obtain research funding for my own research program from VA, National Institutes of Health and private foundations, but all of my applications were rejected as unworthy of funding.

The collaboration with Vezeridis was productive for almost 10 years. We were assigned part of a laboratory in the old temporary research building where a team of technicians, research fellows, Vezeridis and I carried out a new series of exploratory experiments. The facilities and equipment were modest, but the Providence VA built a new Animal Research Facility where we and other investigators were able to carry out our animal experimentation. Our research grant enabled me to purchase some equipment for organic synthesis of new homocysteine thiolactone derivatives for testing in animal models. I decided to resume my experimental investigation of these compounds that had been halted by loss of laboratory facilities and key staff at Massachusetts General Hospital in 1977. During these years, Vezeridis made some enigmatic comments and references to my treatment by Baruj Benacerraf, the Chairman of Pathology at Harvard Medical School.

My first objective for my research program at the Providence VA was to continue study of model compounds synthesized from homocysteine thiolactone to determine which molecular features of the hypothetical derivative are required to prevent growth of transplanted malignant neoplasms in animals. I was able to synthesize new derivatives of homocysteine thiolactone by reaction with maleic anhydride and with maleyl imide. The maleyl homocysteine thiolactone amide showed no activity against growth of transplanted breast cancer in mice. However, the maleimide homocysteine thiolactone amide showed some anti-cancer activity. When I incorporated this compound into a liposomal preparation made from stearylamine, cholesterol, and phosphatidyl choline, we observed a dramatic effect on cancer growth. This compound, purified by re-crystallization, when delivered in liposomes to mice with transplanted breast cancer or rhabdomyosarcoma (a malignant tumor of muscle), caused a 65-89% reduction in tumor size after 2 weeks of treatment. In addition, 70% of the animals with rhabdomyosarcoma had no evidence of residual cancer following treatment with this compound in liposomes! Our results were published in *Proceedings of the Society for Experimental Biology and Medicine* in 1985 [8].

Encouraged by our spectacular results with maleimide homocysteine thiolactone amide, I next explored the reaction between oxalyl chloride, a reactive bifunctional reagent, and homocysteine thiolactone. This reaction yielded an interesting dark brown black oil that could not be crystallized. There was no effect on growth of transplanted breast cancer in mice. In looking for ways to crystallize oxalyl homocysteine thiolactone, I found that complex formation with rhodium trichloride, an easily available transition metal complex, yielded a red-brown powder that resisted crystallization. Treatment of mice with this substance dissolved in lipid vehicle resulted in a prominent 50% reduction of growth of transplanted breast cancer. In one animal, a new malignant tumor, a leiomyosarcoma, was found to have developed in the intestine, indicating that the rhodium trichloride oxalyl homocysteine thiolactone complex was both carcinogenic and also inhibitory to cancer growth [9].

My conclusion from the results of these experiments with the maleimide homocysteine thiolactone amide and with the rhodium trichloride oxalyl homocysteine thiolactone amide was that the unknown compound in normal cells that prevents cancer growth contains an amide nitrogen atom adjacent to the carbonyl of homocysteine thiolactone. Furthermore, complexation with a transition metal ion, rhodium trichloride, enhanced activity and may be involved in inhibition of cancer growth. The well known chemotherapeutic compound, cisplatin, formed from platinum, chloride and ammonium ions, is widely used in cancer chemotherapy because of its inhibitory effects on human cancer, supporting the idea that the unknown derivative may contain a transition metal complex for suppressing cancer growth. Our previous results showing inhibition of tumor growth by arachidonoyl homocysteine thiolactone amide indicated that a conjugated double bond system in the molecule enhances anti-cancer activity.

Because of success in crystallizing homocysteine thiolactone perchlorate and homocysteine thiolactone pyridoxal enamine that I had studied with Pierre Clopath, I sought collaboration with Gene Carpenter, an X-ray crystallographer at the Brown University Chemistry Department. Crystals of these two compounds yielded molecular structures on analysis of X-ray diffraction patterns. The result with the perchlorate salt showed that the ring structure of homocysteine thiolactone perchlorate was identical with that of the hydrochloride salt [10]. Our studies in mice with transplanted breast cancer showed that homocysteine thiolactone perchlorate increased tumor size and caused cell death within the growing tumors. Later experiments showed that this salt is co-carcinogenic in mice, increasing the number of lung tumors induced by ethyl carbamate, a known carcinogen in strain A mice. The other compound, homocysteine thiolactone pyridoxal enamine, had no effect on growth of transplanted breast cancer in mice [11].

In the last series of experiments that Pierre Clopath and I conducted before leaving Massachusetts General Hospital in 1978, we found that the amide formed from retinoic acid, the acid form of vitamin A, and homocysteine thiolactone had a significant inhibitory effect on breast cancer growth in mice. In repeating these experiments with synthesis of thioretinamide, Vezeridis and I were gratified to find significant inhibition of cancer growth, confirming our earlier unpublished results [12]. In a later collaboration with a Master's degree student, Michal Kazimir and his mentor Ray Wilson of Baylor University in Waco, Texas, they significantly improved my method of synthesis of thioretinamide, obtaining pure thioretinamide in high yield [13].

These results with thioretinamide, together with the earlier results with maleimide homocysteine thiolactone amide and rhodium trichloride oxalyl homocysteine thiolactone indicated that the unknown compound for which we were searching most probably contained a conjugated double bond system adjacent to an amide group of homocysteine thiolactone and complexed with a transition metal ion. The most significant transition metal ion in homocysteine and methionine metabolism is the cobalt atom of cobalamin, vitamin B12. Some previous results with synthetic analogues of cobalamin, published earlier from Russia, suggested effects of this class of compound on cellular oxygen metabolism. For these reasons, I searched for a complex between deoxyadenosyl cobalamin, a coenzyme form of vitamin B12, and thioretinamide. I was gratified to find evidence, using spectral changes, of complex formation between two molecules of thioretinamide and one molecule of cobalamin. I named this new complex thioretinaco, which is an abbreviation for the full name, N-homocysteine thiolactonyl retinamido cobalamin. This complex proved to be inhibitory to growth of transplanted breast cancer in mice [14]. In another experiment a single injection of thioretinaco into transplanted human adenocarcinomas transplanted in athymic (nude) mice caused a marked 50% inhibition of tumor growth in 12 days [15]. Thioretinamide was also effective in counteracting the carcinogenic effect of urethane (ethyl carbamate), a carcinogen which induces lung tumors in mice. Our spectral evidence showed that two molecules of thioretinamide bind to the cobalt atom of cobalamin, forming an octahedral complex.

In a collaborative study with Angelina Carvalho, Chief of Hematology at the Providence VA Medical Center, we studied the effect of several homocysteine thiolactone derivatives on the aggregation of normal human platelets. When I synthesized the free base of homocysteine thiolactone from the hydrochloride salt of the compound by neutralization with equimolar sodium hydroxide in the presence of chloroform-methanol, this oil produced a profound effect on platelets, causing intense aggregation at extremely low concentrations. Thioretinamide also caused aggregation of platelets at higher concentrations. We concluded that homocysteine thiolactone has the capacity to activate platelets, contributing to intravascular blood coagulation and the acute inflammatory response [16].

In further experiments with the free base of homocysteine thiolactone, we found that painting this oily substance on the shaved skin of normal mice produced a chronic inflammatory reaction with ulceration of the epidermis and marked thickening and induration of the underlying dermis. Histopathologic study of these pronounced changes revealed proliferation of blood vessels and nerves, an angiogenic response, accompanied by intense chronic inflammation with infiltration of the tissues by lymphocytes, histiocytes and plasma cells [17]. Adjacent to the inflamed area, small venules contained recent thrombi within the lumen. The margin of the epidermis adjacent to the ulcerated area showed a marked dysplastic cellular reaction, and in two animals the dysplasia was accompanied by foci of well differentiated squamous cell carcinoma invading dermis and subcutaneous adipose tissue. In addition, injection of homocysteine thiolactone free base into peritoneum or into muscle caused necrosis of intestinal wall and fatal peritonitis or focal necrosis of muscle with formation of epidermal cysts containing metaplastic squamous cells. In the animals with intramuscular injections of the free base, we found areas of necrosis in liver and kidneys, along with congestion of lung capillaries and fibrin thrombi within pulmonary arterioles. All of the animals with peritoneal injections of homocysteine thiolactone free base died within 48 hours, and a fraction of animals receiving intramuscular injection of the substance also died within several days. These experiments showed that the normal amino acid homocysteine thiolactone in the free base form, confirmed by NMR spectroscopy of the synthetic preparation, caused intense chronic inflammation of normal tissues, angiogenesis, proliferation of nerves and fibrous tissue, intravascular coagulation, dysplasia of epidermal cells, and invasive cancer of the squamous cells of the epidermis.

In a study of cultured cancer cells and normal fibroblasts, Michael Vezeridis, George Tzanakakis, and I examined the effects of homocysteine thiolactone, thioretinamide, thioretinaco and thioco, the complex formed from cobalamin and homocysteine thiolactone free base, on growth and glycolysis within these cells [18]. We showed that several of these compounds inhibited cellular growth of both malignant and normal cells in culture and promoted lactic acid synthesis by anaerobic glycolysis. These results corroborated our findings of anti-neoplastic and anti-carcinogenic activity in mice with transplanted breast cancer and in mice treated with ethyl carbamate to induce lung tumors. In general, these experiments showed a fundamental relationship of our compounds to the abnormalities of oxidative metabolism in malignant tissues studied by Otto Warburg and other biochemists in the early 20th century. This study was the final result of my collaboration with Michael Vezeridis over a 10 year period from 1982 to 1992. When Vezeridis applied for a third renewal of his research grant supporting these studies, the grant was not funded by the granting agency, effectively ending our experimental collaboration. All of my own applications for grant support to continue these studies were either rejected or not funded because of the disbelief in the importance of our results by the reviewers of the applications.

In the early 1980s I began correspondence with a fascinating physician from Mt. Pleasant, Texas, John Marion Ellis, who had published interesting studies of vitamin B6 and carpal tunnel syndrome. This syndrome is characterized by painful disability of the fingers and thumb caused by pressure of the ligaments of the wrist on blood vessels and nerves supplying the hand. In the 1920s John Ellis' father was a physician in Texas and Arkansas who participated in the conquest of pellagra by niacin therapy. Pellagra is a vitamin deficiency disease caused by dietary deficiency of niacin, as demonstrated conclusively by Joseph Goldberger in the 1920s. The cause of pellagra had been unknown before Goldberger's studies, and the dramatic cure of this devastating disease by niacin therapy was regarded as miraculous by Ellis's father.

When John Ellis returned to Mt. Pleasant, Texas after the Second World War to practice medicine, he had been influenced by his training in the Army and at Washington University School of Medicine in St. Louis, Missouri. When Ellis entered practice in the late 1940s, he noticed that carpal tunnel syndrome, the painful deterioration of nerves and muscles of the hand, was more common among the rural poor in the early spring. In the late winter and early spring, many of these residents of the Deep South had little access to fresh vegetables and fruits, subsisting on corn grits and meat simmered all day on the coal and wood stoves in their homes. Influenced by his father's experience with pellagra among the rural poor, Ellis suspected that a vitamin deficiency might be responsible for this seasonal occurrence of carpal tunnel syndrome. When he treated some of the patients with carpal tunnel syndrome with multivitamins, he noticed improvement of their symptoms. Because of his training in medical research at Washington University, he decided to administer individual vitamins by intravenous injection, one by one, to determine which vitamin in the multivitamin preparation was responsible for the improvement in carpal tunnel syndrome. In these early studies Ellis found that injection of synthetic vitamin B6 (pyridoxine) in doses of 50 milligrams per day alleviated symptoms and signs of the disease in 80-90% of his patients [19].

To study the biochemical basis for the clinical improvement of carpal tunnel syndrome by vitamin B6, Ellis contacted the prominent vitamin biochemist at the University of Texas in Austin, Karl Folkers. In their collaboration Ellis and Folkers demonstrated that many patients with carpal tunnel syndrome have low levels of vitamin B6 in the blood, as determined by assay of amino transferase enzymes that require this vitamin as a coenzyme. In controlled clinical trials, they conclusively showed improvement in the symptoms of carpal tunnel syndrome with vitamin B6 therapy [20].

When I invited John Ellis to visit the Providence VA Medical Center to present his findings with carpal tunnel syndrome, he and his wife spent several days giving seminars and discussing their results. Ellis's wife Lillian was a noted medical illustrator and artist who presented the abnormalities of carpal tunnel syndrome in brilliant diagrams and drawings for her husband's scientific papers. Ellis, Folkers and I suspected participation of homocysteine in the etiology of carpal tunnel syndrome, and we made some preliminary collaborative attempts to gain evidence for this hypothesis. Unfortunately, Folkers became ill and died during this period, and I was unable to secure funding for this project. One surgical resident in orthopedics in the Brown Medical School program became interested in conducting a controlled double blind trial of vitamin B6 therapy in carpal tunnel syndrome, but the collapse of my collaboration with Ellis and Folkers and his surgical mentor's opinion of the project prevented completion of this study. Hand surgeons have little interest in promoting vitamin B6 therapy for this common condition that can be alleviated by surgical release of the ligaments of the carpal tunnel.

A fascinating by-product of my collaboration with John Ellis followed a comment he made to me concerning his use of vitamin B6 to treat carpal tunnel syndrome and related rheumatic disorders of nerves, muscles and ligaments of the hands and arms. He said "my patients have fewer heart attacks than the patients of other doctors in Mt. Pleasant because of my use of vitamin B6 therapy." I encouraged Ellis to undertake an epidemiological study of his patients to prove this statement. He made an exhaustive study of the records of his patients to determine how many of them had suffered chest pain, heart attack, or other signs of acute coronary syndrome. He determined that his patients had experienced a dramatic decrease in risk of myocardial infarction, compared with patients treated by other physicians in the community. Ellis had given 50-200 milligrams per day of pyridoxine to almost all of his adult patients over a 30 year period, amounting to an average of 3,259 patients per year, about 13% of the entire population of the community. The other physicians in the community had not used vitamin B6 therapy during the study period. Ellis found no evidence of neuropathy or other adverse effects of vitamin B6 therapy over this 30 year period, except for rare cases of photo-sensitivity. In addition, Ellis studied death records and longevity of his patients dying at home or in nursing homes and determined that his patients treated with vitamin B6 lived about 8 years longer than patients treated by other physicians in the community. These results of this retrospective epidemiological study were published in *Research Communications in Molecular Pathology and Pharmacology* in 1995 [21].

Stimulated by the results of my collaboration with John Ellis, I decided in 1989 to conduct a study of arteriosclerosis occurring in autopsies of our VA patients at Providence over the past ten years. The degree of arteriosclerosis found at autopsy in a continuous, unselected series of 194 cases was classified as minimal, mild, moderate or severe. The clinical records of these cases were studied for evidence of hypertension, diabetes, kidney failure or elevated blood cholesterol levels. The findings showed that two thirds of the patients dying with severe arteriosclerosis had no evidence of hypertension, kidney failure, diabetes or elevated plasma cholesterol. Although serum cholesterol was correlated with risk of arteriosclerosis in the entire study, the average cholesterol level in those with the most severe disease was only 186 milligrams per deciliter, well within the normal range. Homocysteine determination was not available because clinical testing had not yet been developed in the 1970s and early 1980s. I concluded from this autopsy study that important factors, other than known risk factors, were important in the pathogenesis of arteriosclerosis in the majority of VA patients. I suggested that further study of homocysteine metabolism in these patients would help to explain the origin of the disease. My study was published in the *American Journal of the Medical Sciences*, the oldest medical journal in the US, in 1990 [22]. I chose this journal for publishing this study partly because the famous cardiologist, Paul Dudley White, in his discussion with our class at Harvard Medical School, said that he was a faithful reader of this journal.

In an attempt to develop an assay for homocysteine thiolactone in human plasma, I tried an extraction method using organic solvents, followed by thin layer chromatography. Although the control experiments were successful, demonstrating homocysteine thiolactone by chromatography, the experiments with human plasma were unsuccessful. The initial finding of large amounts of homocysteine thiolactone in plasma could not be substantiated by repeat experiments, using lipoprotein fractions separated by ultracentrifugation. The source of contamination by large amounts of homocysteine thiolactone in plasma in the original study could not be determined, and I published a retraction of these findings in *Research Communications in Molecular Pathology and Pharmacology* in 1989 [23,24]. I suspected that the source of this contamination was some sort of human error, unintentional or intentional. Some years later Jakubowski and his research team developed a successful, sophisticated assay for homocysteine thiolactone, demonstrating its presence in human plasma and urine [25].

Using my assay for extraction of homocysteine thiolactone by organic solvents, I decided to study tissue samples from human tumors removed during surgical therapy. Three cases of thymoma and colon carcinoma were studied with this method, and appreciable amounts of homocysteine thiolactone were demonstrated by amino acid chromatography of the extracts, varying from 17 to 124 micromoles per kilogram of fresh tissue [23]. Two additional human tumors, malignant fibrous histiocytoma and polypoid colonic adenocarcinoma failed to reveal detectable quantities of homocysteine thiolactone. These studies supported my previous suggestion in the *Cancer Research* article of 1976 that malignant cells contain increased levels of homocysteine thiolactone [26].

In 1985 a physician from Arizona contacted me concerning new studies on homocysteine and coronary heart disease that were conducted at the National Institute of Food and Nutrition in Warsaw, Poland. After correspondence with the Director of the Institute, Wictor Szostak, and his staff scientist, Andrzej Olszewski, I received an invitation to travel to Warsaw as a visiting scientist in 1986. When my wife Annina and I arrived at the airport in Warsaw, our passports and visas were perused by soldiers in uniform who telephoned the Institute to verify the purpose of our trip. We were admitted for a ten day visit through a locking iron gate, reminding me of Winston Churchill's famous description of the separation of Eastern from Western Europe by an "iron curtain."

Our visit to Warsaw was memorable, and the Polish scientists and staff of the Food and Nutrition Institute were most hospitable and gracious. We were treated to tours and visits to the Royal Palace, reconstructed in Old Warsaw, Wilanow Palace, Chopin's summer residence, and evening visits to the beautifully restored Opera House for ballet and opera performances, where we were seated in the Government boxes. We also visited a church service in a rebuilt cathedral in Warsaw that had been destroyed by a Nazi tank in 1939, and a part of the tank was imbedded in the wall of the reconstructed church as a reminder of that attack on Warsaw in the Second World War. Annina was accompanied by a charming endocrinologist, Magda Bialkowska,whose excellent English was most helpful in describing life in communist Poland.

On one occasion we were invited to an elegant dinner party at the Director's residence, where Wictor Szostak described their experiences during the frightening martial law period declared during the previous year at Christmas time. The protests by Lech Walesa and the Solidarity movement in Gdansk, Poland, in the early 1980s had provoked the Soviet Army, encamped around Warsaw. General Jaruzelski confronted the Soviet Commander and said that if Russian troops entered Warsaw, "the Polish Army would fight." On another occasion during martial law, all of the Institute staff was told to stay home during the Christmas holidays. On New Year's Eve during martial law Wictor Szostak responded to a knock on his door to find a uniformed, armed Polish soldier only looking for a holiday drink of vodka. Fortunately, after this confrontation, Soviet troops did not enter Warsaw, and the Solidarity movement led to relaxation of Communist rule, allowing the Nutrition Institute to resume their studies of nutrition and public health.

At my seminar at the Nutrition Institute in Warsaw, Wictor Szostak introduced me as "the father of homocysteine." Their research group had become interested in studying patients with atherosclerosis for evidence of abnormal homocysteine metabolism. Through a grant supported by Konrad Bloch during his prior visit to Warsaw, the young investigator Andrzej Olszewski purchased a state-of-the-art Beckman Amino Acid Analyzer. He developed a method for determining plasma homocysteine by acid hydrolysis of plasma, followed by column chromatography to separate homocystine and homocysteine cysteine disulfide. Using this method, Olszewski had demonstrated increased concentrations of homocysteine in plasma in patients with vascular disease [27]. The enzymatic methods and fluorescence polarization methods for determining plasma homocysteine bound to albumin, developed later in the 1980s in Japan, South Africa, and Norway, were not yet commercially available for comparison with Olszewski's method.

My visit to Poland was productive, since a number of studies were subsequently conducted in collaboration with Olszewski and the Nutrition Institute research group. Homocysteine concentrations were determined in plasma lipoprotein fractions from patients with hyperlipidemia and atherosclerosis, showing that LDL and HDL both contain homocysteine that was released by the acid hydrolysis of Olszewski's method. The ratio of homocysteine in LDL to that in HDL was found to be elevated in patients, compared with normal controls, showing a correlation between homocysteine bound to LDL and susceptibility to arteriosclerosis [28]. Plasma glucosamine was also found to be elevated in patient samples, correlating with elevation of plasma homocysteine, cholesterol and triglycerides [29].

In an intervention study of 12 survivors of acute myocardial infarction, treatment with pyridoxine, folic acid, cobalamin, choline, riboflavin and the antioxidant troxerutin for 3 weeks produced pronounced 65-80% reductions in plasma homocysteine, cholesterol, triglycerides and LDL, the first such study in the medical literature [30]. In another intervention study of 15 hyperlipemic men, fish oil supplements 12 grams per day were found to decrease serum homocysteine levels, as determined by acid hydrolysis and chromatography, by 36-48%. There was no effect of olive oil supplements in the same dose on serum homocysteine levels, and neither fish oil nor olive oil affected levels of cholesterol, HDL or LDL. The conclusion of this study is that protection against arteriosclerosis afforded by dietary fish consumption may be related to lowering of serum homocysteine levels by the n-3 polyunsaturated fatty acids of fish oils [31].

Through a traveling Fulbright Scholarship, Andrzej Olszewski and his wife Wanda were able to spend two years in America, one year working in my laboratory at the Providence VA Medical Center and one year in a biochemistry laboratory at the National Institutes of Health in Bethesda. We conducted a feeding experiment with rabbits showing that, in agreement with our earlier results, homocysteine thiolactone hydrochloride in the synthetic diet increased plaques in the aortas of these animals. The synthetic diet with butter as a source of fat produced prominent deposition of fats and cholesterol in the arterial plaques, converting them from fibrous plaques to fibrolipid plaques. Administration of thioretinamide or thioretinaco increased plasma homocysteine, determined by the acid hydrolysis method, and increased arterial plaques in aorta and arteries in the major organs of the animals. When corn oil was used in the synthetic diet, homocysteine levels were lower than the butter diet, correlating with the observed protection against arterial plaques [32].

In a collaborative study with Marek Naruszewicz, Eva Mirkiewicz, and Andrzej Olszewski of the Food and Nutrition Institute in Warsaw, our team studied the effect of homocysteine thiolactone on the properties of normal human LDL [33]. We confirmed the earlier finding of French investigators that homocysteine thiolactone reacts with the free amino groups of apoB protein of LDL. When we used increased concentrations of homocysteine thiolactone in our experiments, we observed that the LDL became aggregated and susceptible to spontaneous precipitation. When the thiolated LDL aggregates were exposed to cultured human macrophages in cell culture, the macrophages phagocytosed the aggregates, as visualized by gold-labeled LDL in phagolysosomes by electron microscopy. These macrophages became foam cells with greatly increased cholesterol and cholesterol esters in the cytoplasm. This discovery suggests that aggregates of LDL, caused by exposure to increased levels of homocysteine, become phagocytosed by macrophages of arterial wall, leading to foam cell formation and cholesterol deposition in developing arteriosclerotic plaques.

In another collaborative study with the physiology graduate student Michal Kazimir and Professor Ray Wilson of Baylor University, an improved method of synthesis of thioretinamide and thioretinaco was developed and proven by NMR spectroscopy and elemental analysis [13]. Using this method, thioretinamide was synthesized in high yield in a highly pure form. In experiments with homocysteine injections in rats, these preparations of thioretinamide and thioretinaco, and vitamin B12 all suppressed arterial plaque formation in branches of the aorta induced by homocysteine thiolactone injections. This experiment was significant because of the observed anti-atherogenic effects of these compounds, compared with the increased atherogenic effects of the compounds used in Olszewski's experiments. The results of Kazimir and Wilson pointed to the possibility that our earlier preparations of thioretinamide and thioretinaco may have been contaminated with unreacted homocysteine thiolactone, explaining the disparity with our results, showing an increased atherogenic effect.

With the conclusion of the 9 year research grant supporting Michael Vezeridis's study of the biology of metastasis, there were no longer collaborative research funds available to support exploration of homocysteine in cancer, arteriosclerosis and cellular function. Because of this development in 1991, I decided to turn my attention to developing a theoretical framework that could begin to explain our experimental exploration of the homocysteine field. I can remember pondering the molecular details and trying to work out a theory explaining our results during my 70 minute commute by car between my home in Winchester, Massachusetts and the VA Medical Center in Providence. I spent this time considering a molecular theory of atherogenesis, carcinogenesis, aging and cellular function and decided to write a second monograph to develop these ideas. I felt that a comprehensive molecular theory to explain my results would constitute a significant contribution to understanding the origins of cancer, arteriosclerosis, aging, and abnormal cellular function.

During 1992 I received a call from a friend and colleague, Harold White, a pathologist and amateur violinist with whom I had played string quartets a decade earlier. White had worked as a pathologist in the Boston area, spending some time at the VA Medical Center in West Roxbury some years earlier. He then accepted a position as Medical Director of the Research Laboratories of General Motors Corporation in Michigan. In this position White had investigated the effects of ozone on lung tissues in mice. He found that ozone caused cellular proliferation of lung cells and alveolar damage. Further experiments showed that interferon inducers protected against ozone injury and interferon antibodies enhanced ozone injury [34].

In my earlier reading of the biochemical literature on oxidative phosphorylation, I found reports by T. Wieland from Germany and Henry Lardy at the University of Wisconsin implicating oxidized sulfur amino acids in model systems of ATP synthesis from ADP and phosphate [35,36]. I was amazed to find that the most active compound supporting ATP synthesis in these model systems was homocysteine thiolactone! Trying to conceive of a connection with these earlier reports, I suddenly realized that ozone and oxygen could theoretically stabilize a complex formed between thioretinaco and ATP. Working with bond distances and bond angles of these constituents, I conceived of a complex that would provide energy for removing ATP synthesized on mitochondrial membranes (Figure 11). ATP is known to be synthesized from ADP and phosphate by an ATPase located on the F1 enzyme complex of mitochondrial membranes. This theoretical complex with thioretinaco, ozone and oxygen could supply the energy needed to release synthesized ATP from binding to the F1 complex (Figure 12).

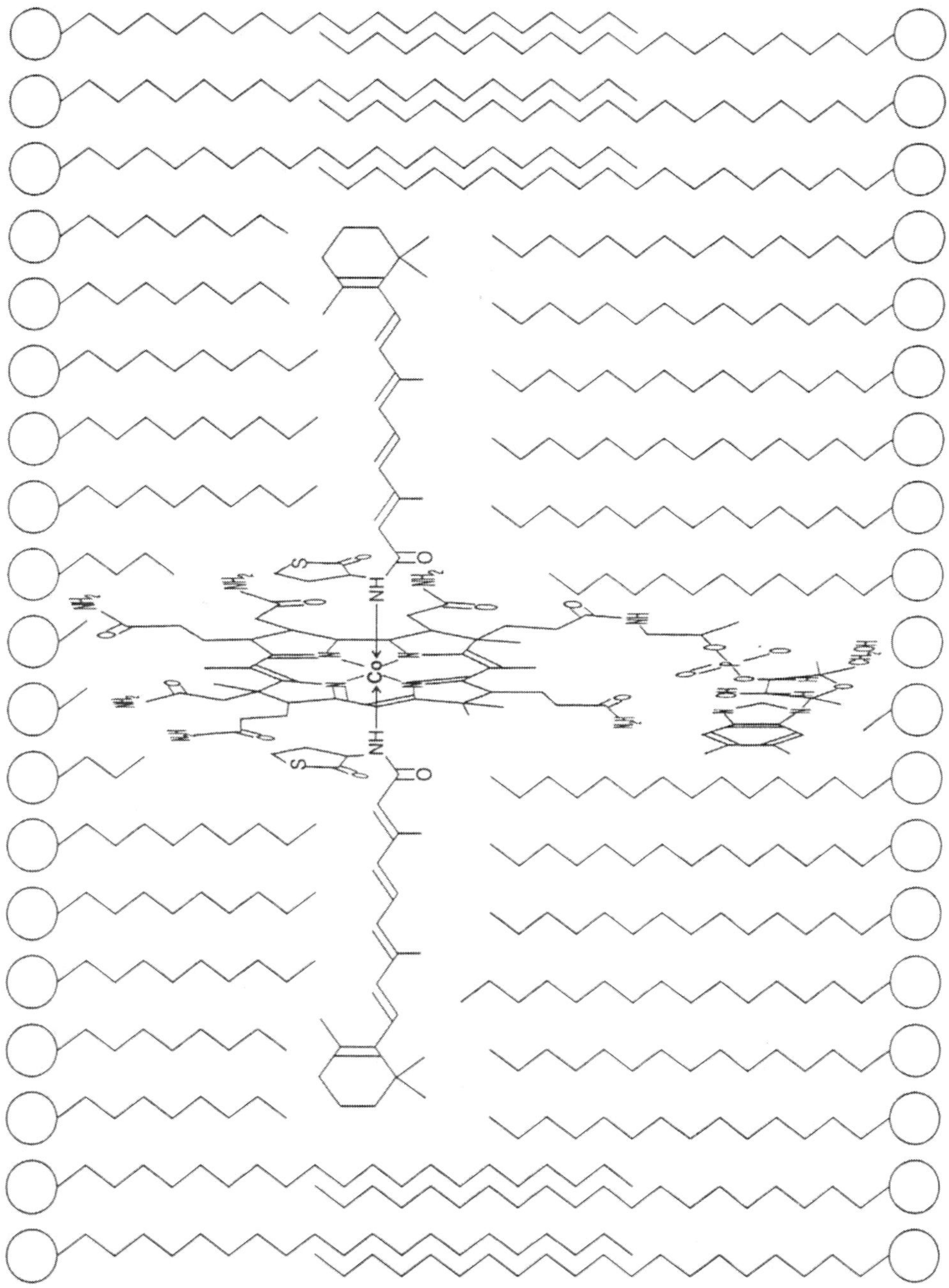

Reprinted from Annals of Clinical and Laboratory Science, 1994, Volume 24, page 40 by permission of the Institute for Clinical Science, Inc.

Figure 11. Thioretinaco, formed from cobalamin and thioretinamide, is bound to the lipid bilayer of mitochondrial and microsomal membranes by interaction of the two thioretinamide groups with the hydrophobic core of the membrane.

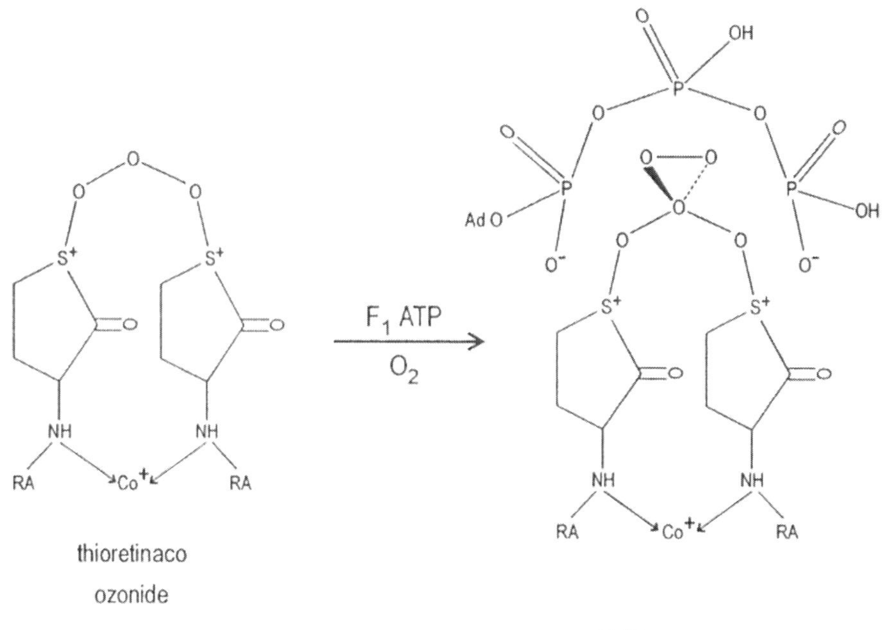

Reprinted from Annals of Clinical and Laboratory Science, 1994, Volume 24, page 42 by permission of the Institute for Clinical Science, Inc.

Figure 12. Thioretinaco ozonide oxygen complex is formed from thioretinaco ozonide, oxygen, and ATP from the F1 complex of mitochondrial membranes.

Earlier conjectures by EC Slater had envisioned a high energy complex, possibly containing oxidized sulfur atoms as sulfonium centers at the site of oxidative phosphorylation [37]. My concept seemed to provide an explanation for Slater's conjectures. During a conference in Boston on ubiquinone several years later, I discussed the possible function of cobalamin complexes in oxidative phosphorylation with Fred Crane, the discoverer of ubiquinone in 1957. He assured me that there was no cobalt detectable in the mitochondria that he had prepared in David Green's laboratory at the University of Wisconsin. On another occasion, I remember meeting Henry Lardy after a nutrition seminar presentation at MIT. When he looked at my molecular theory of activation of thioretinaco by ozone and oxygen and complex formation with ATP, he recommended that "you should publish this theory."

My second monograph, entitled "Chemical Pathology of Homocysteine," was published as a three-part review in *Annals of Clinical and Laboratory Science* in 1994 [38]. The first part, entitled "Atherogenesis," describes the chemistry of homocysteine thiolactone, the discovery of the homocysteine theory of arteriosclerosis by study of children with inherited disorders of methionine metabolism, modification of LDL by homocysteine thiolactone, and the role of homocysteine in the pathogenesis of experimental and human arteriosclerosis.

The second part of the monograph, entitled "Carcinogenesis and homocysteine thiolactone metabolism," summarizes the discovery of abnormal homocysteine thiolactone metabolism in malignant cells, the development of anti-carcinogenic and anti-neoplastic homocysteine thiolactone derivatives, including thioretinamide and thioretinaco, and the theoretical role of homocysteine thiolactone in oxidative metabolism. A center-piece of this section of the monograph is a detailed molecular explanation of the hypothetical function of thioretinaco ozonide in synthesis of ATP by oxidative phosphorylation. Also, the interpretation of the process of carcinogenesis envisions the presumed loss of thioretinaco ozonide from mitochondrial membranes, leading to the over-production of homocysteine thiolactone by malignant cells.

The third part of the monograph, entitled "Cellular function and aging," describes the presumed function of homocysteine and thioretinaco in cell division, tissue growth and function, and cellular respiration. The function of vitamin A and homocysteine in keratinization and squamous metaplasia, dysplasia and megaloblastosis, and in formation and maintenance of connective tissues are related to the newly discovered pathway for sulfate synthesis from the sulfur atom of homocysteine thiolactone, as established by our study of cell cultures from homocystinuric children. Finally, the function of homocysteine thiolactone and thioretinaco in the aging process is described, explaining the increased oxidation of proteins, lipids and nucleic acids found in aging tissues.

My productive years in exile from the medical mainstream contributed to a radically different and novel approach to understanding homocysteine metabolism in arteriosclerosis, cancer and aging. This unanticipated opportunity to develop and understand my initial exploration of homocysteine research occurred during the 20 years following my rejection by the Boston and Harvard medical establishment. Because of my years of preparation and education in medical science, adversity became opportunity.

REFERENCES

[1] Brattstrom LE, Hardebo JE, Hultberg BL. Moderate homocysteinemia – a possible risk factor for arteriosclerotic cerebrovascular disease. *Stroke,* 1984;15:55-59.

[2] McCully KS. Homocysteine theory of arteriosclerosis: development and current status. In: Gotto AMJr, Paoletti R, editors. *Atherosclerosis Reviews*, Volume 11. New York: Raven Press; 1983, pp 157-246. This monograph is the first detailed and comprehensive publication in the medical literature to describe the discovery and early development of the homocysteine theory of arteriosclerosis.

[3] Suzman MM. Effect of pyridoxine and low animal protein diet in coronary artery disease. *Circulation*, 1973;48:Supplement IV-254. This is the first intervention trial in the medical literature demonstrating a beneficial effect of the homocysteine theory of arteriosclerosis in patients with coronary heart disease.

[4] Havlik RJ, Feinleib M. Editors, *Proceedings of the Conference on the Decline in Coronary Heart Disease Mortality*. Bethesda MD: NIH Publication No. 79-1610. This national conference was held on October 24-25, 1978 at the National Heart, Lung and Blood Institute of the National Institutes of Health to examine the factors responsible for the 20% decline in coronary heart disease mortality since 1968. 84 nationally recognized experts in cardiology, epidemiology, nutrition and vascular disease research examined the known or suspected risk factors that could account for this pronounced decline in mortality. Some topics were coronary care facilities, coronary by-pass grafts, medical therapy, smoking, hypertension, physical activity, dietary fat consumption, changes in blood cholesterol, and air pollution. The conclusion of the conference was

"Although there was general agreement that the decline in coronary heart disease is real, the probable cause or causes could not be precisely identified."

[5] Jacques PF, Selhub J, Bostom AG, Wilson PWF, Rosenberg IH. The effect of folic acid fortification on plasma folate and total homocysteine concentrations. *New England Journal of Medicine*, 1999;340:1449-1454. This study analyzed plasma folate and homocysteine concentrations in a group of Framingham Heart Study participants in 1996 and in 1998, before and after fortification of the US food supply with synthetic folic acid. The results showed that plasma folate doubled and plasma homocysteine declined 15% after fortification.

[6] Wang X, Qin X, Demirtas H. Efficacy of folic acid supplementation in stroke prevention: a meta-analysis. *Lancet*, 2007;369:1876-1882. This meta-analysis of almost 17,000 subjects concluded that supplementation with B vitamins including folic acid, vitamin B6 and vitamin B12 significantly reduced the risk of stroke by 18%. They found that a greater beneficial effect was seen in those trials with a treatment duration of greater than 3 years (29% reduction), no prior fortification of grain foods 24 with folic acid (24% reduction), more than 20% decrease in plasma homocysteine concentration (23% reduction), and no prior history of stroke (25% reduction).

[7] Yang Q, Friedman JM, Botto LD. Improvement in stroke mortality in Canada and the United States, 1990 to 2002. *Circulation,* 2006;113:1335-1343. This epidemiological study showed that the decline in mortality from stroke suddenly accelerated in 1998 after fortification of refined grain foods with folic acid was mandated by the Food and Drug Administration in the US and Canada. There was no change in the decline in stroke mortality in the United Kingdom, where folic acid fortification was not mandated.

[8] McCully KS, Vezeridis MP. Antineoplastic activity of N-maleimide homocysteine thiolactone amide encapsulated within liposomes. *Proceedings of the Society for Experimental Biology and Medicine*, 1985;180:57-61.

[9] McCully KS, Vezeridis MP. Antineoplastic activity of a rhodium trichloride complex of oxalyl homocysteine thiolactone. *Cancer Investigation*, 1987;5:25-30.

[10] McCully KS, Boyko ER, Carpenter GB. Homocysteine thiolactone perchlorate: X-ray crystallography of a lipophilic salt. *Chemical-Biological Interactions*, 1985;56:121-124.

[11] McCully KS, Carpenter GB. Structure of pyridoxal homocysteine thiolactone enamine. *Acta Crystallographica*, 1987;C43:2345-2347.

[12] McCully KS, Vezeridis MP. Chemopreventive and antineoplastic activity of N-homocysteine thiolactonyl retinamide. *Carcinogenesis,* 1987;8:1559-1562.

[13] Kazimir M, Wilson FR II. Prevention of homocysteine thiolactone-induced atherogenesis in rats. *Research Communications in Molecular Pathology and Pharmacology*, 2002;5:179-198.

[14] McCully KS, Vezeridis MP. Chemopreventive effect of N-homocysteine thiolactonyl retinamido cobalamin on carcinogenesis by ethyl carbamate in mice. *Proceedings of the Society for Experimental Biology and Medicine*, 1989;191:346-351.

[15] McCully KS, Tzanakakis GN, Vezeridis MP. Inhibition of neoplastic growth by N-homocysteine thiolactonyl retinamido cobalamin. *Research Communications in Chemical Pathology and Pharmacology*, 1989;66:117-122.

[16] McCully KS, Carvalho ACA. Homocysteine thiolactone, N-homocysteine thiolactonyl retinamide and platelet aggregation. *Research Communications in Chemical Pathology and Pharmacology*, 1987;56:349-360.

[17] McCully KS, Vezeridis MP. Histopathological effects of homocysteine thiolactone on epithelial and stromal tissues. *Experimental and Molecular Pathology*, 1989;51:159-170.

[18] McCully KS, Tzanakakis GN, Vezeridis MP. Effect of the synthetic N-homocysteine thiolactonyl derivatives, thioretinamide and thioretinaco on growth and lactate production by malignant cells. *Research Communications in Chemical Pathology and Pharmacology*, 1992;77:125-128.

[19] Ellis JM. Treatment of carpal tunnel syndrome with vitamin B6. *Southern Medical Journal*, 1987;80:882-884.

[20] Folkers K, Ellis JM, Watanabe T. Biochemical evidence for a deficiency of vitamin B6 in the carpal tunnel syndrome based on a cross-over clinical study. *Proceedings of the National Academy of Sciences USA*, 1978;75:3410-3412.

[21] Ellis JM, McCully KS. Prevention of myocardial infarction by vitamin B6. *Research Communications in Molecular Pathology and Pharmacology*, 1995;89:208-220.

[22] McCully KS. Atherosclerosis, serum cholesterol and the homocysteine theory: a study of 194 consecutive autopsies. *American Journal of the Medical Sciences*, 1990;299:217-221.

[23] McCully KS, Vezeridis MP. Homocysteine thiolactone in arteriosclerosis and cancer. *Research Communications in Chemical Pathology and Pharmacology*, 1988;59:107-119.

[24] McCully KS, Vezeridis MP. Homocysteinemia and arteriosclerosis: failure to isolate homocysteine thiolactone from plasma and lipoproteins. *Research Communications in Chemical Pathology and Pharmacology*, 1989;63:301-304.

[25] Jakubowski H. The determination of homocysteine-thiolactone in biological samples. *Analytical Biochemistry*, 2002;308:112-119.

[26] McCully KS. Homocysteine thiolactone metabolism in malignant cells. *Cancer Research,* 1976;36:3198-3202.

[27] Olszewski AJ, Szostak WB. Homocysteine content of plasma proteins in ischemic heart disease. *Atherosclerosis*, 1988;69:109-113.

[28] Olszewski AJ, McCully KS. Homocysteine content of lipoproteins in hypercholesterolemia. *Atherosclerosis*, 1991;88:61-68.

[29] Olszewski AJ, Szostak WB, McCully KS. Plasma glucosamine and galactosamine in ischemic heart disease. *Atherosclerosis*, 1990;82:75-83.

[30] Olszewski AJ, Szostak WB, Bialkowska M, Rudnicki S, McCully KS. Reduction of plasma lipid and homocysteine levels by pyridoxine, folate, cobalamin, choline, riboflavin and troxerutin in atherosclerosis. *Atherosclerosis*, 1989;75:1-6.

[31] Olszewski AJ, McCully KS. Fish oil decreases serum homocysteine in hyperlipemic men. *Coronary Artery Disease*, 1993;4:53-60.

[32] McCully KS, Olszewski AJ, Vezeridis MP. Homocysteine and lipid metabolism in atherogenesis: effect of the homocysteine thiolactonyl derivatives, thioretinaco and thioretinamide. *Atherosclerosis*, 1990;83:197-206.

[33] Naruszewicz M, Mirkiewicz E, Olszewski AJ, McCully KS. Thiolation of low-density lipoprotein by homocysteine thiolactone causes increased aggregation and altered interaction with cultured macrophages. *Nutrition, Metabolism and Cardiovascular Disease,* 1994;4:70-77.

[34] Dziedzic D, White HJ. Quantitation of ozone-induced lung lesion density after treatment with an interferon inducer or an anti-interferon antibody. *Toxicology Letters,* 1987;39:51-62.

[35] Wieland T, Bäuerlein E. N-acetyl-homocystein thiolacton als Vermitter einer oxydativen Synthese von Adenosindiphosphat und Adenosintriphosphat aus Adenosinmonophosphat und Orthophosphat. *Chemische Berichte* 1967;100:3869-3876.

[36] Lambeth DO, Lardy HA. The oxidation of thioethers by bromine: a model system for oxidative phosphorylation. *Biochemistry,* 1969;8:3395-3402.

[37] Slater EC. The mechanism of phosphorylation in the respiratory chain. *Nature,* 1953;172:975-978.

[38] McCully KS. Chemical pathology of homocysteine I. Atherogenesis II. Carcinogenesis and homocysteine thiolactone metabolism III. Cellular function and aging. *Annals of Clinical and Laboratory Science,* 1993;23:477-493, 1994;24:27-59, 134-152.

Chapter 7

REDEMPTION: WORLDWIDE HOMOCYSTEINE RESEARCH CONFIRMS THEORIES

The first inclination that a thaw might be underway in the frozen forces arrayed against my discoveries and theories in the homocysteine field came in the form of an invitation to attend the First International Conference on Homocysteine Metabolism in Ireland in 1995. My classmate from Harvard Medical School and fellow Intern in Medicine at Massachusetts General Hospital, Irwin Rosenberg, who had completed his residency in Internal Medicine and specialized in Gastroenterology, had become interested in the nutritional consequences of folate deficiency in Bangladesh. He had been appointed Director of the Jean Mayer US Department of Agriculture Human Nutrition Research Center on Aging at Tufts Medical School in Boston, where he assembled a prominent team of investigators in the field of human nutrition and disease. Rosenberg was on the Organizing Committee of the International Conference on Homocysteine Metabolism, to be held at Castle Dromoland, Ireland, in 1995. He invited me to present a discussion of the pathological consequences of hyperhomocysteinemia for this conference [1].

To me this invitation was recognition of my role in establishing the importance of homocysteine in human disease through my original study of arteriosclerosis in children with homocystinuria. At the Ireland meeting more than 250 investigators from countries around the world met to discuss the status of the homocysteine field. In the preface to the monograph presenting the proceedings of this meeting, my contribution to the field was acknowledged [2]. "Most agree that it was Kilmer McCully who emphasized the association between homocysteine and the characteristic, premature thrombo-occlusive vascular disease that was sometimes lethal in homocystinuric patients. The index patient with homocystinuria in McCully's report of 25 years ago was a child whose homocystinuria was secondary to an abnormality of cobalamin metabolism that is now designated as Cbl C deficiency." At the Ireland meeting, two other participants, John Lindenbaum and Irwin Rosenberg, and I realized that we were all classmates in the Harvard Medical School Class of 1959. A fourth classmate, George Spaeth, an ophthalmologist in Philadelphia who discovered one of the original cases of homocystinuria, did not attend the Ireland meeting.

At the Ireland Homocysteine meeting in 1995, more than 25 years had elapsed since my first publication in the homocysteine field. My hypothesis concerning the possible role of homocysteine in human arteriosclerosis in 1969 was a challenge to medical investigators to develop evidence supporting or disproving this hypothesis. The first independent confirmation of the homocysteine hypothesis was the Chicago study of autopsy findings in a child with homocystinuria caused by deficiency of methylenetetrahydrofolate reductase [3]. In this 1976 report Kanwar, Manaligod and Wong described arteriosclerotic plaques in the arteries of this 9-year-old girl that are virtually identical with those that I described in homocystinuric children with cystathionine synthase deficiency and methionine synthase deficiency. Their study independently supported my conclusion that homocysteine causes plaques by a direct effect on the cells and tissues of arteries.

Another important study from the 1970s supporting the homocysteine hypothesis was the demonstration of increased blood homocysteine levels following an oral dose of methionine in coronary artery disease patients [4]. This 1976 study by David and Bridget Wilcken demonstrated abnormal homocysteine metabolism for the first time in human arteriosclerosis. The Wilcken team in Australia went on in subsequent studies to demonstrate elevated blood levels of homocysteine in patients with kidney failure, correlating with the known high susceptibility of these patients to rapidly progressive atherosclerosis. They also showed that blood homocysteine levels in women increase after menopause, correlating with increased susceptibility of older women to atherosclerosis.

The important experiment of Lawrence Harker and Russell Ross in 1976 showed that intravenous homocysteine causes arteriosclerotic plaques and arterial thrombosis in baboons [5]. This study added significant experimental evidence to our studies in rabbits showing production of arterial plaques and thrombosis in experimental animals. These studies showed conclusively that homocysteine is atherogenic in animals, supporting the homocysteine theory of arteriosclerosis.

As discussed in the previous chapter, my forced exile from the Boston medical establishment in 1979 had the effect of discouraging other investigators from entering the homocysteine field by casting doubt on the significance of my published discoveries and theories. Meanwhile, proponents of the cholesterol/fat hypothesis held sway over funding of large scale studies of human atherosclerosis. Following the ignominious failure of the Coronary Drug Project of the 1970s because of failure to demonstrate benefit and because of breast cancer in men given female estrogens, other expensive trails attempted to prove the cholesterol/fat hypothesis once and for all. The results of the massive Multiple Risk Factor Intervention Trial (MRFIT) and the even more massive Lipid Research Clinics Trial, each costing in excess of $100M, failed to show that dietary low fat diets, lowering of blood cholesterol by drug therapy, and control of known risk factors like smoking and exercise had a significant effect on human atherosclerosis. The "cholesterol cartel" formed by cholesterol/fat investigators and the pharmaceutical industry became excited by introduction of statin drugs in the 1980s. These drugs had the capacity to lower blood cholesterol levels more reliably and significantly than previous unpalatable drug therapy, used in the MRFIT and Lipid Research Clinics trials. This approach received further encouragement and impetus by awarding of the Nobel Prize in Medicine in 1985 to Michael Brown and Joseph Goldstein for their discovery of defective LDL receptors in patients with familial hypercholesterolemia [6]. These developments emboldened cholesterol/fat investigators to predict the end of coronary heart disease by the year 2000!

It was not until 1984 that the homocysteine field received encouragement from the study by Lars Brattstrom and his team from Sweden, showing greatly increased risk of stroke and cerebrovascular disease in patients with elevated blood homocysteine levels [7]. Soon thereafter, studies from New York, Netherlands, and Ireland showed that elevated blood homocysteine levels conferred increased risk for coronary heart disease and stroke both in unselected populations and in presumed heterozygotes for cystathionine synthase deficiency [8-10]. These studies from the 1980s conclusively showed that elevated blood homocysteine levels independently confer increased risk for vascular disease. In addition these studies also showed that elevated blood homocysteine levels further increase risk by synergizing with known risk factors such as smoking, hypertension, diabetes, kidney failure and dyslipidemia.

The important 1995 Hordaland Homocysteine Study conducted in Bergen and Oslo, Norway, examined plasma homocysteine levels in 16,000 normal men and women aged 40-67 [11]. The results showed significant correlations between plasma homocysteine levels and important known risk factors for cardiovascular disease, including age, male gender, smoking, hypertension, elevated blood cholesterol, and lack of exercise. Adjustment for intake of vitamin supplements, fruits and vegetables strengthened the relation between homocysteine levels and age.

Population and epidemiological studies of homocysteine in vascular disease were made possible by introduction of satisfactory methods for chemical determination of homocysteine in plasma. The original method of amino acid analysis, as developed by Stein and Moore at the Rockefeller Institute in the 1950s and 1960s, was not satisfactory for detecting homocysteine, because the trace amounts of free homocysteine (0.1μM) are co-eluted with large amounts of methionine by column chromatography. More than 95% of homocysteine is chemically bound to albumin and other plasma proteins by disulfide bonds. In order to detect protein-bound homocysteine, the disulfide bond is broken by a strong reducing agent, and the resulting free homocysteine is attached to a fluorescent label for detection during high-performance liquid chromatography. A method for detection of homocysteine by enzymatic reaction coupled with an immunological reaction with an antibody to adenosyl homocysteine was adapted for automated clinical chemical analysis by Mohammed Shipchandler and Edwin Moore of Abbott Laboratories [12,13]. These automated methods proved to be better suited to population studies than Andrzej Olszewski's acid hydrolysis method developed in the early 1980s.

The important 1992 Physicians' Health Study examined 15,000 male physicians aged 40-84 with no history of vascular disease during a 5 year period of observation [14]. Plasma homocysteine levels were measured at the beginning and end of the study. 271 of the men developed myocardial infarction during the observation, and these cases were compared with an equal number of control men without myocardial infarction, matched by age and smoking status. Homocysteine levels were higher in cases than controls, and those men with the highest homocysteine levels had a 3.4 fold increased risk of myocardial infarction, compared with controls. Adjustment for diabetes, hypertension, body weight and total cholesterol/HDL ratio strengthened the association.

The 1993 Framingham Heart Study report examined the relation between the B vitamins, folic acid, vitamin B6 and vitamin B12 and homocysteine levels in more than 1100 elderly participants aged 67-96 [15]. This study showed a strong correlation between age, B vitamin status and blood homocysteine levels. Low levels of folate, vitamin B6, and vitamin B12 in plasma were associated with elevation of blood homocysteine levels. Two thirds of these elderly participants had deficiencies of one or more of these B vitamins, correlating with deficient dietary intakes of folic acid and vitamin B6. Dietary intakes of vitamin B12 were not correlated with blood homocysteine levels, but those participants with low plasma vitamin

B12 levels from poor absorption of the vitamin had an increased incidence of narrowing of the carotid arteries by arteriosclerotic plaques. These Framingham studies of the elderly who are at high risk of vascular disease directly support the homocysteine theory of arteriosclerosis.

The European Concerted Action Project of 1997 examined 750 cases of atherosclerosis involving heart, brain and legs in 19 centers in 9 European countries, compared with 800 controls of both sexes younger than 60 years [16]. In this study an increased plasma homocysteine level was found to confer an independent risk of vascular disease similar to that of smoking or elevated blood lipids. In addition, elevation of plasma homocysteine substantially increased disease risk in those with hypertension and in those who smoked. In confirmation of the Framingham Heart Study, the levels of folate, cobalamin and pyridoxal phosphate in red cells were inversely related to plasma homocysteine levels. In addition, users of vitamin supplements had a substantially lower risk of vascular disease, compared with non-users.

The 1995 meta-analysis from the University of Washington analyzed data from 27 US studies of homocysteine in arteriosclerotic vascular disease and from 11 US studies of the effects of folic acid on blood homocysteine levels [17]. They concluded that 10% of the population risk of coronary heart disease is attributable to elevation of blood homocysteine in both men and women. They estimated that increased dietary folate, vitamin supplements, and grain fortification with folic acid would prevent an estimated 13,500 to 50,000 coronary heart disease deaths in the US per year.

Because of this flurry of publication in prestigious medical journals in 1995, directly supporting the homocysteine theory of arteriosclerosis, and because my 1969 article in the *American Journal of Pathology* was prominently referenced in these articles, I received a call from Gina Kolata, the *New York Times* science reporter, requesting an interview about my contributions to the homocysteine field. After a telephone interview and a photograph of me taken in my office in the Providence VA Medical Center, a lengthy article with a large photograph of me was published in the July 5, 1995 edition of the *New York Times* [18]. In this article Gina Kolata reported on the First International Homocysteine Conference currently being held in Ireland and described my discovery of the homocysteine theory of arteriosclerosis. She quoted Meir Stampfer, the Director of the Physicians' Health Study, about my discovery that I was "one of those unfortunate cases of people being ahead of their time." My answer was "In my view, I was not ahead of my time, the other [investigators] were behind." She also quoted Irwin Rosenberg, the Director of the Framingham Heart Study on B vitamins, in describing the effect of dietary B vitamins on homocysteine levels "I think we're really expanding our definition of what we mean by diet and heart disease." The article also described the findings of Rima Rozen and her team from McGill University in Montreal that 12% of the population carries a genetic variant of the enzyme (methylenetetrahydrofolate reductase) that leads to elevated homocysteine levels when dietary folic acid is insufficient.

Following my return from the Homocysteine meeting in Ireland and publication of the news story about my work in the *New York Times*, the Editor and Publisher of *Keats Publishing Company* contacted me about writing a book concerning my discovery and development of the homocysteine theory of arteriosclerosis. The proposed book was intended to inform the general reader about the discovery of the theory, its general characteristics, and my personal story of rejection and acceptance. My challenge in writing this book, *The Homocysteine Revolution. Medicine for the New Millennium*, was to explain a complex biochemical, nutritional and medical theory of the origin of heart disease in a way that is comprehensible to the general reader without specialized scientific knowledge and training. With assistance of two editors, Phyllis Herman of *Keats Publishing, Inc.* and Annette Francis of *Bravo Books, Inc.*, I was able to complete the manuscript for publication in 1997. In a book of this length, comprising 233 pages, I was able to explain the origin, discovery, and development of the homocysteine theory of arteriosclerosis for the general reader in a comprehensive fashion for the first time [19].

Andrew Weil, a prominent exponent of integrative medicine, and Walter Willett, Professor of Nutrition at the Harvard School of Public Health, wrote a Foreward and Introduction to *The Homocysteine Revolution.* Weil described the book as "a medical detective story" because of the serendipitous way in which I discovered the homocysteine theory, as explained in Chapter 3. He also described my experience of rejection by the medical establishment as "a telling glimpse into the politics of medical research [which] illuminates the tortuous way in which new ideas gain the attention of the medical establishment." Willett also calls attention to this book that "combines an intriguing plot, in this case a fascinating scientific detective story, with information that can be of great personal value." My experience with rejection by the medical establishment is described more fully in Chapter 5.

Public reaction to publication of *The Homocysteine Revolution* was favorable. The book was accepted by many readers and scientists as a satisfactory explanation of the homocysteine theory of arteriosclerosis. The book is currently still in print 15 years after publication. Following publication of the book, the news article about my research in the *New York Times*, and the multiple studies supporting the homocysteine theory in the *Journal of the American Medical Association* and the *New England Journal of Medicine*, a number of journalists, medical writers, and publishers wrote articles and published interviews in newspapers and magazines. Articles were published in the *Washington Post, Los Angeles Times, Providence Journal, Boston Globe, International Herald Tribune, Reader's Digest, Saturday Evening Post, Time Magazine,* and *Newsweek.* A news item was broadcast by NBC TV Nightly News with Tom Brokaw in March 1995. Later in 1997 a segment was broadcast on TV 20/20 Newsmagazine with Dr. Timothy Johnson, a former colleague of mine at Massachusetts General Hospital. Also in 1997 I made television appearances on The Today Show with Katie Couric, and on Fox News.

Not only were the news media interested in the new evidence supporting the homocysteine theory of arteriosclerosis, the prestigious British medical journal *Nature Medicine* contacted me in 1996 to write a Commentary on Homocysteine and Vascular Disease [20]. I this short review I summarized the status of the homocysteine theory, citing much of my own work in the field. I discussed the need for improved methods for estimating LDL-homocysteine aggregates and the homocysteine in lipoproteins to improve risk assessment. I also discussed the epidemiological study by John Ellis demonstrating prevention of myocardial infarction and increased longevity through vitamin B6 supplementation.

In 1998 another prestigious British medical journal *The Lancet* published a profile of my experiences in discovering and investigating the homocysteine theory of arteriosclerosis [21]. The article featured a diagram of homocysteine participation in atherosclerosis and an informal photograph of me at my home in Winchester, Massachusetts. The title of the article was "Kilmer McCully: pioneer of the homocysteine theory."

Because of all the attention to the homocysteine theory in the media and in the medical and scientific press, the New York Times dispatched a journalist and food writer, Michelle Stacey, to Providence for a comprehensive day long interview and discussion about my discovery and advocacy of the homocysteine theory. Her article was published in the *New York Times Magazine* on August 10, 1997 [22]. The article stated that "Homocysteine is the theory of the moment in a notoriously competitive field, and McCully's name is inextricably tied to its ascent. He has been called 'The father of homocysteine' at meetings of leading international figures in cardiology and epidemiology. His book *The Homocysteine Revolution: Medicine for the New Millennium* was published in May." There followed a description of the discovery and development of the theory in simplified but accurate terms. The article also describes the initial rejection of the theory by hospital and academic authorities, ostracism from main stream medicine and the political campaign of harassment against me. The article was illustrated by a full page photograph of me and my microscope taken in my Providence office, as well as in informal photograph of Annina and me in our home garden. The article also describes the antagonism of cholesterol researchers and vested interests at the National Heart Lung and Blood Institute in Bethesda and their determination to ignore or discredit my work on homocysteine. Certainly the impact of this article was profound, informing the interested public on the intricacies of the new theory, the reaction of the establishment, and my experience with academic and medical politics. To this day, friends acquaintances, and interested readers comment to me about how my personal story was publicly revealed by this article.

Following publication of my book *The Homocysteine Revolution* and the article in the *New York Times Magazine* in 1997, my schedule of lectures, trips, and appearances accelerated. There seemed to be an insatiable hunger for information about the homocysteine theory from medical, scientific, and nutritional audiences for my explanation of the homocysteine theory. During the early 1990s I had already been invited to present a lecture at the Massachusetts General Hospital Pathology Department, from which I had been forcefully removed 15 years previously. I was invited to lecture at the Harvard School of Public Health and the Tufts Nutrition Research Center in Boston, whose staff had conducted the important Physicians' Health Study and the B vitamin and homocysteine study of Framingham participants.

Not only was I invited to lecture locally in Providence at Roger Williams Hospital and Miriam Hospital and in Boston at Northeastern University, I also made appearances nationally at the City of Hope Medical Center in Duarte, California, at a national meeting of clinical scientists in Newport, and in international symposia in Brussels, Belgium and meetings in Poland. During the years from 1997 to 2001, I made a total of ten appearances at local hospitals, medical schools and medical centers. At one of these lectures at the Beth Israel Medical Center in Boston, an endocrinologist, Jeffrey Flier, the current Dean of Harvard Medical School, offered a public apology on behalf of the Harvard Medical School faculty for the treatment I had received two decades earlier. During this period I also made presentations at 35 additional venues nationally and internationally, including Grand Rounds discussions, national symposia on vascular disease, and a promotional tour of England and Scotland on behalf of my book.

With a colleague, Stephen Elliott of Milwaukee, I helped to organize and co-chair a national symposium at the 1998 Federation of Societies for Experimental Biology meeting in San Francisco, sponsored by the American Physiological Society. The symposium, Vascular

Biology of Homocysteine, featured national leaders in homocysteine research who were invited to discuss calcium signaling in endothelial cells, homocysteinylated LDL, nitrosohomocysteine, cell signaling and the genetic model of homocystinuria in a mouse lacking cystathionine synthase.

With another colleague, Lesley Klevay of the Grand Forks US Department of Agriculture Human Nutrition Research Center in North Dakota, I helped to organize and co-chair a national symposium at the 2001 Federation of Societies for Experimental Biology and Medicine meeting in Orlando. The symposium Ischemic Heart Disease and Malnutrition, was sponsored by the American Society of Nutritional Sciences and featured national and international speakers discussing fetal influences on heart disease, copper deficiency, homocysteine and vascular disease, iron excess, and trans fatty acids in the pathogenesis of heart disease.

With a colleague in nutrition, Heidi Reber of Vienna, I helped to organize and co-chair an international symposium on Homocysteine as a Risk Factor for Atherosclerosis at the University of Vienna, Austria in 2001. The symposium featured ten speakers from Austria, Germany, Switzerland and me discussing recent results establishing homocysteine as a factor in numerous disease processes, including vascular diseases, endothelial dysfunction, thromboembolism, genetic disorders of homocysteine metabolism, congenital malformations, and children of families with premature heart disease. Most of the presentations were in German, which taxed my study of the language 50 years previously in college, but some were in English. After the symposium, a press conference was held at the Vienna Museum of Natural History, followed by an elegant dinner for the participants and guests. Our visit to Vienna was memorable, first because of the informative symposium, but also because of sightseeing, attending Turandot at the Vienna State Opera, visits to the Vienna General Hospital buildings where medical pioneers like Ignaz Semmelweis, Theodor Billroth, and Carl Rokitansky had made their great medical discoveries, and a guided tour of the University of Vienna Medical History Museum. Our visit to Vienna was altogether a thrilling experience.

In 1998 the important ongoing study of nutrition and health, the Nurses' Health Study, published the results regarding over 80,000 women followed for 14 years [23]. The study reported that deaths and heart attacks among women were most frequent among women with the lowest dietary intakes of vitamin B6 and folate. Among women with the highest dietary intakes of these two B vitamins, the risk of coronary heart disease was 45% lower than the risk of women with the lowest dietary intakes of these vitamins. Moderate alcohol consumption potentiated the beneficial effects of dietary folate and vitamin B6, further reducing the risk of heart disease. The daily amount of folate needed to minimize risk of coronary heart disease was found to be 400 micrograms per day, and the corresponding figure for vitamin B6 was found to be 3 milligrams per day. In my invited editorial comment in the Journal of the American Medical Association, I pointed out that the current recommended dietary intakes of these two B vitamins are too low and need to be revised higher in accordance with the findings of the Nurses' Health Study [24]. I further suggested that increased dietary intakes of these two B vitamins through supplementation, fortification, and better food processing and distribution methods would continue the decline in US cardiovascular disease mortality and morbidity that had begun in the 1960s.

Because of media attention to homocysteine and the many publications in leading medical journals validating key elements of the homocysteine theory of arteriosclerosis, new professional opportunities arose in the 1990s. The new Chair of Pathology at Brown University, Agnes Kane, re-instated my appointment as Associate Clinical Professor of Pathology at Brown University Medical School in 1997. I was also invited to present the Herbert Fanger Memorial Lecture in Pathology at Brown Medical School.

Shortly thereafter, I was asked to consider applying for the position of Director of the VA Boston Area Consolidated Laboratories at the VA Medical Center in West Roxbury, the largest VA Medical Center in New England. Because of their affiliation with Harvard Medical School and Brigham and Womens' Hospital in Boston, I was re-instated as Associate Clinical Professor of Pathology at Harvard Medical School. Through this appointment I renewed cordial relations with the Department of Pathology at Harvard Medical School and its teaching hospitals, Brigham and Womens' Hospital and Massachusetts General Hospital, from which I had been forcefully removed more than two decades previously.

After publication of their book *Beyond Cholesterol* in 1981, I discussed with the authors, Gruberg and Raymond, the consequences of writing my own book on development of the homocysteine theory of arteriosclerosis for the general reader. Stephen Raymond commented to me that "one of the benefits of writing a book for the general public on a scientific/medical topic is the opportunity to meet wonderful people who are interested in your approach." On one of my lecture tours after publication of *The Homocysteine Revolution*, I was invited to make a presentation at Medical Grand Rounds at George Washington University Medical School in Washington DC. In connection with this lecture, Sally Fallon, President of the Weston A. Price Foundation, invited me, Annina, and the other speakers, Leslie Klevay and Uffe Ravnskov, to an elegant dinner party at her home in Washington DC. The food for the dinner was prepared from fresh, nutritious ingredients, according to the *Nourishing Traditions Cookbook*, published by *New Trends Publishing, Inc.* At this event I realized that I had met a knowledgeable group of health enthusiasts with a passionate and informed dedication to understanding and implementing knowledge about nutrition and disease.

I had been aware of the mission of the Price-Pottenger Nutrition Foundation, a group founded in 1965 to popularize and disseminate the concepts and discoveries of these two 20th century American pioneers in human nutrition. Francis Pottenger, Jr., MD was a nutritionally informed California physician who conducted an experimental study of nutrition in more than 900 cats over a ten year period. He inadvertently discovered that substituting cooked meat or heat processed milk in experimental diets produced a progressive decline in vitality and reproduction of these cats, in contrast to the health of cats fed raw meat and raw milk. The deficient cats developed many serious chronic diseases, including parasitic infestations, allergies and skin diseases, softened, decalcified bones, hypothyroidism, personality changes and most of the degenerative diseases encountered in human medicine. Because of progressive decline in reproduction and physical degeneration, kittens of the third generation cats failed to survive six months. Pottenger's cats displayed many of the degenerative diseases occurring when nutritionally depleted foods are consumed by human populations, as discovered by the global nutritional surveys condected by Weston A. Price in the 1930s.

Dr. Weston A. Price DDS was a Canadian dentist who established a thriving dental practice in Cleveland in the early 20th century. He retired from dental practice in 1930 and devoted the last 20 years of his life to the study of nutrition and disease in traditional "primitive" human societies world wide. Because of his many important discoveries and concepts developed by these studies, he has been called the "Charles Darwin of nutrition." From 1930-1939 Price studied 14 isolated human groups that consumed traditional diets in a wide variety of countries, climates, and cultures [25]. These groups included isolated Swiss villagers, Gaelic residents of the Outer Hebrides Islands, Eskimos and Indians of North America, Polynesian South Sea Islanders, African tribes, Australian aborigines, New Zealand Maori, and the Indians of South America. Wherever he went to study these primitive groups, Price found healthy beautiful teeth, freedom from chronic disease, protection against tuberculosis and infectious diseases, and behaviorally stable societies free from crime and mental illness. He found that introduction of "modern" processed foods into these societies produced rampant tooth decay, poorly developed dental arches, decreased reproduction, infectious diseases, mental disturbances, and chronic diseases of physical degeneration within one or two generations.

Not only did Price study nutritional practices and diseases of "primitives," he also studied some of the chemical characteristics of the foods that nourished these groups. His analysis showed that the foods of these "primitive" groups contained four times the quantity of water-soluble vitamins, calcium, magnesium and other minerals and ten times the quantity of fat-soluble vitamins from butter, eggs, fish, shellfish and organ meats, compared with "modern" foods. He studied the practice of primitive groups in supplying foods rich in fat soluble vitamins to young couples, ensuring health pregnancy, easy parturition, and increased infant and maternal survival. He even identified a fat-soluble "X-factor" in spring butter that was potent in promoting successful pregnancy, lactation, and infant health. He showed that this factor had properties of a quinone, and recent research has concluded that this factor is identical with vitamin K2, menaquinone [26]. Vitamin K2 promotes bone heath, prevents osteoporosis and fractures, prevents arterial calcification, and enhances mineral absorption, working in concert with the fat-soluble vitamins A and D. Dietary vitamin K2 has recently been identified as a factor in prevention of aggressive prostate cancer in the Heidelberg Study [27].

The Weston A. Price Foundation was founded by Sally Fallon and Mary Enig in 1999 "to disseminate the research of the nutrition pioneer Weston A. Price, whose studies of isolated non-industrialized peoples established the parameters of human health and determined the optimum characteristics of human diets." The Foundation, like the Price-Pottenger Nutrition Foundation, publishes a newsletter *Nourishing Traditions*, sponsors national and regional meetings, and encourages local chapters nationwide to carry the message of "accurate nutrition instruction, organic and biodynamic farming, honest and informational labeling of foods, prepared parenting and nurturing therapies." Sally Fallon is an enthusiastic promoter of health through traditional foods and the author of *The Nourishing Traditions Cookbook.* Mary Enig PhD is a distinguished biochemist and former director of a laboratory at the University of Maryland specializing in analysis of fats and oils. She was the first scientist to challenge data from industry laboratories, showing that the quantity of trans-fatty acids in commercial oils is much higher than claimed by industry. Her scientific results were attacked by industry representatives, but her work was influential in the movement to ban trans fats from cooking oils because of the deleterious effect of these synthetic fats on susceptibility to heart disease and stroke.

In 2003 the Weston A. Price Foundation invited me to present a comprehensive description of my work on homocysteine metabolism in arteriosclerosis, cancer and diseases of aging at their annual meeting held in Washington DC. At this meeting the Foundation presented their "Integrity in Science Award" in recognition of my research accomplishments and redemption from my scientific exile imposed by the medical establishment. At the same meeting the "Integrity in Science Award" of the Foundation was also presented to the Danish-Swedish physician, Uffe Ravnskov, in recognition of his authoritative and painstaking analysis of the saturated fat and cholesterol hypothesis of the origin of vascular disease.

Uffe Ravnskov (Figure 13) is a Danish physician with specialization in nephrology (kidney diseases) and clinical chemistry, living and working in Lund, Sweden as an independent investigator. When in 1989 the cholesterol campaign was introduced in Sweden, he was surprised because, "having followed the scientific literature about cholesterol and cardiovascular disease…for a number of years, I could not recall any study showing that high cholesterol was dangerous to the heart or the blood vessels, or that any type of dietary fat was more beneficial or harmful than another one." When he "became curious and started to read more systematically, [he found that] anyone who reads the literature in this field with an open mind soon discovers that the emperor has no clothes." He found that "the inaccuracies, misinterpretations, exaggerations and misleading quotations in this research area were so numerous that to question them all demanded a book." The resulting book was *The Cholesterol Myths. Exposing the fallacy that saturated fat and cholesterol cause heart disease,* first published in Sweden in 1991 and in Finland in 1992 [28]. This book made little impact because science journalists lost interest when they consulted researchers or health authorities that were criticized in the book. In Finland the book was criticized by proponents of the cholesterol/saturated fat hypothesis and literally set on fire during a television program.

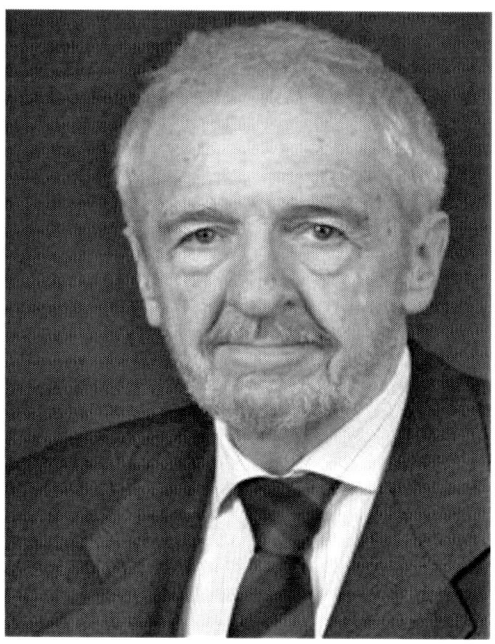

Personal collection of Kilmer McCully.

Figure 13. Uffe Ravnskov is a nephrologist, clinical chemist, author, and independent investigator based in Lund, Sweden. He is founder and webmaster of the www.thincs.org website devoted to the International Network of Cholesterol Skeptics.

Ravnskov's book *The Cholesterol Myths* was first published in English in 2000 by *New Trends Publishing, Inc.*, sponsored by the Weston A. Price Foundation. The message of the book was discussed in speaking tours by Dr. Ravnskov in the US in 2002 and 2003. By singling out 8 common myths about cholesterol, fat and heart disease, the book systematically and conclusively demolishes the principal claims of the hypothesis. He states that "the cholesterol campaign is medical quackery of the first order. In fact, the eminent American physician George Mann called the Diet-Heart idea 'the greatest scientific deception of this century, perhaps of any century.'" The analyses of the published scientific evidence are detailed, clearly explained, and extensively documented by references to the most important studies and publications in the vast medical literature devoted to this subject.

Not satisfied with this landmark book criticizing the fat/cholesterol hypothesis, Uffe Ravnskov recently published two additional books *Fat and Cholesterol are Good for You* and *Ignore the Awkward. How the Cholesterol Myths are Kept Alive* [29,30]. The first book explains the beneficial effects on health of saturated fats and blood lipoproteins and describes how "a steadily increasing number of studies have found that high cholesterol is beneficial, probably because it protects against cancer and infectious disease." These books explain why the cholesterol campaign is immensely harmful, why it led to the current epidemic of obesity and diabetes, and how it encouraged the medicalization of normal physiological functions by pharmaceutical companies. In addition, these books update the revelation of increasingly severe side effects of the cholesterol-lowering statin drugs that cause "lousy memory, weak muscles, sexual failure, and bad temper." These books are exhaustively referenced to the pertinent scientific literature and conclusively demonstrate why the saturated fat/cholesterol hypothesis is outmoded and disproven. The second book explains how statistical distortions and deceptive publication practices prevent the truth about the obsolescence of the cholesterol theory from reaching to medical profession and the general public.

Not only has Uffe Ravnskov published a series of definitive analytical articles on the deficiencies of the cholesterol/fat hypothesis, he became the founding webmaster of a website devoted to the scrutiny and evaluation of the merits of this hypothesis [31]. THINCS.ORG is the website of The International Network of Cholesterol Skeptics, attracting independent-minded investigators and commentators on the causation of heart disease from around the world. Lively discussions and critiques are regularly posted on this website devoted to evaluation of the latest discoveries and the latest assessments of the understanding of heart disease, including results of investigation in the homocysteine field. Ravnskov has received several prizes and awards for his leadership in this field of skeptical inquiry.

Not only was the scientific creditability of my discoveries in the homocysteine field redeemed by the results of scientific investigators worldwide, the public reaction to my book *The Homocysteine Revolution*, and my many appearances in newspapers, magazines, radio and television helped to restore my standing in the scientific and medical community. Through meeting of informed health and nutrition enthusiasts like Sally Fallon and critical scientists like Uffe Ravnskov and Mary Enig, I felt that there was new appreciation of the importance of my discoveries in homocysteine metabolism and their influence on human disease. My position of responsibility within the VA as Medical Director for laboratories of 8 major medical centers in New England restored and redeemed my creditability as a physician specializing in Pathology and Laboratory Medicine. I had indeed progressed a long way since the utter rejection of my professional career by the medical establishment two decades earlier.

REFERENCES

[1] International Conference of Homocysteine Metabolism. *Irish Journal of Medical Sciences*, 1995;164 Supplement 15, pp 1-36. The first international meeting on homocysteine metabolism was held at Castle Dromoland, Ireland July 2-6, 1995. This landmark conference gathered the principal investigators from the USA, Europe and other countries to discuss how disturbances in homocysteine metabolism contribute to many important human diseases.

[2] Graham I, Refsum H, Rosenberg IH, Ueland PM, Shuman JM, editors. *Homocysteine Metabolism: From Basic Science to Clinical Medicine*. Boston: Kluwer, 1997, pp 251-257. This volume contains the full articles based on papers presented at the First International Conference on Homocysteine Metabolism, July 1995 in Ireland.

[3] Kanwar YS, Manaligod JR, Wong WK. Morphologic studies in a patient with homocystinuria due to 5,10-methylenetetrahydrofolate reductase deficiency. *Pediatric Research*, 1976;10:598-609. This article is the first in the medical literature to report the autopsy findings in a human case of the third major type of human homocystinuria, caused by deficiency of methylenetetrahydrofolate reductase. The demonstration of arterial plaques, steatosis of the liver, and other findings in this case independently supports the conclusion that homocysteine causes arterial plaques and other pathological changes by a direct effect of the amino acid on the cells and tissues of arteries, as reported in cases of cystathionine synthase deficiency and methionine synthase deficiency by KS McCully in the *American Journal of Pathology* in 1969.

[4] Wilcken DEL, Wilcken B. The pathogenesis of coronary artery disease. A possible role for methionine metabolism. *Journal of Clinical Investigation*, 1976;57:1079-1082. This study is the first human study of homocysteine metabolism in coronary heart disease, demonstrating accumulation of homocystine and homocysteine-cysteine disulfide in the plasma following an oral dose of methionine.

[5] Harker LA, Ross R, Slichter SJ, Scott CR. Homocystine-induced arteriosclerosis. Role of endothelial cell injury and platelet response to its genesis. *Journal of Clinical Investigation*, 1976;58:731-741. This report is the first published study to confirm the finding of arterial plaques in experimental animals treated with homocysteine, as first reported by KS McCully and BD Ragsdale in *American Journal of Pathology* in 1970.

[6] Brown MS, Goldstein JL. A receptor-mediated pathway for cholesterol homeostasis. *Nobel Lectures*, December 9, 1985.

[7] Brattstrom LE, Hardebo JE, Hultberg BL. Moderate homocysteinemia – a possible risk factor for arteriosclerotic cerebrovascular disease. *Stroke*, 1984;15:1012-1016.

[8] Boers GHJ, Smals AGH, Trijbels FJM, Fowler B, Bakkeren JAJM, Schoonderwaldt HC, Kleijer WJ, Kloppenborg PWC. Heterozygosity for homocystinuria in premature peripheral and cerebral occlusive arterial disease. *New England Journal of Medicine*, 1985;313:209-715.

[9] Murphy-Chutorian D, Wexman MP, Grieco AJ, Heininger JA, Glassman E, Gaull GE. Methionine intolerance: a possible risk factor for coronary disease. *Journal of the American College of Cardiology*, 1985;6:725-730.

[10] Clarke R, Daly L, Robinson K, Naughten E, Cahalane S, Fowler B, Graham I. Homocysteinemia: an independent risk factor for vascular disease. *New England Journal of Medicine*, 1991;324:1149-1155.

[11] Nygard O, Vollset SE, Refsum H, Stensvold I, Tverdal A, Nordrehaug JE, Ueland PM, Kvale G. Total plasma homocysteine and cardiovascular risk profile: the Hordaland Homocysteine Study. *Journal of the American Medical Association*, 1995;274:1526-1533.

[12] Shipchandler M, Moore E. Rapid, fully automated measurement of plasma homocysteine with Abbott IMx analyzer. *Clinical Chemistry*, 1995;41:991-994.

[13] Refsum H, Ueland PM, Svardal AM. Fully automated fluorescence assay for determining total homocysteine in plasma. *Clinical Chemistry*, 1989;35:1921-1927.

[14] Stampfer MJ, Malinow MR, Willett WC, Newcomer LM, Upson B, Ullman D, Tishler PV, Hennekens CH. A prospective study of plasma homocyst(e)ine and risk of myocardial infarction in US physicians. *Journal of the American Medical Association*, 1992;268:877-881.

[15] Selhub J, Jacques PF, Wilson PWF, Rush D, Rosenberg IM. Vitamin status and intake as primary determinants of homocysteinemia in an elderly population. *Journal of the American Medical Association*, 1993;270:2693-2698.

[16] Graham IM. Plasma homocysteine as a risk factor for vascular disease. The European Concerted Action Project. *Journal of the American Medical Association*, 1997;277:1775-1781.

[17] Boushey CJ, Beresford SAA, Omenn GS, Motulsky AG. A quantitative assessment of plasma homocysteine as a risk factor for vascular disease. Probable benefits of increasing folic acid intakes. *Journal of the American Medical Association*, 1995;274:1049-1057.

[18] Kolata G. New clue to heart disease: a vitamin lack. *New York Times*, July 4, 1995.

[19] McCully KS. *The Homocysteine Revolution. Medicine for the New Millennium.* New Canaan, Connecticut: Keats Publishing, 1997.

[20] McCully KS. Homocysteine and vascular disease. *Nature Medicine*, 1996;4:386-389.

[21] Larkin M. Kilmer McCully: pioneer of the homocysteine theory. *Lancet*, 1998;352:1364.

[22] Stacey M. The Fall and Rise of Kilmer McCully. *New York Times Magazine*, August 10, 1997.

[23] Rimm EB, Willett WC, Hu FB, Sampson L, Colditz GA, Manson JE, Hennekens C, Stampfer MJ. Folate and vitamin B6 from diet and supplements in relation to risk of coronary heart disease in women. *Journal of the American Medical Association*, 1998;279:359-364.

[24] McCully KS. Homocysteine, folate, vitamin B6 and cardiovascular disease. *Journal of the American Medical Association*, 1998;279:392-393.

[25] Price WA. *Nutrition and Physical Degeneration.* 50th Anniversary Edition. New Canaan, Connecticut: Keats Publishing, 1989.

[26] Masterjohn C. Dr. Price's X-factor. *Wise Traditions*, 2007;8:14-32. Weston A. Price found in the 1930s that the combination of cod liver oil and the high-activation X-factor of spring butter oil concentrate was more effective than cod liver oil alone in treating his patients for dental caries and other chronic diseases. Price also implicated his X-factor in calcium metabolism and in prevention of arterial calcification 60 years before other scientists established these activities for vitamin K2.

[27] Nimptsch K, Rohrmann S, Linseisen J. Dietary intake of vitamin K and risk of prostate cancer in the Heidelberg cohort of the European Prospective Investigation into Cancer and Nutrition (EPIC-Heidelberg). *American Journal of Clinical Nutrition*, 2008;87:985-992.

[28] Ravnskov U. *The Cholesterol Myths. Exposing the fallacy that saturated fat and cholesterol cause heart disease.* Washington DC: New Trends Publishing, 2000.

[29] Ravnskov U. *Fats and Cholesterol are Good for you.* Sweden: GB Publishing, 2009.

[30] Ravnskov U. *Ignore the Awkward! How the Cholesterol Myths are Kept Alive.* Lexington KY, 2010.

[31] wwwTHINCS.ORG The International Network of Cholesterol Skeptics is a lively website containing informal and penetrating scrutiny regarding the shortcomings of the cholesterol/fat hypothesis of the origin of heart disease and related disease of aging.

Chapter 8

DEVELOPMENT OF HOMOCYSTEINE RESEARCH

Following redemption of the homocysteine field by hundreds of medical investigators working in laboratories, clinics, and medical centers worldwide, as described in chapter 7, there followed a period of recognition of the significance of the homocysteine theory of arteriosclerosis on the part of some segments of the medical establishment. Professional societies and other groups interested in nutrition, functional medicine, preventive medicine, and integrative or alternative medicine were the most prominent in recognizing the homocysteine field and my contributions over the past 25 years.

Every two or three years, international conferences on homocysteine metabolism were held after the first such conference in Ireland in 1995. Subsequent conferences were held in Nijmegen, Netherlands, in 1998, Sorrento, Italy, in 2001, Basel, Switzerland in 2003, Milan, Italy, in 2005, Saarbruecken, Germany, in 2007, Prague, Czech Republic, in 2009 and Lisbon, Portugal, in 2011. During this period, additional conferences on Hyperhomocysteinemia were held in Saarbruecken, Germany, by Wolfgang Herrmann and his team of the Saarland Medical School of Homburg, Germany every 2 or 3 years. At each of these meetings, 400 or more scientists from countries worldwide met to present their research findings on homocysteine and to discuss progress in the field.

In 1998 Jeffrey Bland of the Institute for Functional Medicine in Gig Harbor, Washington, invited me to present the keynote lecture at the Fifth International Symposium on Functional Medicine in Kona, Hawaii. The meeting was attended by practitioners of nutritional, integrative, and preventive medicine, many of whom were interested in my analysis of B vitamin deficiency and elevated blood homocysteine in prevention of vascular disease. During the meeting, I was surprised and honored to receive the 1998 Linus Pauling Award in Functional Medicine. This recognition was particularly gratifying, not only because of the endorsement of my discoveries in the homocysteine field, but also because the Award honored the memory of the great 20th century scientist, Linus Pauling, who contributed to basic chemistry, biochemistry of proteins, and the concept of orthomolecular medicine, a term coined by Pauling. In fact, I corresponded with Pauling several times about my work on homocysteine. He sent me copies of his books on vitamin C and commented favorably on my discoveries in the homocysteine and vitamin B6 field. I remember meeting Pauling at a celebration of the life and work of the biochemist, Albert Szent-Gyorgi, at a symposium at Boston University in 1976. It was a thrill for me to meet these two prominent scientists, hear them lecture, and shake their hands at this meeting.

Later in 1998 I was invited to present at lecture at the 25th anniversary meeting of the American College for Advancement in Medicine in Phoenix. This meeting gathered practitioners interested in nutrition, preventive medicine and chelation therapy for chronic disease. At this meeting I was awarded the Norman C. Clarke Jr Award, commemorating a founder of chelation therapy. This therapeutic approach is based on intravenous administration of a chelation chemical (ethylene diamine tetra-acetic acid) with a vitamin mixture, intended to chelate heavy metals like lead and mercury for elimination in the urine. The therapy is also intended to promote removal of calcium from arterial plaques by a similar process of chelation. While chelation therapy is effective in mobilizing and excretion of heavy metals, the effect on arterial plaques is controversial. The B vitamins administered in the chelation solution by this therapeutic technique may have a preventive effect on atherogenesis by decreasing homocysteine formation from methionine. At this meeting, there were two interesting presentations regarding the role of infection in arterial plaques, one concerning *Chlamydia pneumoniae,* the respiratory protozoan, and *Porphyromonas gingivalis*, the oral cavity microbe implicated in peri-odontal disease. Both of these organisms have been demonstrated in arterial plaques, pointing to a role for these microbial pathogens in atherogenesis.

As an indication of the increasing interest in the homocysteine theory of arteriosclerosis on the part of the food and nutrition industry, I was invited to the annual convention of the National Nutritional Foods Association (NNFA) in Las Vegas in 1999. At this meeting I was awarded the Burton Kallman Scientific Achievement Prize, named for their former scientific director, in recognition of the significance to nutrition and public health of the homocysteine theory of arteriosclerosis. Established in 1939, the NNFA is the oldest and largest non-profit trade organization dedicated to nutritional foods and the natural products industry. This organization was instrumental in passage of the landmark 1994 Dietary Supplement Health and Education Act (DSHEA), protecting public access to vitamins, minerals, herbals and other supplements. During the presentation of this award, Senator Thomas Harkin of Iowa was also recognized for his support and passage of the DSHEA legislation.

Later in 1999 I was invited to present a lecture at the College of Physicians in Philadelphia, where I was presented with the first Edna G. Kynett Foundation's Cardiology Award of Excellence. During the festivities, I was informed that I was the first pathologist to receive this award. In connection with my visit, the librarian gave me a tour of rare books and archives that are maintained by the College for physicians in Philadelphia. This library was the principal medical library in the city for its 5 medical schools, prior to establishment of their own medical libraries [1]. During this tour, I was able to examine first editions of works by Vesalius, Harvey, Virchow, Rokitansky and Aschoff, all pioneers in the history of medicine. The curator also gave me a tour of the Mutter Medical Museum, also housed at the College. This tour was riveting because of the historic specimens on display in exhibits dedicated to the history of medicine in the United States of America. As a souvenir of my visit to the College, the curator gave me a book on the yellow fever epidemic that occurred in 1793 in Philadelphia, edited by Worth Estes, my classmate from Harvard College and former fellow pathology resident at Massachusetts General Hospital [2]. This visit to the College of Physicians encouraged me to believe that cardiologists and internists were beginning to acknowledge the significance to cardiology practice of the homocysteine theory of arteriosclerosis.

At their annual meeting in 2000, the International and American Association of Clinical Nutritionists (IAACN) invited me to present two lectures, one on the homocysteine link to cardiovascular disease through correction of dietary micronutrient depletion, and the other on chronic infection and cardiovascular disease. After reviewing the discovery of the homocysteine theory of arteriosclerosis and reviewing the evidence supporting the theory, I commented on the possible role of infection by *Chlamydia pneumoniae, Porphyromonas gingivalis, Herpes simplex virus,* and *Cytomegalovirus* in the pathogenesis of arterial plaques. During this meeting I was honored to receive the Lifetime Achievement Award of IAACN, recognizing the importance of my research work in nutrition and disease. The audience consisted of nutritionally oriented physicians, dietitians, and practitioners. Another Lifetime Achievement Award was also presented to Mildred Selig for her work on clinical magnesium deficiency.

Also in 2000 I was chosen to receive the Jim Dinsdale Memorial Award in honor of Jim Dinsdale from the Society for Scientific Exploration. Dinsdale was known for his investigations of the Loch Ness Monster tales from Scotland. This Society gathers a wide range of scientists and explorers interested in explaining "anomalies" to the conventional wisdom in a variety of scientific fields. The meeting in London, Ontario indeed explored topics ranging from homeopathy to electromagnetic field detection to sprouting of seeds in the Orgone Energy Accumulator. My lecture concerned "The Biomedical Significance of Homocysteine [3]." The participants were sympathetic with my experience of rejection by the medical establishment, as described in Chapter 5.

One of the participants, who were interested in my experience of rejection, Joel Kauffman, is a Professor of Chemistry at the University of the Sciences in Philadelphia. Kauffman is a critical observer of the biomedical field and a member of the International Network of Cholesterol Skeptics. In 2006 he published a fascinating book *Malignant Medical Myths: Why Medical Treatment Causes 200,000 Deaths per Year* [4]. In one of the chapters of his book, Kauffman analyzes the fat/cholesterol hypothesis of heart disease causation. In his penetrating analysis, he cites a number of pertinent studies refuting the claims of Big Pharma that cholesterol lowering is beneficial to survival in older subjects. "A 2004 observational study of 150,000 subjects from Austria showed that low cholesterol levels predict premature death of men of all ages, and in women over 50. In the 1990 Quebec Cardiovascular Study of men aged 35-64, total cholesterol levels were not associated with either cardiovascular disease or all-cause mortality. In a 2005 study of Manhattan residents, 2,277 subjects aged 65-98 were followed for 10 years. The chance of dying was twice as great in the lowest quartile of total cholesterol or LDL cholesterol levels, while HDL cholesterol and triglyceride levels were not related to all-cause mortality in this age group." From these and other studies cited in his book, Kauffman concludes "drug advertising claims that higher total cholesterol levels mean quicker death from cardiovascular disease are false – in large groups of people of mixed ages, the older ones will have higher total plasma cholesterol and LDL cholesterol, and older people die sooner than younger ones, not necessarily from cardiovascular disease."

An unusual acknowledgement of my discovery and development of the homocysteine theory came in the form of an invitation to attend an evening celebration in New York, honoring men selected as "Heroes" by *Men's Journal* magazine [5]. The party was hosted by Tom Brokaw of NBC TV and included eleven men from many fields making special contributions. Some of the luminaries honored at this event were Robert Kennedy Jr,

President of Waterkeeper Alliance, Eric Simonson, explorer of Mt Everest, Donovan McNab and Duante Culpepper, professional quarterbacks, two survivors of the World War II sinking of the USS Indianapolis, John Pritchard, Brooklyn Fire Chief, Bono, advocate for Drop the Third World Debt, and Richard Gere, Chairman of the International Campaign for Tibet. In talking with Tom Brokaw at this event, we found that we were both descended from grandfathers who were pioneers in 19th century Dakota Territory. A special issue of *Men's Journal* of May 2001 featured the photographs and descriptions of the accomplishments of each "hero."

Some other recognitions of my contributions were selection to the 20th Century Hall of Fame by *Prevention Magazine*, the Benjamin Franklin Literary and Medical Society Award, and a Special Achievement Award by the *International Journal of Integrative Medicine,* all in 2000. Another special recognition was my selection to receive the 2003 Edward Rhodes Stitt Award from the Association of Military Surgeons of the United States at their annual convention in San Antonio. This national award is given to a laboratory pathologist in the Military or Federal Service of the United States of America in honor of Dr. Stitt, a pathologist and former Surgeon General of the US Navy. After my lecture, several in the audience commented on my determination to "take on the medical establishment."

In 2003 I was contacted by Raymond Wegmann of France, the President and Founder of the Society for Cellular and Molecular Biology in 1949, to be the editor of a Special Theme Issue of the Journal [6]. The result was a published symposium featuring an international panel of authors presenting review articles and original research results in a special issue of the *Journal of Cellular and Molecular Biology*. The subjects included a review of ischemic heart disease as deficiency disease by Leslie Klevay from North Dakota; a study of homocysteine thiolactonase activity of paraoxonase by Heironym Jakubowski and his team from New Jersey Medical School and Poland; a study showing a correlation between homocysteine, C-reactive protein and cardiovascular disease by Wolfgang Herrmann and his team from Homburg, Germany; a study of increased plasma homocysteine from arginine administration in apoE, INOS double knockout mice by Diane Handy, Joseph Loscalzo and their team from Boston University; a study of increased plasma homocysteine as a factor impairing vasodilation by Sandra Heil, Henk Blom and their team from Nijmegen, Netherlands; effects of homocysteine on blood coagulation in hyperhomocysteinemic rats by Lisa Ebbesen of Aarhus, Denmark; a study of inhibition of angiogenesis by homocysteine by Suresh Tyagi of Louisville, Kentucky; a study of homocysteine in abnormal human embryogenesis caused by folate deficiency by Regine Steegers-Theunissen and her team from Rotterdam, Netherlands; the role of homocysteine in aortic dissection by Bette Giusti and her team from Florence, Italy; and the role of homocysteine in restenosis following angioplasty by Olaf Stanger of Salzburg, Austria. This Theme Issue Symposium published in the *Journal of Cellular and Molecular Biology* in 2004 highlighted important advances in homocysteine research both in animal models and in human disease [7].

The next year in 2005, many of the contributors to the Theme Issue on Homocysteine and Disease presented their findings at the 4th World Congress of Cellular and Molecular Biology held in Poitiers, France. These oral presentations were concerned with the inhibition of neural tube formation by homocysteine in chick embryos, the lowering of elevated homocysteine levels by intravenous B vitamin treatment in human kidney failure patients, two studies linking homocysteine with cognitive decline of the elderly, the effect of mental stress and anger on acute elevation of plasma homocysteine, association of homocysteine thiolactonase of HDL with coronary heart disease, up-regulation of glutamate-cysteine ligase, an enzyme involved in glutathionine synthesis, homocysteine levels in exfoliative glaucoma, and the molecular targeting hypothesis for homocysteine in atherogenesis. These presentations offered a current summary of research results in a broad range of homocysteine studies. After the symposium, Annina and I hosted a reception and dinner party for the participants at a nearby elegant French chateau.

The meeting in Poitiers, France was memorable because eleven Nobel laureates in Physiology, Medicine, Physics, and Chemistry attended the conference and were invited guests at special dinners sponsored by the *Society for Cellular and Molecular Biology*. Several important French political figures, including Segolene Royal, from the Poitou-Charentes region, addressed participants of the World Congress. I was able to meet and converse with a number of these distinguished scientists and politicians. On one occasion participants were taken for sight seeing in Rochelle, France, the site of a 17th Century siege and battle between the Catholic King of France and the Protestant residents of the city. Refugees from this battle founded New Rochelle, New York near New York City in the late 17th Century. An elegant reception by the Town Fathers was held in Rochelle to honor the attending Nobel Laureates, acknowledging their visit to the city.

Also in 2005 I was invited to present the keynote address to the 4th International Conference on Hyperhomocysteinemia, held in Saarbruecken, Germany [8]. In this lecture I described the history of the development of the homocysteine theory of arteriosclerosis, starting with the description of arterial plaques by Andreas Vesalius (1514-1564) and other anatomists of the 16th Century. I briefly reviewed the development of the concept of arteriosclerosis by description of calcification and fibrosis of arterial plaques in the 17th and 18th Centuries, followed by the concepts of atherogenesis by inflammation, fat deposition, intimal damage and degeneration of the arterial wall by the two pioneers of pathology in the 19th Century, Carl von Rokitansky (1804-1878) of Vienna and Rudolf Virchow (1821-1902) of Berlin. The contemporary version of the inflammatory origin of atherosclerosis is the "response to injury" hypothesis, advocated by Russell Ross (1929-1999). I also described the experiments of Wladimir Sergius Ignatowsky (1880?-1935?) and Nicolai Anistchkow (1885-1964) of St. Petersburg in production of arterial plaques in rabbits. These experiments led to the protein intoxication and cholesterol deposition theories of atherogenesis, as described in Chapter 4. I also summarized my own discovery of the homocysteine theory of arteriosclerosis, as described in Chapter 3.

In 2005 on the occasion of my 50th reunion of the Class of 1955 from Harvard College, I participated in a special medical symposium "Keeping the young elderly healthy" at the 2005 Harvard Commencement ceremonies. At this symposium, several of my classmates and I discussed how improved nutrition, exercise, and life-style improvements can increase longevity and improve health. My contribution was published as part of a supplement in *The American Journal of Clinical Nutrition* entitled "Homocysteine, vitamins, and vascular disease prevention [9]." In this lecture I described the epidemic of coronary heart disease in the 20th Century, which seemed to reach a peak in the 1950s when I was a medical student and intern in medicine. I recounted my discovery of the homocysteine theory of arteriosclerosis, as explained in Chapter 3, and I concluded with some recommendations taken from my book *The Heart Revolution* about the effectiveness of B vitamin supplements in lowering homocysteine levels in those classmates of mine at increased risk of vascular disease.

In 2007 I was invited to serve as the Chairman of the opening plenary session of the 6th World Congress of Homocysteine Metabolism, held in Saarbruecken, Germany. During this meeting, scientists and epidemiologists discussed recent developments in the homocysteine field and focused on the difficulties in using B vitamin supplements for prevention of recurrent disease in patients who have survived stroke or heart attack. I also described my discovery of the homocysteine theory of arteriosclerosis at the Dean's Hour lecture at the University of North Dakota in Grand Forks in 2007 and as keynote lecturer for Research Day at the Albert Einstein Medical Center in Philadelphia in 2008.

Because of the plausibility and evidence supporting the homocysteine theory of arteriosclerosis, as described in previous chapters, a number of intervention trials were started in the 1990s to determine whether B vitamin supplements can decrease vascular disease and its complications in human subjects. The first of these trials to show positive results was the Swiss Heart Study conducted in 553 coronary angioplasty patients treated in the University Hospital in Bern from 1998 to 1999 [10]. Moderate daily doses of folic acid (1 mg), vitamin B12 (400 μg), and vitamin B6 (10 mg) for 6 months significantly reduced the rate of restenosis following angioplasty, compared to placebo. The diameter of coronary artery lumen was determined by angiography. Blood homocysteine levels were reduced from 11 μM to 7 μM, and the rate of restenosis was reduced from 48% to 40%, a significant difference. Follow-up after 1 year of observation showed reduction in major adverse events, defined as death, nonfatal myocardial infarction, and revascularization [11]. The positive effect was more pronounced in small arteries subjected to angioplasty, and a study of patients with stents placed after angioplasty showed no benefit of supplemental B vitamins [12].

Several large trials of B vitamin therapy studied the effect of homocysteine lowering in patients who had survived stroke, heart attack, or who had kidney failure. In all of these trials (VISP, HOPE2, NORVIT, HOST), the patients to be studied were at an advanced stage of vascular disease. Some hope for success came from a small uncontrolled trial of stroke survivors in which B vitamin therapy seemed to halt the progression of narrowing of the carotid artery, as reported by David Spence, a neurologist from London, Ontario [13]. Several other studies from different countries also showed a beneficial effect of B vitamin supplementation on progression of carotid artery plaques and thickening of renal arteries.

The principal finding of the large interventional trials with B vitamin supplementation was that advanced vascular disease is not reversed in subjects who have survived heart attack (NORVIT), stroke (VISP), kidney failure (HOST), or generalized arteriosclerosis (HOPE2). Secondary prevention of recurrent adverse events by moderate doses of folic acid, pyridoxine and cobalamin is ineffective in preventing recurrent myocardial infarction, stroke, gangrene, and in promoting increased survival of subjects with advanced disease. In these trials the participants generally received a variety of drugs and vitamin supplements that may have obscured the potential benefit of B vitamin supplementation. Some trials were conducted in populations consuming diet already fortified with folic acid (VISP, HOST, HOPE2), so additional B vitamins would not be expected to offer additional benefit.

Some support for this assertion comes from an efficacy analysis of the VISP trial by David Spence and his team [14,15]. He showed that exclusion of subjects with kidney failure, subjects with malabsorption of vitamin B12, and subjects with high levels of vitamin B12 from non-study supplementation yielded significant reductions in stroke, coronary disease, and all-cause mortality from B vitamin intervention over a 2 year period. The excluded participants in this analysis would not have been expected to respond to B vitamin intervention, because they were already receiving adequate B vitamins or were unable to absorb B12 normally.

In the HOPE2 trial 5522 patients with advanced vascular disease or diabetes were followed for five years while taking folic acid, vitamins B6 and B12 in populations with or without folic acid fortification of the food supply [16]. Homocysteine lowering was significant in non-fortified participants, but overall the lowering of homocysteine was not statistically significant at 2 years and at 5 years in the total sample. Although there was no reduction in coronary events in this trial, the total incidence of strokes was reduced by 25% at five years, a statistically significant reduction. The study authors dismissed this important finding for unknown reasons, claiming that it might have been a chance finding.

The NORVIT trial was conducted in 3749 survivors of heart attack that were observed for 3 years following B vitamin supplementation with folic acid, vitamins B12 and B6 in moderate doses in a complex trial design of four groups [17]. No reduction in recurrent heart attacks or mortality was observed during this relatively short observation period. There was a suggestion of increased recurrence of myocardial infarction in the subgroup receiving B12, folic acid and pyridoxine, but the placebo group had a significantly increased rate of angioplasty and by-pass grafting, possibly affecting the outcome.

In the HOST study of 2000 subjects with advanced kidney failure and high risk of vascular disease, B vitamin intervention lowered homocysteine levels but had no effect on stroke, myocardial infarct, gangrene, or mortality [18]. Although I participated in the Executive Committee of this trial, the anticipation that B vitamin therapy could affect the course of underlying kidney failure in these subjects was unfounded, as I suggested during the planning of the study. The major disturbances in oxidative metabolism and endothelial dysfunction in kidney failure patients could not reasonably be expected to be reversed by increased doses of B vitamins in subjects already receiving low dose B vitamin supplementation.

The overall impact of these major intervention trials was to discourage practicing physicians from measuring plasma homocysteine in their vascular disease patients and from using B vitamin supplementation to lower homocysteine levels in an attempt to reverse or prevent progression of their disease. The secondary prevention approach seemed to be a dead end of little use, and one physician at the VA Medical Center in Boston commented to me that "homocysteine is dead."

Careful statistical analysis of published studies of primary prevention trials, however, tells a different story. The meta-analysis of 8 intervention trials with supplemental folic acid, involving a total of almost 17,000 subjects, as reported in Lancet in 2007, concluded that this approach "significantly reduced the incidence of stroke by 18% [19]." The authors further found that a greater beneficial effect was seen in those trials with a treatment duration of greater than 3 years (29% reduction), a decrease in concentration of homocysteine greater than 20% (23% reduction), no fortification or partially fortified grain foods (24% reduction) and no history of stroke (25% reduction). They also commented that the earlier meta-analysis by another group of investigators also showed a significant reduction in stroke if the VISP trial was excluded from the analysis, because the VISP trial was conducted in subjects with a history of stroke [20].

In their analysis and comment in the *British Medical Journal*, David Wald and his team of investigators examined evidence from patients with homocystinuria, evidence from genetic polymorphism studies [of C677T homozygotes], and randomized controlled trials of homocysteine lowering by B vitamin supplementation [21]. They concluded that the "estimate from the trials is consistent with a short term protective effect of 12% on ischaemic heart disease events and 22% [protective effect] on stroke, or a larger long term effect." The authors pointed to a dose response relation in the genetic studies as "particularly relevant in suggesting a causal effect [of homocysteine on heart disease]." A recent meta-analysis by Robert Clarke, a leader in the epidemiological study of homocysteine, and his team at Oxford University, concluded, however, that publication bias has over-estimated the effect of this polymorphism on risk of coronary heart disease from moderate homocysteine elevation [22].

Additional evidence for the efficacy of homocysteine lowering by folic acid in stroke prevention comes from the decision of the US Food and Drug Administration to require fortification of enriched flour and other grain foods by folic acid in 1998. The original impetus for this decision came from the observation of increased risk of neural tube birth defects in mothers with dietary deficiency of folic acid. Intervention studies showed that folic acid supplementation decreased these birth defects in supplemented mothers. After the FDA mandate to add folic acid to flour in an amount sufficient to supply 100 micrograms per day, the Framingham Heart Study showed that blood folate levels doubled and homocysteine levels fell 15% after 1998 in participants studied before and after fortification [23]. An important study from the Centers for Disease Control and Prevention (CDC) showed that the decline in stroke mortality accelerated in 1998 in the US and Canada, but not in the United Kingdom where folate fortification was not instituted [24]. This statistical study analyzed mortality from stroke in populations and concluded that "folic acid fortification helps to reduce deaths from stroke." In a commentary, the American Heart Association projected that there would be a 36% decline in coronary heart disease deaths and a 34% decline in stroke deaths in the US in the decade starting in 1999, based on 2005 statistics from the CDC.

In their review of the decline in deaths from heart disease and stroke in the US from 1900 to 1999, the US Department of Health and Human Services showed that age-adjusted death rates for total cardiovascular disease and stroke reached a peak in 1955 of over 400 per 100,000 in the population [25]. Thereafter the rate declined steadily to under 200 per 100,000 by the end of the 20th Century. Changes in risk factors that are cited to explain this precipitous decline are reduced incidence of hypertension from 37% to 23%, reduction in smokers from 42% to 24%, and reduction in blood cholesterol from 220 mg/dL to 203 mg/dL. Interestingly, the percentage of dietary total fat calories dropped only slightly from 36% to 34%, the percentage of dietary saturated fat calories was almost unchanged from 13% to 12%, and the percentage of overweight persons increased from 24% to 35%. The report also cited improvements in medical care, including advances in diagnosis and treatment, more effective medications for hypertension and elevated blood cholesterol, more cardiovascular disease specialists, improved emergency medical services for heart attack and stroke, and an increase in coronary care units, as factors in the decline in cardiovascular deaths in the 20th Century.

As described in Chapter 6, the National Institutes of Health Conference on the Decline in Cardiovascular Mortality in 1979 was the first to recognize and study the possible causes of this dramatic decline in the number one killer of Americans in the second half of the 20th Century [26]. The conclusion of this conference was that the probable causes for the decline could not be attributed to the known risk factors for cardiovascular disease, even though encouraging trends were found in treatment of hypertension, decreased smoking, and improved medical and surgical care of cardiovascular disease patients. Certainly the slight changes in dietary fat calories and almost unchanged percentage of saturated fat calories could not explain the continuing decline in mortality in the follow-up data 20 years after the original NIH conference. The important addition of synthetic pyridoxine (vitamin B6) and synthetic folic acid to the food supply in the form of fortification of cereals and in vitamin supplements explains why the decline in mortality began in the 1960s and continued to the end of the century because of lowering of homocysteine levels in the population. Neither the 1979 NIH conference nor the 1999 report of the Department of Health and Human Services cited these important dietary changes as a factor in decline in vascular disease mortality [27].

In a recent collaborative study, my colleague Uffe Ravnskov and I have proposed a new hypothesis that explains how cholesterol, homocysteine, and infections conspire to produce vulnerable plaques in arteries that by rupturing cause thrombosis and arterial occlusion, leading to heart attack, stroke and gangrene of the legs [28]. This hypothesis explains how known risk factors for arteriosclerosis cause aggregation of lipoproteins, inactivation of micro-organisms, and the inflammatory changes in artery wall that are known to participate in plaque formation. According to this hypothesis, lipoprotein complexes with micro-organisms and autoantibodies to lipoproteins containing homocysteine and oxidized fats and cholesterol lodge in the small blood vessels nourishing the walls of arteries in areas of high pressure. Obstruction of these *vasa vasorum* by these complexes causes cell death, rupture of capillaries, hemorrhage into plaques, and creation of foam cells from monocytes, leading to pustules of arterial wall, known as vulnerable plaques. Endothelial dysfunction from elevated blood homocysteine contributes to trapping of aggregates of homocysteinylated lipoproteins and microbes by narrowing the lumens of *vasa vasorum*.

We have learned that cholesterol plays a minor role in creation of plaques, at least in younger men, and that homocysteine elevation increases the formation of plaques and risk of disease in animals and in human populations, through dietary deficiency of B vitamins, genetic factors, and altered metabolism of methionine. However, there are many other factors that are known to increase risk of vascular disease. In particular, mental and emotional stress, smoking, aging, male gender, postmenopausal status in women, diabetes, kidney failure, hypothyroidism, and high blood pressure are all important determinants of disease risk. Surveys, case control studies, and experimental studies have shown that each of these factors increases homocysteine levels in animals and man. How do these diverse factors conspire to produce vulnerable plaques in the arteries that by rupturing cause hemorrhage, thrombosis with occlusion, and death of heart, brain and other tissues in patients with vascular disease?

A century ago the cause of arteriosclerosis was generally considered to originate from "direct irritation of [arterial] tissue by infection or toxins." Bacteria and viruses were considered as the main cause of atherosclerosis, because of increased plaques in patients dying of typhoid fever and other infections. Sir William Osler, the Canadian pathologist and physician who became the Regius Professor of Medicine at Oxford and a leading physician of his time, described the vulnerable plaque as a pustule. More recently, much evidence has been reported to support the role of infections in vascular disease. In particular, cardiovascular mortality increases during influenza epidemics. A third of patients with acute myocardial infarction or stroke have had an infectious disease immediately before onset. Bacteriemia and periodontal infections are associated with an increased risk of cardiovascular disease. Serological markers of infection are elevated in patients with cardiovascular disease. And coronary arteries are found to be narrowed in children who died of infectious diseases.

Beginning in 1939 and in the next decade, investigators discovered that lipoproteins function as a nonspecific immune system that is capable of inactivating a wide variety of bacteria, viruses, protozoans and their toxins. Lipoproteins form complexes with these organisms that render them inactive, and macrophages in the tissues are capable of phagocytosis of these complexes, leading to formation of foam cells that destroy these organisms. The lipopolysaccharides and lipoteichoic acids of these organisms bind with lipoproteins, probably because of their lipophilic properties, rendering them inactive. Some examples of organisms that are inactivated this way are *Salmonella*, the cause of typhoid fever and other gastrointestinal infections, *Herpes simplex, Rotavirus* and *Cytomegalovirus*, the cause of ubiquitous viral infections, *Chlamydia pneumoniae,* a respiratory pathogen, and *Staphylococcus aureus,* an important cause of boils, carbuncles, and pneumonia.

Beginning in the 1970s investigators found evidence of a wide variety of micro-organisms in human atherosclerotic plaques, as demonstrated by immunohistochemistry, polymerase chain reaction for DNA fragments, and electron microscopy. Only in the case of *Chlamydia pneumoniae* were investigators able to culture viable organisms directly from plaques. In most cases, only remnants of micro-organisms are found, and viable organisms cannot be cultured from plaques. Using sophisticated DNA technology, a recent report from Germany demonstrated the presence of 50 different micro-organisms in human plaques, and the average number was 12 per plaque. Arteries without plaques contained no microbial remnants. Many common organisms form complexes with lipoproteins, such as *Escherichia coli, Staphylococcus, Streptococcus, Salmonella, and rotavirus.* The same organisms are demonstrated in plaques, suggesting an infectious origin of plaques. Recent experimental and clinical evidence support the causal role of microbes in formation of vulnerable plaques, as discussed in a review article by Ravnskov and McCully in *The American Journal of the Medical Sciences* [29].

Homocysteine participates in the aggregation of lipoproteins by reacting with the protein to form cross-linkages, leading to aggregation, spontaneous precipitation and phagocytosis by macrophages to form foam cells. Thus in persons with elevated homocysteine levels, there is an increased ability of lipoproteins to form aggregates, leading to foam cell formation from macrophages by phagocytosis. In addition, lipoproteins containing homocysteine have altered antigenic structure, leading to the formation of antibodies that complex with lipoproteins. A similar process has been identified with lipoproteins within foam cells, since oxidation reactions create modified or oxidized lipoproteins that incite autoantibody formation. In the presence of invading micro-organisms, the complexes with lipoproteins theoretically become enlarged and subject to precipitation and phagocytosis by macrophages.

Figure 14 illustrates our concept of the creation of vulnerable plaques within arteries. In the case of a massive invasion of micro-organisms, or when the immune system is impaired, the complexes of micro-organisms with lipoproteins, enhanced by the effect of excess homocysteine, obstruct the *vasa vasorum,* the small arterioles, venules and capillaries that normally nourish the wall of the artery. Obstruction of the blood flow causes ischemia of the artery wall (lack of blood supply), increasing the tendency to cell death and rupture of the capillaries. These large complexes are phagocytosed by macrophages to form foam cells that accumulate, initially in the adventitia, but then migrating into the intima, where lipoproteins, inflammatory cells, and lipid deposits, including cholesterol, accumulate. This process is probably increased and enhanced in cases where autoantibodies are formed to homocysteinylated lipoproteins and oxidized lipoproteins. The result is a vulnerable plaque that by rupturing causes thrombosis, obstruction of the arterial lumen, and death of the heart, brain, kidney or other tissue supplied by the artery. The *vasa vasorum* are functionally end arteries, since blood flow ceases at the point where the pressure within these blood vessels is opposed by the pressure within the arterial lumen. Thus, the process of plaque formation is potentially enhanced in areas of increased blood pressure, such as disrupted laminar flow, turbulence, angulation of arterial lumen, and increased systemic pressure. In fact, these are the areas in the arteries where vulnerable plaques are most commonly observed.

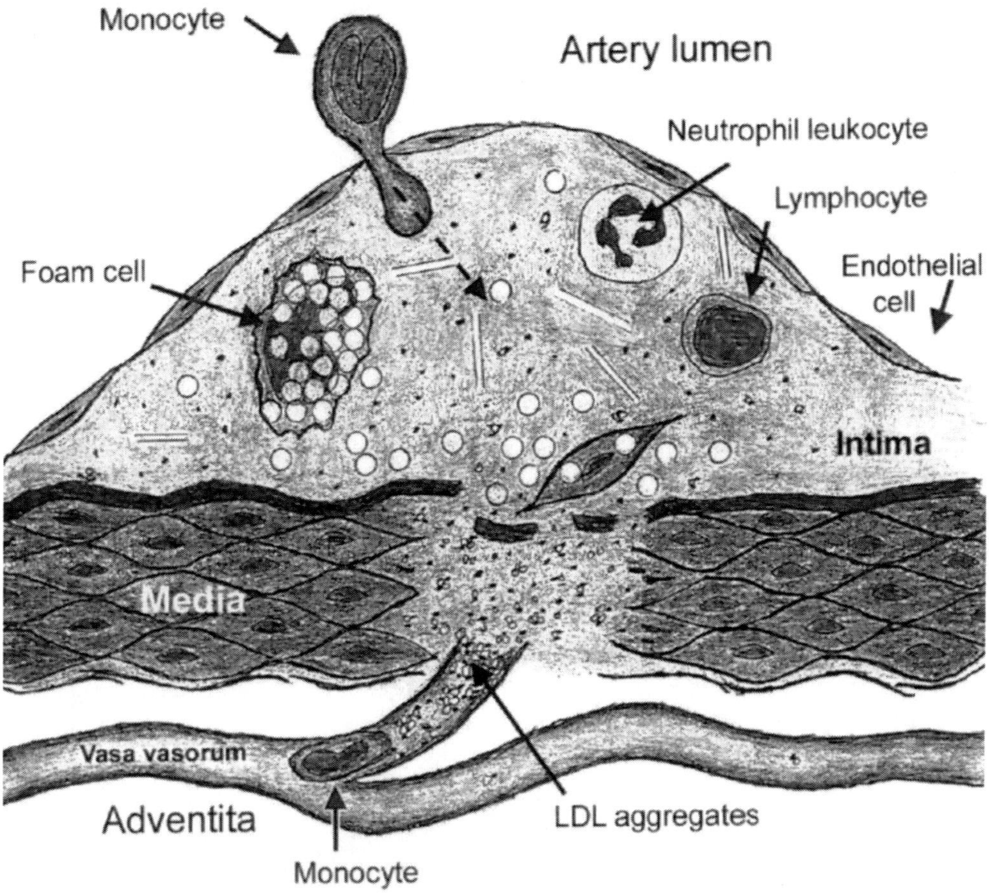

Reprinted from Annals of Clinical and Laboratory Science, 2009, Volume 39, page 9 by permission of the Institute for Clinical Science, Inc.

Figure 14. Development of the vulnerable plaque. The small globules inside the *vasa vasorum* and in the vulnerable plaque represent lipoproteins; the black dots represent microbes, endotoxins, anti-oxLDL autoantibodies, and anti-thiolated-LDL autoantibodies; the large globules at the basal part of the vulnerable plaque and inside the macrophages represent lipid droplets. The right capillary represents a normal healthy artery containing a few microbes and lipoproteins that are able to traverse the lumen without obstruction or adherence. The left capillary represents an artery with severe microbial invasion, in which microbial products and autoantibodies form aggregates with lipoproteins, obstructing the lumen, leading to ischemia, microbial growth, and inflammation. A monocyte enters the plaque from the arterial lumen by diapedesis between endothelial cells. Another monocyte enters the plaque via *vasa vasorum*, leading to formation of foam cell macrophages within the plaque. With an intact immune system, the inflammatory area heals and is converted to a fibrous plaque. With an insufficient immune system, microbes escape into the tissue and create a micro-abscess, the vulnerable plaque.

One can readily understand that our interpretation explains many of the observations about vulnerable plaques and the pathophysiological processes found in vascular disease. It explains how risk factors, such as stress, B vitamin deficiency, elevated blood pressure, smoking, and kidney failure lead to increased disease risk through formation of homocysteinylated lipoprotein aggregates. It explains the resistance of persons with elevated lipoprotein levels to infectious diseases. It explains how cholesterol becomes deposited in plaques. It explains the inflammatory process and the release of inflammatory cytokines, C-reactive protein, fever, leukocytosis, and the frequent occurrence of bacteriemia and sepsis in myocardial infarction complicated by shock. It explains the observation of microbial remnants in plaques. And it explains the inflammatory nature of cardiovascular disease.

Endothelial dysfunction, an abnormality of the endothelial cells lining all blood vessels, is generally considered to be the earliest manifestation of vascular disease. Many factors lead to endothelial dysfunction, including stress, elevated blood homocysteine, and antagonism of the actions of the vasodilator, nitric oxide, on blood vessel walls [30]. Other factors leading to endothelial dysfunction are kidney failure, smoking, hypertension, and diabetes, all of which promote arterial plaques. Another factor leading to endothelial dysfunction is deficiency of ascorbic acid (vitamin C), as shown by deposits of fats in the lining tissues of the arteries of guinea pigs deprived of this vitamin. As shown by our early studies, experimental scurvy in guinea pigs causes abnormal metabolism of homocysteine, leading to accumulation of the free form of the amino acid. Endothelial dysfunction in human subjects with atherosclerosis is reversed by intravenous doses of vitamin C, potentially ameliorating the earliest stages of plaque formation.

Morphologically, endothelial dysfunction is characterized by vacuolization, cytoplasmic swelling, and hyperplasia of endothelial cells, all of which are observed in children with homocystinuria. Constriction of the lumen of *vasa vasorum*, supplying blood flow to the arterial wall, by these changes in endothelial cell morphology would be expected to enhance trapping of lipoprotein complexes with micro-organisms, with lipoprotein aggregates containing homocysteine, and with autoantibodies to LDL containing homocysteine or oxidized fats. Thus formation of arterial plaques and creation of vulnerable plaques are dependent upon numerous pathophysiological factors leading to endothelial dysfunction, elevated blood homocysteine, infection and inflammation.

Suggestions for prevention and therapy of vascular disease readily follow from our interpretation of the origin of vulnerable plaques. Risk factors that lead to elevated homocysteine levels need to be addressed by smoking cessation, dietary B vitamins, stress reduction, and control of diabetes and hypertension. The immune system needs to be enhanced by intake of vitamin A, vitamin D, pyridoxine, and other factors that are needed for proper immune function. Appropriate antibiotic therapy is needed in heart attack and stroke patients who have evidence of active infection. Dietary improvement is needed to supply the nutrients that are needed to minimize homocysteine elevation, to supply anti-microbial medium chain saturated fats, and to support anti-oxidant function [31]. Attempts to prevent cardiovascular disease and prolong life may be more successful by understanding the fallacies of the "diet-heart" hypothesis and determining what is harmful to the immune system and what may strengthen it.

REFERENCES

[1] Bell WJJr. *The College of Physicians of Philadelphia. A Bicentennial History.* CantonMA: Science History Publications, USA, 1987.

[2] Estes JW, Smith BG. *A Melancholy Scene of Desolation. The Public Response to the 1793 Philadelphia Yellow Fever Epidemic.* CantonMA: Science History Publications, USA, 1997.

[3] McCully KS. The biomedical significance of homocysteine. *Journal of Scientific Exploration,* 2001;15:5-20.

[4] Kauffman JM. *Malignant Medical Myths. Why Medical Treatment Causes 200,000 Deaths in the USA Each Year, and How To Protect Yourself.* West ConshohockenPA: Infinity Press, 2006.

[5] Men's Journal, May 2001. The Heroes Issue.

[6] McCully KS. Homocysteine and Disease: Basic and Clinical Aspects. *Cellular and Molecular Biology*, 2004;50:875-988.

[7] McCully KS. Homocysteine and Disease Symposium. *Cellular and Molecular Biology*, 2005;52:53-58.

[8] McCully KS. Hyperhomocysteinemia and arteriosclerosis: historical perspectives. *Clinical Chemistry and Laboratory Medicine*, 2005;43:980-986.

[9] McCully KS. Homocysteine, vitamins and vascular disease prevention. *American Journal of Clinical Nutrition*, 2007;86(suppl):1563S-1568S.

[10] Schnyder G, Roffi M, Pin R, Flammer Y, Lange H, Eberli FR, Meier B, Turi ZG, Hess OM. Decreased rate of restenosis after lowering of plasma homocysteine levels. *New England Journal of Medicine*, 2001;345:1593-1600.

[11] Schnyder G, Roffi M, Flammer Y, Pin R, Hess OM. Effect of homocysteine-lowering therapy with folic acid, vitamin B12 and vitamin B6 on clinical outcomes after percutaneous coronary intervention. *Journal of the American Medical Association*, 2002;288:973-979.

[12] Lange H, Suryapranata H, DeLuca G, Borner C, Dille J, Kallmayer K, Pasalary MH, Scherer E, Dambrink JH. Folate therapy and in-stent restenosis after coronary stenting. *New England Journal of Medicine*, 2004;350:2673-2681.

[13] Petersen JC, Spence JD. Vitamins and progression of atherosclerosis in hyper-homocyst(e)inemia. *Lancet*, 1998;351:263.

[14] Spence JD, Bang H, Chambless LE, Stampfer MJ. Vitamin intervention for stroke prevention trial. An efficacy analysis. *Stroke,* 2005;36:2404-2409.

[15] Toole JF, Malinow MR, Chambless LE, Spence JD, Pettigrew LC, Howard VJ, Sides EG, Wang CH, Stampfer MJ. Lowering homocysteine in patients with ischemic stroke to prevent recurrent stroke, myocardial infarction and death. *Journal of the American Medical Association*, 2004;291:565-575.

[16] The Heart Outcomes Prevention Evaluation (HOPE)2 Investigators. Homocysteine lowering with folic acid and B vitamins in vascular disease. *New England Journal of Medicine*, 2006;354:1567-1577.

[17] Bonaa KH, Njolstad I, Ueland PM, Schirmer H, Tverdal A, Stigen T, Wang H, Nordrehaug JE, Arnesen E, Rasmussen K. Homocysteine lowering and cardiovascular

events after acute myocardial infarction. *New England Journal of Medicine*, 2006;354:1578-1588.

[18] Jamison RL, Hartigan P, Kaufman JS. Effect of homocysteine lowering on mortality and vascular disease in advanced chronic kidney disease and end-stage renal disease: a randomized controlled trial. *Journal of the American Medical Association*, 2007;298:1163-1170.

[19] Wang X, Qin X, Demirtas H, Li J, Mao G, Huo Y, Sun N, Lin L, Xu X. Efficacy of folic acid supplementation in stroke prevention: a meta-analysis. *Lancet*, 2007;369:1876-1882.

[20] McCully KS. Reply to EZ Soliman and OA Shalash. *American Journal of Clinical Nutrition*, 2008;87:1070-1071.

[21] Wald DS, Morris JK, Law M, Wald NJ. Folic acid, homocysteine and cardiovascular disease: judging causality in the face of inconclusive trial evidence. *British Medical Journal,* 2006;333:1114-1117.

[22] Clarke R, et al for the MTHFR Studies Collaboration Group. Homocysteine and coronary heart disease: meta-analysis of MTHFR case-control studies, avoiding publication bias. *PLOS Medicine*, 2012;9:1-11.

[23] Jacques PF, Selhub J, Bostom AG, Wilson PWF, Rosenberg IH. The effect of folic acid fortification on plasma folate and total homocysteine concentrations. *New England Journal of Medicine,* 1999;340:1449-1454.

[24] Yang Q, Botto LD, Erickson JD, Berry RT, Sambell C, Johansen H, Friedman JM. Improvement in stroke mortality in Canada and the United States, 1990 to 2002. *Circulation*, 2006;113:1335-1343.

[25] Decline in deaths from heart disease and stroke in the US 1900-1999. *Morbidity and Mortality Weekly Reports*, 1999;48:649-656.

[26] Havlik RJ, Feinleib M, Editors. *Proceedings of the Conference on the Decline in Coronary Heart Disease Mortality*. Bethesda MD: NIH Publication No. 79-1610.

[27] Kung HC, Hoyert DL, Xu J, Murphy SL. *National Vital Statistics Reports*, 2008;56:1-18.

[28] Ravnskov U, McCully KS. Vulnerable plaque formation from obstruction of *vasa vasorum* by homocysteinylated and oxidized lipoprotein aggregates complexed with microbial remnants and LDL autoantibodies. *Annals of Clinical and Laboratory Science*, 2009;39:3-16.

[29] Ravnskov U, McCully KS. Infections may be causal in the pathogenesis of atherosclerosis. *American Journal of the Medical Sciences*, 2012; *In press*. This review discusses the contradictions to the cholesterol hypothesis, the association of cardiovascular disease with infections, and new pathological evidence for the presence of Chlamydia pneumonia, mycoplasma pneumonia, and archaeal organisms in arterial plaques.

[30] McCully KS. Chemical Pathology of Homocysteine IV Excitotoxicity, oxidative stress, endothelial dysfunction and inflammation. *Annals of Clinical and Laboratory Science*, 2009;39:219-232.

[31] Kabara JJ. *Fats are good for you and other secrets. How saturated fat and cholesterol actually benefit the body*. Berkeley CA: North Atlantic Books, 2008.

Chapter 9

THE HEART REVOLUTION

Not long after publication of my first book *The Homocysteine Revolution* in 1997, I was encouraged to write a second book for the general reader explaining how to apply the homocysteine theory to prevention of disease, promotion of optimal health, and increased longevity. This new book, *The Heart Revolution. The B Vitamin Breakthrough that Lowers Homocysteine, Cuts Your Risk of Heart Disease, and Protects Your Health*, was designed as an expanded, reader-friendly account of the homocysteine approach to prevention of heart disease [1]. With the collaboration of my daughter, Martha McCully, who is experienced in editing, writing and publishing, as Beauty Editor of *Allure Magazine* and Executive Editor of *InStyle Magazine*, we embarked upon an extended, simplified explanation of how proper eating of a nutritious diet, combined with moderate exercise, smoking cessation and avoidance of processed foods, can lead to enhanced health through an improved style of living. This book was published in 1999 as a hardback, and an updated soft cover version containing a six week program of implementation and suggested recipes for healthful meals was published in 2000. The book, like *The Homocysteine Revolution*, is still in print 10 years after publication. Martha's contribution to the new book was invaluable because of her ability to convey descriptive, memorable phrases, words, and organization that appeal to readers without a scientific, medical or technical background. Another strategy of the book was to suggest a list of helpful practical hints and tips to illustrate the point of each chapter.

The Heart Revolution is intended to present a comprehensive, enlightened view of the origin of arteriosclerosis, heart disease and stroke, the most important causes of death and disability in developed countries today. This approach offers practical, life-saving advice concerning improved nutrition and life style changes for prevention of vascular diseases. *The Heart Revolution* offers an alternative to the traditional advice of the pharmaceutical-agribusiness-medical establishment views of prevention and treatment of these diseases, based on the "diet-heart" hypothesis. *The Heart Revolution* places dietary fats and cholesterol in a proper perspective, while emphasizing all factors known to participate in causation of disease. Thus *The Heart Revolution* is a balanced approach that is based on proven factors in prevention of arteriosclerosis.

Critical review of the cholesterol/fat hypothesis by Uffe Ravnskov, Joel Kauffman and other authorities disclosed many fallacies and contradictions that invalidate the traditional approach [2,3]. As elegantly explained in *The Cholesterol Myths* by Ravnskov and *Malignant Medical Myths* by Kauffman, the low fat diet, advocated by the American Dietetic

Association, the US Department of Agriculture, the American Diabetes Association, the US Food and Drug Administration, the National Cholesterol Education Program, the American Medical Association, the American Heart Association, Health Canada, and the UK National Advisory Committee, amounts to a high carbohydrate diet. This dietary recommendation is largely responsible for the ominous increase in diabetes, obesity, and metabolic syndrome observed in the US during the past quarter century. The discredited Food Pyramid of the US Department of Agriculture advocates 6-11 daily servings of bread, cereal, rice and pasta, providing an unreasonably high carbohydrate intake.

The Framingham Heart Study showed a half century ago that dietary cholesterol does not determine blood cholesterol levels [4]. Instead the liver and intestines produce adequate cholesterol from acetate to supply the needs of the body, as shown by the observation that strict vegetarians who consume no dietary cholesterol have adequate blood cholesterol levels, albeit lower than consumers of meat, seafood and dairy foods. Dietary saturated fats, including butter, lard and tropical oils are beneficial to health, whereas transfats are deleterious, as shown by Mary Enig in her book *The Oiling of America* [5]. Monolaurin, a saturated medium chain monoglyceride fat, is particularly beneficial in combating infections, as shown by Jon Kabara in his book *Fats are Good for You* [6]. As discussed in Chapter 8, lipoproteins form a non-specific immune system that effectively prevents infections by bacteria, viruses, and protozoan micro-organisms and helps to prevent formation of vulnerable plaques in arteries. The immune system is strengthened by an adequate dietary supply of micro-nutrients, including vitamins A, B, C, E, D, and K, further enhancing protection against invading micro-organisms.

As explained by the critical reviews by Ravnskov and by Kauffman, low cholesterol levels are associated with increased susceptibility to infections, heart failure, cancer and other life-shortening conditions. Thus the strategy to lower blood cholesterol levels by drug therapy is misguided, crippling the normal defense of the body against life threatening diseases. Indeed the much touted statin drugs are ineffective in prolonging life in primary prevention trials of normal subjects. The trivial reduction of adverse events, amounting to 1-3% absolute risk reduction, in statin trials of subjects with established vascular disease, is counteracted by an increase in cancer deaths, as shown in the CARE and PROSPER trials. As shown by critical analysis, the cholesterol/fat hypothesis is effectively disproven by published data from many sources. As described in Ravenskov's book *The Cholesterol Myths*, many proponents of the "diet-heart" hypothesis are guilty of bias in interpretation of trial results and epidemiological studies through selection of data and bias in citation of medical literature references.

According to Ancel Keys, former professor of physiology and nutrition in Minnesota and now deceased, the earliest epidemiological investigation relating cholesterol to human atherosclerosis was conducted by the Dutch physician, CD DeLangen, who reported his experience working with patients in Java [7]. In 1916 DeLangen reported that Javanese natives have low levels of cholesterol in the blood, possibly explaining the rarity of atherosclerosis, phlebothrombosis and gallstones in this Asian population. In contrast, Javanese stewards on Dutch ships in Java, who consumed the rich Dutch diet, had increased levels of cholesterol in their blood, and DeLangen advocated a low cholesterol diet for prevention of atherosclerosis, based on these observations.

Keys later became the leading advocate of what was known as the "diet-heart" hypothesis, relating coronary heart disease to dietary consumption of fats and cholesterol.

Keys and his colleagues studied mortality rates from coronary heart disease from countries around the world, reporting an association with dietary fat available for consumption in the *Seven Countries Study* [8]. However, as pointed out by Ravnskov [2], when similar data from 22 countries, available to Keys, are considered, the association becomes almost non-existent. For example, the mortality rate in Finland was almost 7 times higher than in Mexico, although fat consumption was identical. Subsequently authoritative critical review of the *Seven Countries Study* by statisticians Smith and Pinckney revealed "a massive set of inconsistencies and contradictions," leading to the conclusion that the "study cannot be taken seriously by the objective and critical scientist [9]."

The longest running study of cardiovascular disease in a population was initiated in Framingham, Massachusetts in 1948 and continues to this day [4]. This landmark longitudinal study identified important major risks for cardiovascular disease, especially smoking, lack of exercise, age, male gender, high blood pressure, and elevated blood cholesterol levels in younger men. In spite of the great emphasis on blood cholesterol levels, the Framingham Heart Study made several critical observations that refute the "diet-heart" hypothesis. In the first place, as previously discussed, dietary cholesterol has no relation of cholesterol levels in the blood, and dietary cholesterol has no relation to the risk of developing cardiovascular disease. This observation was confirmed by multiple large studies from Chicago, Puerto Rico, Honolulu, Netherlands, Ireland, and the massive Lipid Research Clinics study of US citizens. The next astounding finding is that elevated blood cholesterol is not a risk factor for women of any age or for men over age 47. Furthermore, both total mortality and cardiovascular mortality in Framingham participants increases in those with LOW blood cholesterol levels. This finding has been confirmed by multiple studies from Canada, Sweden, Russia and New Zealand. These contradictory findings have been ignored, distorted, and incorrectly reported by supporters of the "diet-heart" hypothesis.

The massive Multiple Risk Factor Intervention Trial (MRFIT) screened 360,000 US men to find those with the highest risk of developing cardiovascular disease. Approximately 12,000 overweight, hypertensive, smokers with elevated blood cholesterol levels were recruited for this 7 year trial, involving consumption of a low fat diet, smoking cessation, exercise and anti-hypertensive drugs. At the end of the trial, blood pressure was down, smoking decreased, and average blood cholesterol levels were down 7%. When the results of this $100M trial were analyzed, 115 in the treatment group had died of heart disease, compared with 124 in the control group, an insignificant difference. Looking at mortality from all causes, there were 265 deaths in the treatment group, compared with 260 in the control group. In looking at the failure of this massive and expensive trial, the investigators found minor benefits of smoking cessation, no benefit of lowering blood pressure, and no effect of lowering blood cholesterol levels by 2% compared with the control group.

In the even more massive $150M Lipid Research Clinics (LRC) trial, 4000 participants with very high blood cholesterol levels were selected from almost half a million US men. After significant lowering of cholesterol levels for 7 years by the resin cholestyramine, 190 men had suffered non-fatal heart attacks in the treatment group, compared with 212 in the control group. As for fatal heart attacks, the figures were 1.7% compared with 2.3%, a difference of 0.6%, or 12 individuals. The investigators misleadingly expressed these differences as relative risk reductions of 19% and 30% by throwing out the denominators of their fractions.

In the later trials with statin drugs that lower blood cholesterol levels more effectively than the unpleasant resin cholestyramine, a similar statistical approach was taken to increasing the apparent effet on reducing cardiovascular mortality and adverse events. In an analysis of 6 major statin trials (EXCEL, 4S, WOSCOPS, CARE, AFCAPS, LIPID) by Ravnskov in *The Cholesterol Myths*, the reduction of cardiovascular mortality ranged from -19% to -41% when expressed as relative risk reduction, but from -0.12% to -3.5% when expressed as absolute risk reduction [2]. This statistical manipulation to make results more impressive illustrates Mark Twain's aphorism: "There are lies, damn lies, and statistics." Thus a multi-billion dollar drug industry depends upon using misleading statistical interpretation of trial data showing trivial differences between treated and control groups.

Another way of looking at absolute risk reduction is to consider the number needed to treat (NNT) to achieve one positive outcome. In the case of antibiotic therapy for pneumonia, the NNT is 1.1, meaning that 10 of 11 patients treated are cured, or a 90% success rate. The NNT for a successful medication is generally considered to be 2 to 4, meaning a 25% to 50% success rate. In the recent ENHANCE trial of Vytorin, a combination of simvistatin and ezetimibe prescribed to lower blood cholesterol, the NNT is 67, meaning that a positive outcome is observed in only one of 67 participants when taken for 5 years [10,11]. This number corresponds to a 2% success rate, or a 98% failure rate, a dismal and unacceptable outcome. In addition, Vytorin failed to prevent intimal-medial thickening, as assessed by ultrasound, contradicting the claim that cholesterol lowering by this medication prevents the early stages of atherosclerosis. These results further call into question the claims for a preventive effect of cholesterol lowering on arteriosclerosis.

The gigantic MONICA study, sponsored by the World Health Organization, analyzed the relation between cardiovascular mortality and blood cholesterol in 27 countries, in much the same way as the *Seven Countries Study*. The results are similar, showing that countries like Japan and China have lower cardiovascular mortality and low cholesterol levels, and countries like Finland have high mortality and high cholesterol levels. Yet countries like France, Germany, Switzerland, and Luxembourg have a low cardiovascular mortality rate and a high blood cholesterol value. This so-called "French paradox" is not a paradox at all, when examination of the data reveals great disparities in mortality between different regions with the same cholesterol levels. Similarly the residents of Corfu have a 5 fold greater mortality than residents of Crete, despite identical dietary practices and identical cholesterol levels. Residents of the North Karelia region of Finland have a cardiovascular mortality rate of 493/100,000, and those in Fribourg France have a rate of 102/100,000, yet the cholesterol levels are identical at 245 mg/dL in both regions.

The National Cholesterol Education Program (NCEP) is a quasi-governmental body sponsored by members of the National Heart, Lung and Blood Institute, the American Heart Association, and other supporters of the "diet-heart" hypothesis. This body recommends a low fat, high carbohydrate diet to prevent heart disease, in spite of the increasing incidence of diabetes, obesity and hypertension in the US that is linked to consumption of this diet. The NCEP consistently advocates programs of extreme lowering of blood cholesterol levels by drug therapy, in spite of solid evidence of increased risk of mortality from heart failure, cancer, cirrhosis, and other diseases in older subjects with low blood cholesterol levels. In 2002 the NCEP recommended lowering the acceptable level of Low Density Lipoprotein (LDL) in the population by statin drug therapy, in spite of the fact that 8 of the 9 members of the advisory panel had a direct conflict of interest by accepting payments from the pharmaceutical industry. The NCEP has popularized the concept that LDL is "bad cholesterol" and HDL is "good cholesterol" in spite of the marginal and sometimes contradictory data distinguishing these fractions from total blood cholesterol. The NCEP also advocates "aggressive cholesterol lowering" in the general population in spite of the fact that no cholesterol lowering trials have demonstrated reduced mortality or sudden death from such treatments in the otherwise normal population.

The Heart Revolution, in contrast to the traditional "diet-heart" approach, emphasizes control of factors that produce vascular disease by causing elevation of blood homocysteine and alterations of methionine and homocysteine metabolism [1]. Because the B vitamins, folic acid, pyridoxine and cobalamin, are all involved in normal metabolism to prevent excessive production of homocysteine, the homocysteine theory of arteriosclerosis implicates dietary deficiencies of these vitamins in human arteriosclerosis, heart attacks, strokes, and amputations from vascular disease. Because the sensitive vitamins folic acid and pyridoxine are destroyed by traditional methods of food processing, such as milling of grains, canning, extraction of sugars and oils from whole foods, and addition of chemical additives to bleach or preserve foods, this theory helps to explain the large increase in vascular disease in the early and mid 20th century in the US. Similarly, the decline in mortality from cardiovascular disease beginning in the 1950s can be attributed to addition of the synthetic B vitamins pyridoxine and folic acid to the food supply by fortification of processed foods. Important support for the homocysteine theory was provided by the Framingham Heart Study, which showed that deficiencies of these B vitamins are widespread in older participants, leading to elevation of blood homocysteine levels and increased risk of arterial plaques.

Many hundreds of published studies by investigators worldwide have now proven that elevated blood homocysteine levels are associated with increased risk of heart disease, stroke, peripheral vascular disease, and with decreased longevity in diverse populations. In 1998 the US Food and Drug Administration mandated addition of folic acid to refined flour, rice and other grain foods, the first such action since niacin, thiamin, riboflavin and iron were mandated for addition to refined grain foods in 1941. One of the rationales for adding folic acid is the demonstration that deficiency of dietary folate is implicated in susceptibility to birth defects of the neural tube type. An additional rationale, not officially cited by the FDA, was the hope that vascular disease incidence and complications might also be prevented in the US. Studies have indeed shown that birth defects have decreased about 16% in the US and up to 78% in Canada in Newfoundland since fortification of grain foods by folic acid. In a recent study by the Centers for Disease Control and Prevention in Atlanta, the declining incidence of mortality from stroke accelerated in 1998 in the US and Canada, but no change was found in the United Kingdom, where folic acid fortification is not mandated [12]. In 2007 a meta-analysis, as reported in Lancet, concluded that trials yielding significant reduction in blood homocysteine levels from folic acid, pyridoxine and cobalamin over a 3 to 5 year period produced significant reductions in mortality from stroke [13]. Trials studying participants with a history of advanced vascular disease, heart attack and stroke, have been less successful, as explained in Chapter 8. The Swiss Heart Study showed that restenosis following coronary angioplasty was benefited by B vitamins, but a later trial with stented patients showed no benefit.

During the past decade a series of epidemiological studies provided direct evidence that inadequate dietary intake of folate and vitamin B6 increases the incidence of cardiovascular disease. In 1998 the Nurses' Health Study of 80,000 women reported that those participants with the lowest dietary consumption of folate and vitamin B6 had a significantly increased incidence of myocardial infarct (heart attack) and death from heart disease during a 14 year follow up period [14,15]. The preventive effect of increased folate and vitamin B6 consumption was potentiated by moderate alcohol intake. The European Prospective Investigation into Cancer and Nutrition (EPIC) studied 22,345 healthy participants from Potsdam, Germany for almost 5 years [16]. An increased dietary consumption of folate was associated with a decreased incidence of myocardial infarction in this study. In a 2008 study from Japan, 40,803 healthy subjects were followed for 10 years; those subjects with the highest dietary intakes of folate and vitamin B6 had the lowest incidence of coronary heart disease and myocardial infarction [17]. In 2009 the Northern Sweden Health and Disease Study followed 73,879 healthy participants for up to 13 years, showing that those with the highest dietary consumption of folate had the lowest incidence of myocardial infarction [18]. Elevated plasma homocysteine levels correlated with increased incidence of coronary heart disease and with low dietary consumption of folate. These large prospective epidemiological studies all provide direct evidence to support the homocysteine theory of arteriosclerosis by showing that vascular disease is caused by deficient consumption of folate and vitamin B6, leading to increased blood homocysteine levels. In contrast to the inability of high dose B vitamins to reverse advanced vascular disease in the VISP, HOPE2, NORVIT, and HOST trials, as described in Chapter 8, these recent prospective studies of healthy populations prove that dietary folate and vitamin B6 intake are important factors determining the incidence of heart disease.

Deficient dietary consumption of folate and vitamin B6 is only one of the more than 100 conditions known to produce elevation of blood homocysteine and increased risk of vascular disease. Well established risk factors for vascular disease, including aging, male gender, post-menopausal status in women, smoking, hypertension, diabetes and kidney failure have long been known to increase blood homocysteine levels. The common (12%) genetic condition, involving homozygosity for the TT genotype of methylenetetrahydrofolate reductase, leads to increased blood homocysteine and vascular disease risk in populations with limited consumption of dietary folate. Many drugs lead to elevation of blood homocyteine levels by antagonizing the functions of folate, vitamin B12 and vitamin B6 in the body [19]. Some commonly used drugs include methotrexate for cancer therapy or rheumatoid arthritis, phenytoin (Dilantin), carbamazepine, or valproic acid for anti-epileptic therapy, estrogen analogues (Tamoxifen) for cancer therapy, nitrous oxide for anesthesia, and azaribine for psoriasis are all examples of drugs that cause elevation of blood homocysteine. In the case of azaribine, the FDA banned the use of this drug because of increased incidence of thrombosis, heart disease and stroke observed in patients given this therapy for psoriasis. Cyclosporine and other immunosuppressive drugs for organ transplantation and acute phase response to infections, cholesterol lowering drugs such as cholestyramine, colestipol, and nicotinic acid, and thiazide diuretics have all been found to cause elevation of blood homocysteine levels.

Some other conditions leading to elevation of blood homocysteine are leukemia, metastatic cancer, hypothyroidism, Alzheimer's dementia, autoimmune diseases such as lupus erythematosus, ulcerative colitis, myelodysplasia, and rheumatoid arthritis, schizophrenia, depression, osteoporosis and hip fracture. One can appreciate that many medical conditions and diseases other than B vitamin deficiency are associated with elevated blood homocysteine levels. For this reason, a physician's detailed clinical analysis is needed to determine the probable cause for elevation of blood homocysteine in individual cases.

Since publication of *The Heart Revolution* in 1999, a number of nutritional and environmental hazards to health have been described and clarified. Among these hazards are dietary glutamate and other excitotoxins, fluosilicic acid used for fluoridation of drinking water, and the phytoestrogens, phytates, and multiple toxic proteins of soy foods.

In a remarkable book *Excitotoxins. The Taste that Kills*, Russell Blaylock recounts the pioneering experiments of Lucas and Newhouse in 1957, demonstrating toxicity of injected glutamate on the retinal cells of infant mice [20]. He also describes the systematic studies by John Olney in 1969, demonstrating neuronal damage to the brain cells of newborn mice by glutamate, aspartate, and sulfur amino acids, including homocysteine and homocysteic acid. Blaylock explains how the food industry conceals the addition of glutamate and other excitotoxins to processed foods by using hydrolyzed plant proteins, protein extracts, and "natural flavorings," all of which contain glutamate, aspartate, and cysteine. Glutamate and these other food additives enhance the flavor of processed foods, increasing food consumption, leading to obesity, as shown by a recent study from China. In newborn mice glutamate and other excitotoxins damage the hypothalamic centers controlling appetite and hormonal function, leading to massive obesity, stunted growth, and female sterility in the experimental animals. Homocysteine has recently been discovered to activate the same receptors in brain cells (NMDA receptors) as glutamate, causing excitation and neuronal damage [21]. Homocysteine is also used by the food industry as a flavoring agent for processed foods.

In his review of the literature on excitotoxins, Blaylock points out that dietary glutamate causes higher blood levels of glutamate in human subjects than in monkeys, mice or rats. He also notes that developing human brain, human brain injury, and aging brain increase the potential susceptibility to neurotoxicity by dietary excitotoxins because of reduced integrity of the blood brain barrier. Blaylock further suggests that dietary exposure to glutamate, Aspartame, and cysteine may exacerbate important human neurodegenerative diseases, including Alzheimer's dementia, amyotrophic lateral sclerosis (ALS), Parkinson's disease, and Huntington's chorea. Dietary intake of glutamate, aspartate, and cysteine from hydrolyzed protein extracts, flavorings, and seasonings in processed foods is unknown because of a lack of a labeling requirement by the US Food and Drug Administration. Blood homocysteine levels are elevated in several chronic neuropsychiatric disorders such as Alzheimer's dementia, schizophrenia, cognitive dysfunction, and multiple sclerosis. Activation of glutamate receptors by elevated blood homocysteine resulting from developmental, dietary, and aging factors may affect the progression and exacerbation of these disorders.

As described in Chapter 2, my interest in biochemistry and experimental psychology led me to propose an experiment to study the toxic effects of the metabolic poison fluoroacetate on rat behavior in 1953. The toxicologist Phyllis Mullenix used a similar approach in 1994, using computer-enhanced analysis of photographic images of rat behavior to demonstrate a profound effect of fluoride on learning responses. In his book *The Fluoride Deception* Christopher Bryson describes the efforts of the US Atomic Energy Commission, the aluminum and fertilizer industries, and the US Public Health Service to conceal the toxicity of fluoride, leading to fluoridation of drinking water in the 1940s in the US [22]. One of the strategies of the military-industry-government cabal was to discredit the seminal discoveries of PF Moller and Kaj Roholm, the Danish toxicologists who originally discovered the toxic properties of fluorine compounds in the 1930s [23]. Among the toxic effects of fluorine compounds on human and animal tissues are deformities, hardening, and fibrosis of bones and joints, leading to "poker spine," fibrosis of lung, damage to skin and gastrointestinal tract, and increased risk of cancer. Roholm himself was a scientific martyr, dying an early death from cancer in 1948 because of his exposure to fluorine compounds.

One of my classmates at Harvard College in the 1950s, Roger Masters, became a distinguished Professor of Government at Dartmouth College. He was interested in applying scientific investigation and concepts to human behavior, as manifested in political behavior, delinquency in childhood, and criminal behavior. With his collaborator, the environmental engineer Myron Coplan, Masters published a series of studies on fluoridation of drinking water by fluosilicic acid and sodium fluosilicate [24,25]. These toxic byproducts of the fertilizer and aluminum industries are used to provide fluoridation of drinking water in 90% of fluoridated US communities. These compounds dissociate into fluoride ion when diluted in water. Masters and Coplan discovered that fluoridation of drinking water with these compounds correlates with criminal behavior, lead poisoning, and alcohol and drug abuse. The blood lead levels of children are higher in Massachusetts communities where silicofluorides are used for fluoridation, compared with communities where sodium fluoride is used. Silicofluorides increase absorption of lead, manganese, and other heavy metal intoxicants. Increased blood lead levels are correlated with alcohol and drug abuse and higher crime rates in communities across America. From this multifactorial approach, Masters and Coplan conclude "when otherwise unexplained geographical and historical differences in rates of crime are analyzed from this perspective, environmental pollution and the use of silicofluorides in water treatment seem to play a critical role in triggering social dysfunction." These findings help to explain why the United States has crime rates that are much higher than those of other industrial nations, why violent crime peaked in 1991 and has begun to decline, and why some US cities have more violent crime than others.

Recently a highly significant development occurred on March 23, 2006, when a National Academy of Sciences panel unanimously recommended lowering the Maximum Contaminant Level of 4 ppm of fluoride in drinking water. The twelve person panel reviewed the fluoride literature over a 3 year period and concluded that 4 ppm could jeopardize children and adults in areas of the country where natural fluoride is high in water supplies. The panel cited dental fluorosis and increased risk of bone fractures as adverse health effects of excess fluoride ingestion. Members of the panel warned that the Abstract and Conclusion sections of the report, still to be released, do not agree with the findings in the body of the report. Fluoride is ubiquitous in the environment, and common food and drink, prepared with fluoridated water contain appreciable concentrations of fluoride. Some commonly consumed products with increased fluoride are tea, wine and beer.

My long standing interest in the toxic effects of fluorine compounds on biochemical processes culminated in the publication of the fourth installment of my second monograph, The Chemical Pathology of Homocysteine [21]. In this review I compared the molecular structure of oxygen difluoride, an extremely toxic gas, to that of ozone, a component of thioretinaco ozonide. My suggestion is that oxygen difluoride is capable of displacing ozone from thioretinaco ozonide, thereby inhibiting cellular respiration, oxidative metabolism and ATP synthesis.

Because of the extreme toxicity of oxygen difluoride, one of the most toxic gases known, this compound was investigated in World War I as a chemical weapon. The effectiveness of oxygen difluoride is limited, however, by the decomposition of the compound by traces of water vapor or humidity in the atmosphere. This compound is also suspected of causing injuries and deaths in the Manhattan Project in World War II because of its production from elemental fluorine and atmospheric oxygen in the synthesis of uranium hexafluoride.

In my review I explain that fluoride is a toxic anion that stimulates oxygen consumption and increases superoxide production in resting white blood cells called neutrophils. Intracellular calcium ions are required for superoxide production of neutrophils during phagocytosis of micro-organisms by these white blood cells. The effect of fluoride on superoxide production is reversible in these cells, causing superoxide production in the presence of fluoride, decreasing superoxide production when fluoride is removed, and restoring superoxide production when fluoride is again added. Viability of neutrophils is maintained during superoxide formation. These experiments show that superoxide radical production by white blood cells is modulated by fluoride, providing a means for producing intracellular oxidative stress. In white blood cells oxidative stress is an essential process by which phagocytosed microbes are inactivated and killed.

Fluoride has been known as a metabolic inhibitor for many years, causing inhibition of oxidative metabolism and decreased ATP synthesis. Fluoride is believed to inhibit the activity of many enzymes by disrupting the molecular structure of proteins by interfering with normal hydrogen bonding [26]. In addition, the effects of fluoride on chromosomal structure, genetic damage, and carcinogenesis may by attributable to inhibition of the enzyme systems that repair damaged DNA.

The effect of fluoride in the induction of cellular oxidant stress is attributable to interaction of fluoride ions with the amide groups of thioretinaco ozonide, the postulated center for oxidative metabolism and ATP synthesis. Conformational change in the binding of thioretinamide groups to the cobalt of thioretinaco by hydrogen bonding with fluoride would be expected to inhibit the binding of superoxide and other oxygen radicals to the active site of oxidative phosphorylation, resulting in inhibition of ATP synthesis and accumulation of oxygen radicals within cells.

In 1996 a colleague, Steven Zeisel, invited me to participate in the 7th International Congress on Phospholipids in Brussels, Belgium. The meeting was devoted to the topic of "choline, phospholipids, health and disease." My presentation "Homocysteine and vascular disease: the role of folate, choline and lipoproteins in homocysteine metabolism" focused on the metabolic controls of homocysteine formation from the methyl groups of choline and betaine through an alternative pathway for conversion of homocysteine to methionine [27]. In this presentation I also suggested a new molecular interpretation of the observed aggregation of extracellular proteoglycans in skin cultures from children with homocystinuria. The meeting was sponsored by the American Oil Chemists Society and by several large companies involved in the production and marketing of soy foods and products. These companies were Archer, Daniels, Midland of Illinois, Central Soya Company of Indiana, and Riceland Foods of Arkansas, and companies from several European Countries. At this meeting I perceived an intense motivation by these representatives of the agribusiness-nutrition complex to promote and market foods and other products derived from soybeans.

Soy products from soybeans are an immense industry in the US and many other countries. Soybean oil, particularly in its hydrogenated form containing transfats, is ubiquitous in processed foods because of its abundant cheap supply, its resistance to rancidity, and its promotion of "shelf life" of food products. Soy protein, a highly processed protein extract devised by food chemists is widely used as a "meat extender" and "meat substitute" in processed foods. Soy lecithin containing choline is widely used in processed foods as an emulsifier. Also, as previously explained, hydrolyzed soy protein extract is widely used as a flavoring agent in processed foods because of its content of glutamate, aspartate, cysteine and other excitotoxins. In addition food chemists and industry scientists have heavily promoted the use of phytoestrogens of soy, including genistein, diadzin and other isoflavones as preventive nutraceuticals for prevention of menopausal symptoms, heart disease, stroke and cancer. The reasons for the wide use of soy products in processed foods are the abundant, cheap supply and the high protein and oil content of soybeans. The soy industry has lobbied the US Food and Drug Administration for permission to make health claims for the supposed efficacy of soy foods in prevention of disease.

Through my affiliation with Sally Fallon of the Weston A. Price Foundation, I was asked to review the manuscript of an important new book *The Whole Soy Story* by nutritionist Kaayla Daniel of Santa Fe [28]. In reading the manuscript I recalled that soy protein, which is notoriously deficient in methionine, was used in the early experiments at the Harvard School of Public Health [29]. A soy protein extract and cholesterol were fed to monkeys, showing that arterial plaques were observed after several months of feeding. Supplementation of the monkey diet with added methionine decreased arterial plaques in the animals. In human studies, dietary deficiency of protein causes elevation of blood homocysteine levels, as shown in West Africans with goiter and protein malnutrition and in elderly Baltimore school-teachers. The Belgian nutritional scientist, Yves Ingenbleek, has traced the elevation of blood homocysteine to decreased formation of adenosyl methionine and down regulation of cystathionine synthase, because of methionine deficiency in vegetarian African populations [30]. Adenosyl methionine (SAMe) is the co-enzyme that regulates the conversion of homocysteine to methionine and cystathionine. Deficient formation of adenosyl methionine leads to decreased conversion of homocysteine to cystathionine and decreased inhibition of methylation of homocysteine to methionine, resulting in elevation of plasma homocysteine levels. Thus the Harvard monkeys fed a diet of soy protein developed arterial plaques most likely because of elevated blood homocysteine resulting from dietary methionine deficiency, decreased adenosyl methionine formation, and down regulation of cystathionine synthase and the transsulfuration pathway.

The Whole Soy Story is a remarkable book because it clearly documents many of the adverse health effects of soy foods. The ancient Chinese realized the usefulness of soybean crops as a means of enriching soil for other crops, now known to be secondary to nitrogen fixation by the bacteria in the roots of this legume. The Chinese considered soybeans inedible until 2500 years ago, when many Asian cultures discovered that fermentation would eliminate digestive distress, bloating and gas associated with eating freshly cooked soybeans. The fermented food products *chaing*, better known by the Japanese word "miso," natto, tempeh, and soy sauce, were introduced between 1000 and 1600AD. Tofu was invented in 164BC in China by treating cooked soybeans with *nigari*, a form of magnesium chloride found in seawater. According to Daniels "East Asian countries all developed distinct soybean cuisines, but shared a reliance on fermentation, precipitation or both. Except for monasteries, during famines and among the very poor, Asians consumed soy foods only in small amounts as condiments or seasonings, not as substitutes for animal foods like fish or pork."

The Whole Soy Story describes a litany of toxic effects on human health, caused by constituents of soybeans. Some of the most important of these adverse effects are hypothyroidism from goitrogenic isoflavones, decreased fertility and precocious puberty from phytoestrogens, allergic reactions to soy proteins, flatulence from soy carbohydrates, poor digestion from protease inhibitors, poor iron, zinc and calcium absorption from phytates, gastrointestinal disturbances from lectins and saponins, kidney stones from oxalates, brain toxicity from magnesium, aluminum and fluoride, and antifertility effects in women and men. All of these myriad toxic effects of soy constituents are exhaustively discussed with references to the medical and scientific literature. My quote for the Introduction and Book Jacket is "*The Whole Soy Story* is a devastating and authoritative indictment of the safety of soy foods and a 'must read' for consumers who are under the misconception that soy foods promote health. Convincingly argued and extensively supported by the medical and scientific literature, it exposes the misleading propaganda used by the soy industry to promote the supposed benefits of this inferior food." In addition, many of the effects of hypothyroidism and deficiency of dietary methionine induced by soy foods help to promote arteriosclerosis by causing elevation of blood homocysteine levels.

The Heart Revolution is a way of life for promotion of health, prevention of disease and increased longevity through improved nutrition, avoidance of toxins, avoidance of dietary additives, avoidance of unnecessary prescription drugs, moderate exercise and stress reduction. Through this strategy, based on current knowledge of prevention of cardiovascular and other chronic diseases, the outlook is for increased longevity with improved cognitive function, lower risk of heart attack, stroke, and cardiovascular disease, reduced risk of osteoporosis and fracture, in radiant good health.

References

[1] McCully KS, McCully ME. *The Heart Revolution. The Extraordinary Discovery that Finally Laid the Cholesterol Myth to Rest.* New York: Harperperennial, 2000. The soft cover edition of The Heart Revolution includes a six week plan for implementing the recommendations for adopting the principles of the homocysteine theory of arteriosclerosis for promotion of health. This edition contains a number of favorite family recipes for daily living that illustrate the main nutritional tenets of the theory.

[2] Ravnskov U. *The Cholesterol Myths. Exposing the Fallacy that Saturated Fat and Cholesterol Cause Heart Disease.* Washington DC: New Trends Publishing, 2000. Uffe Ravnskov, a Danish nephrologist and clinical chemist, practiced medicine in Sweden and later became an independent investigator with an interest in the cholesterol/fat hypothesis concerning the origin of vascular disease. Ravnskov's contributions are discussed in Chapter 7.

[3] Kauffman JM. *Malignant Medical Myths. Why Medical Treatment Causes 200,000 Deaths in the USA Each Year, and How to Protect Yourself.* West Conshohocken PA: Infinity Publishing, 2006, pp 45-77. Joel Kauffman, Professor of Chemistry at University of the Sciences in Philadelphia, analyzes 11 cherished dogmas of the medical and public health establishment. He concludes that the advice to the public concerning these myths is based on unsound and unsupported science and may be

responsible for as many as 200,000 deaths in the USA annually. The myths described in this book include (1) aspirin therapy for prevention of vascular disease, (2) the ineffectiveness of low carbohydrate diets for losing weight, (3) the use of cholesterol lowering statin drugs for prevention of mortality, (4) drug therapy for moderate hypertension, (5) prolongation of lifespan by moderate alcohol consumption, (6) exercise to extend lifespan, (7) the ineffectiveness of intravenous EDTA chelation therapy for atherosclerosis, (8) the danger of low dose ionizing radiation, (9) prologation of life by annual mammography in women, (10), improved rates of cancer survival from early detection and therapy, and (11) water fluoridation to prevent caries. In each case the author analyzes extensive published studies in the medical literature for critical evidence to support these myths, and in each case he finds that the evidence is lacking, contradictory, or otherwise non-supportive. Further comments are published in my review of this book in *Journal of Scientific Exploration* 2006;20:622-629.

[4] Levy D, Brinks S. *A Change of Heart. How the Framingham Heart Study Helped Unravel the Mysteries of Cardiovascular Disease.* New York: Knopf, 2005. This book describes the establishment of the Framingham Heart Study in 1948 and many of the principal findings published over the years. Chapter 13 "Renegade on the Trail of the Unknown" is devoted to a description of my contributions to the homocysteine theory of arteriosclerosis and my interaction with the investigators of the Framingham Heart Study.

[5] Enig, MG. *The Oiling of America.* Washington DC: New Trends Publishing, 1999. In this book the distinguished biochemist and investigator at the University of Maryland, Mary Enig, describes her discovery of excessive quantities of transfats in processed foods and the efforts of the food industry to discredit and suppress her findings.

[6] Kabara JJ. *Fats Are Good for You and Other Secrets. How Saturated Fat and Cholesterol Actually Benefit the Body.* Berkeley CA: North Atlantic Books, 2008. Doctor Kabara is a biochemist and student of George Leroy and Konrad Bloch of the University of Chicago. Kabara devoted his career to investigating the beneficial properties of saturated fats in the nonspecific immune system against microbial infections. He identified monolaurin, a mono-glyceride of the medium chain saturated fatty acid lauric acid, as the most potent of these natural fats in natural resistance to infectious diseases.

[7] Keys A. Coronary heart disease – The global picture. *Atherosclerosis*, 1975;22:149-192.

[8] Keys A. *Coronary Heart Disease in Seven Countries.* American Heart Association Monograph #29, 1970.

[9] Pinckney ER, Smith RL. Statistical analysis of Lipid Research Clinics Program. *Lancet,* 1987;8531:503-504.

[10] Peskin BS, Sim D, Carter MJ. The failure of Vytorin and statins to improve cardiovascular health: bad cholesterol or bad theory? *Journal of American Physicians and Surgeons*, 2008;13:82-87.

[11] Kastelein JJP, Akdim F, Stroess ESG. Simvistatin with or without ezetimibe in familial hypercholesterolemia. *New England Journal of Medicine*, 2008;358:1431-1443.

[12] Yang Q, Botto LD, Erickson JD, Berry RT, Sambell C, Johansen H, Friedman JM. Improvement in stroke mortality in Canada and the United States, 1990 to 2002. *Circulation*, 2006;113:1335-1343.

[13] Wang X, Qin X, Demirtas H, Li J, Mao G, Huo Y, Sun N, Lin L, Xu X. Efficacy of folic acid supplementation in stroke prevention: a meta-analysis. *Lancet*, 2007;369:1876-1882.

[14] Rimm EB, Willett WC, Hu FB, Sampson L, Colditz GA, Manson JE, Hennekens C, Stampfer MJ. Folate and vitamin B6 from diet and supplements in relation to risk of coronary heart disease in women. *Journal of the American Medical Association*, 1998;279:359-364.

[15] McCully KS. Homocysteine, folate, vitamin B6 and cardiovascular disease. *Journal of the American Medical Association*, 1998;279:392-393.

[16] Drogan D, Klipstein-Grobusch K, Dierkes J, Weikert C, Boeing H. Dietary intake of folate equivalents and risk of myocardial infarction in the European Prospective Investigation into Cancer and Nutrition (EPIC)—Potsdam Study. *Public Health and Nutrition*, 2006;9:465-471.

[17] Ishihara J, Iso H, Inone M, Iwasaki M, Okada K, Kita Y, Kobuko Y, Okayama A, Tsugane S for the JPHC Study Group. Intake of folate, vitamin B6 and vitamin B12 and the risk of CHD: the Japan Public Health Center-Based Prospective Study Cohort I. *Journal of the American College of Nutrition*, 2008;27:127-136.

[18] VanGuelpen B, Hultdin J, Johansson I, Witthoft C, Weinehall L, Eliasson M, Hallmans G, Palmqvist R, Jansson JH, Winkvist A. Plasma folate and total homocysteine levels are associated with the risk of myocardial infarction, independently of each other and of renal function. *Journal of Internal Medicine*, 2009;266:182-195.

[19] Ueland PM, Refsum H. Plasma homocysteine, a risk factor for vascular disease: plasma levels in health, disease and drug therapy. *Journal of Laboratory and Clinical Medicine*, 1989;114:473-501.

[20] Blaylock RL. *Excitotoxins. The Taste that Kills.* Albuqurque NM: Health Press NA, 1997.

[21] McCully KS. Chemical Pathology of Homocysteine. IV. Excitotoxicity, oxidant stress, endothelial dysfunction, and inflammation. *Annals of Clinical and Laboratory Science*, 2009;39:307-320.

[22] Bryson C. *The Fluoride Deception.* New York: Seven Stories Press, 2004.

[23] Roholm K. *Fluorine Intoxication: A Clinical-Hygiene Study, with a review of the literature and some experimental investigation.* London: HK Lewis, Ltd, 1937.

[24] Masters RD, Coplan MJ. A dynamic, multifactorial model of alcohol, drug abuse, and crime: linking neuroscience and behavior to toxicology. *Social Science Information*, 1999;38:591-624.

[25] Masters RD, Coplan MJ. Water treatment with silicofluorides and lead toxicity. *International Journal of Environmental Studies*, 1999;56:535-449.

[26] Yiamouyiannis J. *Fluoride the Aging Factor. How to Recognize and Avoid the Devastating Effects of Fluoride.* Delaware OH: Health Action Press, 1993.

[27] McCully KS. Homocysteine and vascular disease: the role of folate, choline and lipoproteins in homocysteine metabolism. In SH Zeisel, BJ Szuhaj, editors. *Choline, Phospholipids, Health and Disease.* Champaign IL: ACOS Press, 1998, pp 117-130.

[28] Daniel KT. *The Whole Soy Story. The Dark Side of America's Favorite Health Food.* Washington DC: New Trends Publishing, 2007.

[29] Mann GV, Andrus SB, McNally A, Stare F. Experimental atherosclerosis in cebus monkeys. *Journal of Experimental Medicine*, 1953;98:195-218. This experiment was described to the Harvard Medical School Class of 1959 during a first year nutrition clinic presentation in 1955 by Frederick Stare, the Chairman of Nutrition at Harvard. My interest in experimental atherogenesis was first awakened by this study because of my previous experience in the biochemistry laboratory of Konrad Bloch at Harvard.

[30] Ingenbleek Y, McCully KS. Vegetarianism produces subclinical malnutrition, hyperhomocysteinemia and atherogenesis. *Nutrition*, 2012;28:148-153. This nutritional study of vegetarian subjects in Chad documents hyperhomocysteinemia in protein energy malnutrition secondary to loss of lean body mass from low dietary intake of sulfur and methionine. According to 2010 WHO estimates, half of coronary heart disease mortality occurs worldwide in vegetarian populations with dietary methionine deficiency. Plasma levels of lipoproteins are normal and dietary intake of folate and vitamin B6 are adequate, B12 is marginal, and other conventional risk factors are not elevated.

Chapter 10

HOMOCYSTEINE AND CANCER

The human scourge of cancer has been known since antiquity, as the word "cancer" is derived from the Latin word for "crab." To the eyes of ancient physicians the growth of malignant tumors, particularly breast cancer in women, suggested the appearance of a crab during its progression to advanced disease. To this day all physicians, from medical school days through years of medical practice, confront the ravages of this often fatal disease in their patients. Although the fatal outcome of cancer was appreciated for many centuries, only in the 19th century did the cellular and tissue origin and the spread of cancer become understood through introduction of the new techniques, concepts and discoveries in the modern era of medicine. In particular, the methods of gross and microscopic study of the anatomy of cancer tissues and cells in the mid to late 19th century revealed the nature of malignant growth of cancer tissue, as medical scientists and physicians understand the process today.

When studying the cells and tissues of malignant tumors, the medical student, resident or fellow soon learns the basic appearance and behavior of the disease in their patients. The internist, surgeon, radiologist, dermatologist, or sub-specialist learns the gross appearance of early or advanced cancer cases by inspection, dissection, and imaging of malignant tissues. The pathologist learns the gross and microscopic appearance of malignant tissues through study of biopsy specimens, surgically resected tissues, or autopsy tissues of deceased patients. Physicians soon learn that malignant growth can originate in any tissue or organ of the body. The gross appearance of the primary malignant growth recapitulates, to a greater or lesser extent, the normal architecture of the tissue from which the cancer originates. During progression of cancer, the growth of the tissue at the primary site enlarges and invades surrounding tissues and organs. Finally malignant cells spread through blood vessels, lymphatics, or along surfaces of organs to produce secondary growths known as metastases. In the final stages of the disease, the malignant cells and tissues invade widely within normal tissues and organs. Death results from a variety of causes, such as hemorrhage from an invaded artery or vein, perforation of an abdominal organ, infection of an affected organ, growth within the skull causing pressure on normal brain structures, or widespread growth in many tissues, causing weight loss (cachexia) and wasting (atrophy) of normal organs and tissues.

Study of the microscopic appearance of malignant cells and tissues through examination of specimens that are fixed, imbedded in paraffin, sectioned, stained and mounted on glass slides reveals characteristic histopathological abnormalities that are shared to a greater or lesser extent by cancers arising in different tissues of the body. Analysis of cytologic features of cytopathology of washings, brushings, or needle aspiration of malignant cells reveals many of the characteristic abnormalities found in cancer cells by histopathological techniques. In general, malignant cells have enlarged nuclei with irregular aggregated chromatin representing abnormal DNA and nuclear proteins. The nuclei vary in size and shape (pleomorphism), and the intensity of staining is increased (hyperchromasia). There are frequent mitotic figures representing dividing cells in which individual chromosomes can be observed. The nuclear membranes become abnormal, showing irregular contours and shapes, folding (nuclear grooves), occasional nuclear inclusion bodies, and enlarged prominent nucleoli. The cytoplasm of malignant cells is usually diminished in quantity, resulting in an increased nucleo-cytoplasmic ratio. The cytoplasm may contain specialized proteins or cellular products, such as mucin or keratin that are found in the cells of origin of the primary tumor. Groups of malignant cells may form structures relating to the tissue of origin, such as glands, ducts, or keratin pearls. Giant cells containing multiple nuclei are sometimes present. Cytogenetic studies reveal irregular numbers of chromosomes with abnormal numbers (aneuploidy), distribution or morphology in almost all cancer types. Abnormal attachment between chromosomes (translocation) or missing pieces of chromosomes (deletion) are frequently observed.

Physicians and medical scientists knew little about the underlying causes of cancer until the late 18th century, when Percival Pott discovered that cancer of the scrotum was frequent in men who worked as chimney sweeps, clearing the soot and tar from chimneys in early industrial England. This association between an occupational exposure and cancer was noticed before the advent of modern medicine. Little more was discovered about cancer causation for another century, when other examples of exposure to industrial toxins were associated with the occurrence of cancer. The first experimental production of cancer by a chemical carcinogen was reported in 1915, when Yamagiwa and Itchikawa in Japan were able to cause skin cancer by application of coal tar to the shaved skin of animals. By 1940 British chemists had identified a series of polycyclic hydrocarbon compounds from coal tar that are highly active in producing skin cancer in animals. One of my chemistry professors at Harvard, Louis Fieser, was a leading chemist in identification of the chemical structure of carcinogenic hydrocarbons in the 1940s.

In reading James Miller's account of his masterful investigation of the electrophilic (electron withdrawing) properties of chemical carcinogens, I was impressed by his isolation of the homocysteine derivative of the potent synthetic carcinogen, acetylaminofluorene (AAF) [1]. Moreover, his team identified the role of a sulfate transferase enzyme in the carcinogenic process induced by this compound [2]. Detailed study of the effect of chemical carcinogens by Isaac Berenblum and other scientists revealed that an initiation phase of carcinogenic compounds in target tissues was followed by a prolonged promotion phase, often lasting months, to produce the maximum yield of experimental cancers in animals [3]. The carcinogenic chemical was often modified in the liver to a more active intermediate form, and characteristic electronic features of the active forms were identified by French scientists. The nature of the molecular processes involved in initiation and promotion of carcinogenesis by chemical compounds remained obscure, even though many investigators suspected interaction with DNA as the critical event in carcinogenesis.

Following the discovery of X-rays by Wilhelm Conrad Roentgen in 1895 and the discovery of the radioactivity of uranium by Antoine Henri Becquerel in 1896, early investigators with these new energy sources suffered radiation burns of skin, malignant tumors, and leukemia. Two prominent investigators, Walter Bradford Cannon, who used X-rays to study gastrointestinal motility and function, and Marie Sklodowska Curie, who with her husband isolated the radioactive element radium, both died of malignant diseases. Cannon died of a malignant tumor of skin, mycosis fungoides, and Curie died of aplastic anemia, a form of early leukemia.

In the early 20th century the therapeutic effect of X-rays and ionizing radiation from radium on cancer were recognized and introduced by oncologists of that period. During Marie Curie's visit to the United States in the 1920s, she was hailed as a savior because of the expectation that radiation therapy by radium would be effective in treating cancer. In subsequent years, of course, the whole field of radiation therapy was developed because of the therapeutic effect of ionizing radiation on cancer growth that was observed by the early pioneers in the field.

Ultraviolet light is a non-ionizing form of radiation, which nevertheless is capable of inducing skin cancer, most prominently from chronic sun exposure in susceptible individuals. Ionizing radiation produces a massive release of free radicals from oxygen within tissues, but how this intense oxidizing effect induces cancer, on the one hand, and how it cause selective destruction of cancer cells during radiation therapy is less clear. Most explanations of these effects over the years have speculated about the effects of ionizing and ultraviolet radiation on the DNA of chromosomes as a cause of the carcinogenic and therapeutic effects of radiation. Enzyme systems within cells are capable of repairing radiation damage to DNA, providing the ability of normal cells to recover from the effects of radiation. Radiation therapy also produces a response of connective tissues, producing a characteristic increase in fibrous tissue in areas exposed to radiation.

Some support for the view that radiation carcinogenesis affects DNA comes from the observation that ionizing radiation is mutagenic in micro-organisms, causing genetic mutations, and that many, but not all, carcinogens are mutagenic. The most widely useful test of mutagenicity of chemicals was developed by Bruce Ames, whom I met at the National Institutes of Health in 1960 while working with Maxine Singer and Giulio Cantoni. Ames developed his test for mutagenicity by utilizing a mutant of Salmonella, the bacterium that causes gastrointestinal infections [4]. He used this test to demonstrate that many foods contain mutagenic chemicals, some of which are carcinogenic in test animals. Observations like these have led many investigators to assume that cancer formation from normal cells is related to mutation of genes produced by the effects of chemical carcinogens and ionizing radiation.

A century ago in 1909 the Danish investigators, V Ellerman and O Bang, succeeded in transmitting the disease, erythro-myeloblastic leukemia, by a sub-microscopic filterable virus in chickens. The significance of this discovery was questioned initially because in that period there was some doubt that leukemia was indeed a form of cancer. However, in 1911 Peyton Rous of the Rockefeller Institute in New York succeeded in transmitting the first solid cancer, a sarcoma of chickens, by a filtered virus. Over the next half century investigators succeeded in transmitting a variety of malignant or benign tumors in animals by filterable viruses. These tumors included fibromas and papillomas of rabbits (Shope), chicken lymphomatosis (Furth), breast cancer in mice transmitted by a filterable virus in milk (Bittner), frog kidney cancer (Lucke), and leukemia and parotid gland tumors by polyoma virus in mice (Gross) [5].

Over the past century a number of human tumors, such as warts and genital papillomas, were found to be transmitted by filterable viruses. And today human cancer of the cervix is known to be related to infection by several specific types of genital herpes virus, currently identified in patients by newly developed molecular testing methods. Other examples of human cancers, such as Merkel cell skin cancer and Kaposi sarcoma in AIDS patients, are known to be related to infection by specific types of herpes viruses [6]. In the 1970s the investigators Howard Temin and David Baltimore found that cultured human cells, transformed by Rous sarcoma virus, contain a persistent provirus, associated with an enzyme reverse transcriptase that transcribes the RNA of the tumor virus into the DNA of the transformed cells. It was clear from all of these studies that cancer can be induced in animals and humans by a variety of oncogenic viruses. However, a convincing explanation of exactly how the molecular changes induced by these oncogenic viruses, chemical carcinogens, or radiation injury can produce cancer cells from normal cells has not been forthcoming [7].

Many other factors affect development of human cancer. Some of these factors are (1) hormones affecting cancer development in responsive tissues like breast, endometrium, or prostate, (2) infectious agents such as hepatitis B and hepatitis C viruses, Shistosomiasis of bladder or colon, *Helicobacter pylori* of stomach, (3) drugs such as anabolic steroids in liver, statin drugs in skin, breast and other organs, (4) chronic irritation and inflammation, such as skin cancer from burns or osteomyelitis, colon cancer from ulcerative colitis, (5) physical agents like asbestos in lung and pleura causing mesothelioma or gallstones leading to gallbladder cancer, or (6) chemical agents like acid reflux in esophagus leading to esophageal cancer, and chemical carcinogens in cigarette smoke causing cancer of lung, mouth, larynx, bladder or kidney. The molecular explanations of how these diverse factors promote cancer development in different tissues are quite murky and unconvincing. Added to this list are many rare genetic cancer syndromes that are clearly inherited, such as retinoblastoma of eye in children, multiple basal cell skin cancers in adults, xeroderma pigmentosum and skin cancer, Wilms tumor of kidney in children, and many others. Most human cancers, however, are not directly inherited, even though inherited cancer genes like BRCA1 and BRCA2 do increase the risk of human cancer.

An early advance in understanding how altered metabolism may explain cancer development was made by the German biochemist Otto Warburg. In his early 20th century studies of oxygen metabolism and cellular respiration in 1924, Warburg discovered that abnormal production of lactic acid from glucose in the presence of oxygen is a characteristic pattern of metabolism in most malignant tumors and in embryonic tissues [8]. In the 19th century Louis Pasteur had discovered that oxygen prevents lactic acid formation from glucose in micro-organisms. Warburg's studies suggested that an abnormality of oxygen metabolism underlies most if not all cancer development [9].

Warburg's discoveries and theories about the metabolic origin of cancer were questioned in the 1940s and 1950s by the American biochemist Sidney Weinhouse. He argued with Warburg about inconsistencies and contradictions in some of Warburg's findings and pointed out that lactic acid production in the presence of oxygen is characteristic of the metabolic pattern of respiration of embryonic and regenerating tissues [10]. Warburg's concept is that carcinogenic agents, whether they are chemical carcinogens, ionizing or ultraviolet radiation, oncogenic viruses, inflammation or other factors cause "an irreversible injury of cellular respiration." Exactly how or why diverse carcinogenic agents produce abnormal cellular respiration in cancer was not clear to Warburg, and other investigators were subsequently unable to explain the molecular basis for Warburg's findings. His concept seems to suggest that respiratory poisons and carcinogens cause loss of some substance that is essential to cellular respiration. Once lost from cancer cells, this substance cannot be replaced by cellular metabolism, and the molecular nature of this substance remains obscure.

The elucidation of the molecular structure of DNA and its function in genetic inheritance in 1953 by James Watson, Francis Crick, Maurice Wilkins, and Rosalind Franklin electrified the biomedical research community worldwide. The concept of transcription of genetic information from DNA of chromosomes to messenger RNA of cytoplasm and its conversion of the genetic code into the sequence of amino acids of protein molecules became known as the "central dogma." The power of these discoveries and concepts seemed to point the way for investigators of cancer to a new and promising field that might explain how altered processing of genetic information might affect carcinogenesis and explain the origin of cancer cells. The effort to understand Warburg's discovery of abnormal oxygen metabolism in cancer tissues fell into disfavor, as the younger generation of cancer investigators enthusiastically took up the challenges of the new field of molecular biology.

Otto Warburg died in 1970 at the age of 87, and his critical discovery was neglected in the stampede to understand how the new field of molecular biology could explain the many factors responsible for development of cancer. In a recent *New York Times* editorial my former mentor, James Watson himself, called for re-investigation and renewed efforts to understand the Warburg effect in cancer cells [11]. He pointed to progress in this field by the recent studies of the ability of cancer cells to accumulate glucose and other nutrients within cytoplasm, although "a definitive explanation of Warburg's observation has remained elusive [12]."

A new chapter in the study of cancer causation began in 1946 when DH Copeland and WD Salmon discovered that a diet that is deficient in the amino alcohol, choline, causes formation of malignant tumors of the liver, lungs and other tissues when fed to animals over prolonged periods [13]. Choline is a component of the phospholipid lecithin, a normal constituent of lipoproteins and fats in the body, and is also found in acetyl choline, an essential neurotransmitter in the central nervous system. The ability of diets that are deficient in choline to cause fat deposition and cirrhosis of the liver was discovered in the 1920s and 1930s in the aftermath of the discovery of insulin in 1922. The amino acid methionine, and the B vitamins folic acid and cobalamin (vitamin B12), were also found to prevent fat deposition in the livers of animals fed a diet that is deficient in choline.

Both choline and methionine prevent malignant tumors in animals fed a diet deficient in choline, possibly by preventing loss of an essential compound needed to prevent malignant transformation of normal tissues. The interpretation of these experiments was questioned because of possible aflatoxin contamination of the peanut meal used to formulate the experimental diet. However, chemically defined diets that are deficient in choline and methionine and contain no chemical carcinogens produce malignant tumors in animals [14]. This same diet that is deficient in choline and methionine was shown in 1952 to cause arterial plaques in the arteries of rats, pointing to a fundamental connection between cancer and arteriosclerosis, involving the metabolism of methionine. The biochemical reason that choline, methionine, folic acid and vitamin B12 have the capacity to prevent fat deposition and cancer formation in liver in choline-deficient animals is believed by many scientists to be related to the ability of these substances to engage in transfer of one carbon methyl groups, a process studied by DuVigneaud and others in the 1930s, termed transmethylation [15].

Subsequent to these early studies of nutritional induction of cancer in animals, many other lines of evidence were found to demonstrate abnormal metabolism of methionine and homocysteine in malignant cells. Unlike normal cells, most cultures of cancer cells require methionine and cannot use homocysteine and folic acid for their growth and survival in culture. The reason for this requirement is not clearly understood by scientific investigators. For a number of years scientists have known that the DNA of malignant tumors contains reduced levels of methyl groups, derived from methionine. Moreover, tumors contain increased activity of enzymes needed for methylation of transfer RNA, and some tumors were found to contain increased quantities of methyl groups attached to the nucleotides of transfer RNA. The aerobic glycolysis and production of lactic acid by cell cultures transformed by oncogenic viruses, the Warburg effect, is decreased by added methionine in the culture medium of these transformed cells [16]. These observations suggest, as I pointed out in my 1994 monograph, The Chemical Pathology of Homocysteine, that "intracellular deficiency of a metabolite of methionine is involved not only in the carcinogenic process but also in the control of cellular respiration [17]."

More recently, elevation of blood homocysteine levels has been demonstrated to be a risk marker for cancer, including leukemia and metastatic breast cancer [18]. Multiple reports indicate a characteristic elevation of blood homocysteine levels in patients with oral cancer, ovarian cancer, colon cancer, and breast cancer. In a recent epidemiological study, dietary deficiency of folic acid and vitamin B6, vitamins needed for normal metabolism of methionine and homocysteine, was found to increase risk of colon cancer [19]. The experimental studies of abnormal methionine metabolism in animals with cancer and in cell cultures of malignant cells, therefore, are likely to pertain to common forms of cancer as they occur in human populations.

Toward the end of my two years of studying transfer RNA in Giulio Cantoni's laboratory at the National Institutes of Health in 1960, I read a memorable issue of *Proceedings of the National Academy of Sciences of the USA* in the NIH library. In addition to an article on genetic coding by Marshall Nirenburg and an article on DNA synthesis by Severo Ochoa, this issue contained an intriguing article on cancer research written by the great Hungarian biochemist, Albert Szent-Gyorgi. His article described his efforts to develop a theory of cancer based on inhibitory and stimulatory substances extracted from calf thymus, aorta and other normal tissues. The substance "retine" was found to decrease cancer growth in experimental transplanted tumors, and the substance "promine" was found to increase the growth of tumors in these animals. Szent-Gyorgi was never able to purify and identify these substances, and he eventually was forced to give up this line of research.

Some years later in 1975 I attended a symposium at Boston University in honor of Szent-Gyorgi's 82d birthday [20]. Also in attendance were colleagues and admirers, including Linus Pauling, Hans Krebs, Charles Huggins, and his nephew Andrew Szent-Gyorgi. During the lecture Szent-Gyorgi described his efforts to extract inhibitory substances from normal tissues that would retard cancer growth. He showed a dramatic picture of the highly colored extract from normal tissues, and he pointed out that this colored substance was not present in cancer tissue. After the lecture I was able to shake hands with and greet Szent-Gyorgi and Linus Pauling, two of my personal scientific heroes. Although Szent-Gyorgi's ideas and research work on cancer therapy never came to fruition, I was intrigued by the possibility that normal tissues might lose a growth-regulatory molecule during carcinogenesis and cancer formation.

My own personal involvement as an investigator in cancer research began in 1966, when I started a series of experiments aimed at growing organ cultures of human tumors on chick embryos, as described in Chapter 3. Although I was able to demonstrate incorporation of radioactive amino acids into the proteins of surviving tissue fragments of human tumors maintained in these organ culture, there was no indication that this method could have a more general or productive application to study of human tumors.

Later in 1968 I declined an offer to collaborate with Judah Folkman in studying angiogenesis produced by cancer tissues in this organ culture system. By that time, I had made my critical observation of arteriosclerosis in the arteries of children with homocystinuria caused by different inherited enzyme deficiencies of methionine metabolism. I decided to devote all of my energy and resources to investigation of homocysteine metabolism in arteriosclerosis. However, my interest in understanding homocysteine metabolism in cancer gradually developed through comparison of homocysteine metabolism in cell cultures of malignant cells, in comparison with cell cultures from children with homocystinuria, as described in Chapter 4.

As pointed out by James Watson in his recent editorial in the *New York Times*, scientists have learned a great deal about the genetics of cancer since the discovery of DNA structure in 1953. Indeed the discovery of proto-oncogenes by Harold Varmus and Michael Bishop in the 1970s opened new understanding about how oncogenic viruses affect genetic expression in cancer cells. As described in Varmus' recent book, Varmus and Bishop discovered a mutated viral gene v-src within normal cells infected by Rous sarcoma virus [21]. "The name [v-src], pronounced 'sark' was chosen to indicate the ability of Rous sarcoma virus, and its transforming gene, to induce sarcomas in animals." Following the experiments of Steven Martin on temperature sensitive mutants of Rous sarcoma virus, Varmus and Bishop concluded that "a normal cellular gene, closely related to the viral oncogene, src, was present in the genomes of normal cells." Later studies showed that the v-src protein is a protein kinase, an enzyme that transfers a phosphate group from ATP to amino acids in cellular proteins. According to Varmus, "When the proto-oncogenes are converted into oncogenes by mutation, the [protein kinase] enzymes they encode become stronger," increasing the ability of this enzyme to add phosphate groups to the tyrosine amino acids of proteins. Thus the cellular enzyme c-src is converted to an activated form v-src that is more effective in protein phosphorylation.

Yet these penetrating insights into how oncogenic viruses affect genetic expression do not explain how human oncogenic viruses alter the metabolic apparatus of normal cells to produce cancer cells. As Harald Zur Hausen points out, infection of human cells with human oncogenic viruses is followed by a long period of latency before cancer cells are detected [6]. Indeed most individuals infected by human oncogenic viruses, for example Epstein-Barr virus, hepatitis B virus, or human papilloma virus, never develop cancer. In those individuals in which transformed or dysplastic cells progress to malignancy, the fundamental changes in metabolism, like aerobic glycolysis, the Warburg effect, and dependency upon methionine for growth, are not explained by the transformation of proto-oncogenes to oncogenes within cancer cells.

The recent success of anti-cancer drugs like Gleevec, Iressa, Tarceva, Herceptin, and Velcade is attributable to increased understanding of the multiple cell signaling pathways within normal cells and how they are altered in cancer cells. Gleevec is an inhibitor of the Bcr-Abl oncoprotein, a tyrosine kinase involved in a cell signaling pathway that is abnormal in human leukemia cells of the myelocytic series of white blood cells. This compound induces remissions in 90% of patients with early myelocytic leukemia. Gleevec also induces remissions in medulloblastoma, a highly malignant brain tumor in children, and in gastrointestinal stromal tumors (GIST) in adults. Unfortunately, resistance to therapy with Gleevec develops during treatment, leading to eventual recurrence of these cancers.

Two other cell signaling antagonists, Iressa and Tarceva, act on the receptor for epidermal growth factor (EGF-R), which is expressed in many human cancers. These drugs cause partial remissions and slight increases in life expectancy, particularly in lung cancer and brain cancer cases. Herceptin is a genetically engineered antibody to Her2Neu protein, which is an EGF receptor encoding protein overexpressed in some cases of breast cancer. Herceptin is engineered from human and mouse antibody to this protein, and passive immunization with this synthetic antibody can lead to remissions and increased survival in breast cancer cases. The anti-cancer drug Velcade is partially effective against the bone cancer, multiple myeloma, by inhibiting the effectiveness of intracellular proteosomes, the organelle responsible for degradation of proteins within cell cytoplasm. Like Gleevec and these other recently studied anti-cancer molecules, the remissions from cancer cell signaling antagonists are temporary, and patients eventually succumb to their cancers.

As described in Chapter 4, investigation of homocysteine metabolism in cancer cells and the effect of new molecules synthesized from homocysteine thiolactone on growth of cancers in animals became a key component of my research program in the 1970s and 1980s. Although subjects with homocystinuria do not have an increased susceptibility to cancer, many of them develop accelerated growth and tall stature in childhood. In our experiments with normal rabbits and guinea pigs and with hypophysectomized rats, my research team found that homocysteic acid stimulates growth of normal animals and causes a growth response in animals lacking a pituitary gland and treated with thyroid hormone. The growth response was traced to increased release of a growth-stimulating plasma factor, insulin-like growth factor, which is synthesized in the liver. In our experiments with cultured skin cells from children with homocystinuria, we observed altered cellular behavior, including loss of contact inhibition of growth and increased formation of sulfated matrix proteins that resembles growth of cultured cancer cells. In analysis of homocysteine thiolactone metabolism in these cell cultures, our research team demonstrated a previously unknown pathway for conversion of the sulfur atom of homocysteine to sulfate [17]. Using cultured cancer cells induced in animals by chemical carcinogens or by oncogenic viruses, we discovered that cancer cells are totally unable to metabolize homocysteine thiolactone to sulfate [22]. As a consequence, cancer cells over-produce homocysteine thiolactone from methionine and this reactive homocysteine molecule becomes attached abnormally to cellular proteins.

In my article in *Cancer Research* in 1976 I hypothesized that cancer cells have lost a molecule containing homocysteine thiolactone that is present in normal cells and required for conversion of homocysteine thiolactone to sulfate [22]. Our research design was to synthesize new chemical derivatives of homocysteine thiolactone and test them for their ability to retard growth of transplanted cancers in animals. By studying the molecular features of these new compounds, we expected to identify the essential characteristics of the unknown molecule that is lost during conversion of normal cells to cancer cells.

As described in Chapter 4, our first success in this new line investigation came in 1977, when our research team demonstrated that the amide synthesized from arachidonic acid and homocysteine thiolactone strongly inhibited growth of transplanted breast cancer in mice. In addition we found that pre-treating animals with pyridoxal homocysteine thiolactone enamine, a molecule formed from vitamin B6 and homocysteine, also inhibited growth of breast cancer in mice. Many of the other molecules synthesized from homocysteine thiolactone and fatty acids had little or no effect on growth of cancer in mice. This promising line of research was interrupted for almost ten years following my ostracism from Boston medicine in 1979, as described in Chapter 5. It was not until 1985 that I was able to resume these investigations at the VA Medical Center in Providence.

Working in the old research building at the Providence VA, I had access to some basic equipment and supplies in collaboration with Michael Vezeridis of the Surgical Service. As described in Chapter 6, I was able to synthesize thioretinamide from retinoic acid and the free base form of homocysteine thiolactone. We observed significant inhibition of growth of transplanted cancer fragments in mice when this compound was given in a variety of vehicles. In 1988 I succeeded in synthesizing a complex from two molecules of thioretinamide and one molecule of adenosyl cobalamin, the coenzyme form of vitamin B12. This complex, thioretinaco, is active in preventing chemical carcinogenesis of lung tumors by urethane in mice and also in inhibiting growth of human pancreatic carcinoma in immune deficient mice when injected directly into the growing tumors [23]. Both thioretinamide and thioretinaco also inhibited growth of human pancreatic carcinoma growing in cell cultures.

As described in Chapter 6, in 1994 I published my monograph on the Chemical Pathology of Homocysteine in which I explained my molecular theory of how thioretinaco ozonide produces ATP by oxidative phosphorylation in normal cells [17]. This detailed theory was developed during my 20 year period of exile in Providence. The experiments of Kazimir and Wilson, which were published in 2002, provided independent confirmation of molecular structure and an improved method of synthesis of thioretinamide and thioretinaco [24]. Their results showed that both of these molecules inhibit arteriosclerosis in rats injected with homocysteine thiolactone. The origin of homocysteine thiolactone from methionyl transfer RNA aminoacyl synthase and the production of homocysteine thiolactone by malignant cells in culture were published by Heironim Jakubowski in 1993 [25]. Jakubowski's results confirmed our discovery of homocysteinylated proteins and suggestion of excess production of homocysteine thiolactone in cancer cells, as predicted in my article in *Cancer Research* in 1976.

In the discussion of the development of cancer cells in my 1994 monograph I emphasize that the theoretical loss of thioretinaco ozonide from the membranes of mitochondria by the action of electrophilic chemical carcinogens, oncogenic viruses, ionizing radiation, aging, and reactive oxygen species from metabolism is the key process in conversion of normal to malignant cells [17]. As a consequence of this loss of thioretinaco ozonide, the metabolism of malignant cells is shifted to a primitive mode of metabolism in which large quantities of glucose are converted to lactic acid during ATP synthesis, since the ability of mitochondria to generate ATP from oxidative metabolism is lost. This theory explains how the concept of Otto Warburg that injury to respiration, increased synthesis of lactic acid, and conversion to aerobic glycolysis occur because of loss of thioretinaco ozonide from mitochondria.

Another consequence of the presumed loss of thioretinaco ozonide from cell membranes during carcinogenesis is increased conversion of methionine to homocysteine thiolactone and failure of oxidation of homocysteine thiolactone to sulfate in malignant cells. Overproduction of homocysteine thiolactone leads to widespread reaction of homocysteine with amino groups of proteins, glycosaminoglycans, deoxyribonucleic acid, and ribonucleic acid to form peptide bound homocysteine groups. This process leads to formation of new antigens from proteins, diffuse abnormalities of cellular membranes by alteration of glycosaminoglycans, oxidation of unsaturated fatty acids and cholesterol of cell membranes, aggregation and alteration of DNA of chromosomes, and altered small inhibitory RNA molecules, affecting genetic expression.

All of these biochemical changes produced by excessive homocysteine thiolactone synthesis from methionine are manifested in abnormally aggregated chromosomes and irregular chromatin, diffusely abnormal cellular membranes, and alterations of growth and differentiation of malignant cells and tissues, as shown by induction of skin cancer by topical application of homocysteine thiolactone in mice. Thus the abnormalities of nucleoproteins of cancer cells are interpreted as a secondary effect of the consequence of loss of thioretinaco ozonide from cell membranes during carcinogenesis. In this sense, cancer originates from abnormal methionine metabolism, in which a vital molecule, derived from homocysteine thiolactone, retinoic acid and cobalamin, cannot be replaced by biochemical synthesis of thioretinaco ozonide within cells affected by carcinogenic processes.

Many scientific investigators in the cancer field assume that genetic changes and chromosomal abnormalities are the principal etiologic factors in carcinogenesis. My formulation of the process of carcinogenesis attributes the primary etiologic factor in carcinogenesis to loss of thioretinaco ozonide from mitochondrial membranes, and the genetic, membrane, growth and differentiation abnormalities observed in malignant cells and tissues are interpreted as secondary to this primary change. This view is in accord with Warburg's concept that carcinogens cause an irreversible damage to cellular respiration and with Szent-Gyorgi's concept that carcinogenesis and cancer cell characteristics are caused by a loss of a normal cellular constituent rather than a primary genetic change as the underlying biochemical abnormality in cancer cells. This view is also in accord with James Watson's recent call for increased understanding of the biochemical abnormalities of cancer cells and for testing of "promising drug candidates...that will move through animal testing to the exploratory phases of clinical testing in humans."

The prevailing view of the biomedical/pharmaceutical establishment is that cancer has its primary origin in genetic alteration of normal cells by the process of carcinogenesis. There are a number of observations in the history of cancer research that are difficult to reconcile with this view. In 1975 Beatrice Mintz and Karl Illmensee demonstrated that highly malignant teratocarcinoma cells, passaged for years in ascites cells in the abdominal cavity of mice, yield normal genetically mosaic mice when injected into developing embryonic blastocysts [26]. According to these scientists, "the results...furnish an unequivocal example in animals of a non-mutational basis for transformation to malignancy and of reversal to normalcy." In 1997 Mina Bissell's research team reported that an inhibitory beta1-integrin antibody caused a reversion of the malignant phenotype of human breast cancer cells to normal in three dimensional organ cultures [27]. Tumor cells treated with this antibody produced a significantly reduced number and size of tumors when injected into mice with immune deficiency. In both of these experimental examples, highly malignant cancer cells, either of animal or human origin, were converted to normal tissues either by growth in normal embryonic tissues or by growth in an artificial organ culture system. These experimental results are difficult to reconcile with the concept of a primary genetic origin of cancer cells. However, these results are compatible with the concept that a substance present in embryonic cells or extracellular matrix is capable of converting the metabolic and genetic abnormalities of cancer cells to the corresponding normal properties of non-malignant cells.

The other observation that is difficult to explain by the genetic theory of carcinogenesis is the concept of malignant transformation by a "field effect." For many years pathologists have observed a gradual progression of pre-malignant abnormalities in cells, called dysplasia, leading over a period of months or years to the origin of a malignant tumor. In tissues such as the lining cells of the urinary bladder, the lining cells of the lower esophagus, the lining cells of ducts within the breast, or the cells of adenomas of the colon, dysplastic changes in the cells of these tissues gradually exacerbate and acquire more and more characteristics of malignancy. Finally, after months or years of progression, frankly malignant cancer cells, capable of independent growth, direct invasion of normal tissues or organs, and metastatic spread to organs and tissues throughout the body, arise in one or more areas. If multiple cancers arise in a single dysplastic tissue, they are referred to as "multicentric" in origin.

This gradual progression from dysplasia to malignancy is difficult to reconcile with the concept of a single genetic abnormality as the cause of carcinogenesis. This progression is more compatible with the concept of gradual loss of a vital substance from dysplastic cells during carcinogenesis, finally resulting in malignant transformation when its concentration reaches a critical low quantity within dysplastic cells. I believe that the critical substance theoretically lost from cells during carcinogenesis is thioretinaco ozonide. Presumably the concentration of this molecule within mitochondrial membranes falls to a critical low point, ATP synthesis is inhibited, aerobic glycolysis begins to supply ATP for cellular functions, and excess homocysteine thiolactone begins to accumulate because of failure of its conversion to sulfate. When malignant cells begin to grow at the primary site of origin, the release of homocysteine thiolactone into surrounding tissues stimulates normal connective tissue cells to grow and produce fibrous tissue, a process known as desmoplasia. The interior lining surfaces of arteries supplying malignant tumors frequently develop fibrous arterial arteriosclerotic plaques, presumably caused by release of homocysteine thiolactone from the malignant cells of the primary cancer.

Years ago in 1955 I had an unusual experience that influenced the conduct and outcome of my homocysteine research program years later. After graduation from Harvard College in 1955, my plans for my wedding to Annina and my first year at Harvard Medical School were finalized in early June. Because I needed to earn some money for these events, I applied to the Civil Service Commission in Washington DC for a summer job. Having completed my undergraduate degree in chemistry with high honors, I wanted a more interesting experience that the previous summer's job as a clerk typist for the US Army Signal Corps at the Pentagon. Looking at my qualifications and work history, the personnel recruiter asked whether I would be interested in becoming a patent examiner in the US Patent and Trademark Office in the Department of Commerce. I explained that I was entering medical school in the fall and was only looking for a temporary position. The recruiter explained that I could serve two months and decide later whether to consider a permanent position as a patent examiner or patent attorney.

My first three weeks in the Patent Office consisted of a fascinating introductory training course for new patent examiners. We learned about the history of the Patent Office, from the clause inserted by the Founding Fathers in the US Constitution in 1787 authorizing the Federal Government to grant patents on inventions, to the current laws governing patents, trademarks and copyrights. We also learned about many famous inventors like Thomas Edison, Alexander Graham Bell, and even Abraham Lincoln, who had successfully obtained US patents. We learned about what constitutes a patentable invention and what could be anticipated by an experienced practitioner of the prior art that is not a patentable invention. We learned about devices, processes, new compositions of matter, and other innovations that could be patented. We learned about grounds for rejection of claims in patent applications because of violation of physical laws like perpetual motion machines, what had previously been claimed in prior patents in the field, and what could reasonably be anticipated by an experienced practitioner of the prior art in the field.

After conclusion of the training course, I was assigned to the section concerned with patents of chemical polymers. One of the senior patent examiners became my mentor and helped me with the format of writing an office action in response to a patent application by a chemical corporation developing new types of chemical polymers. In those days before computers, the hard copies of previous patents in the field were kept in carefully labeled drawers for assistance in comparing the claims of the patent application with the claims allowed in previously granted patents. The staff was pleased with my ability to understand and prepare appropriate responses to the claims in the patent applications. They urged me to accept a permanent position as an examiner in the office, but I explained my plans to attend medical school in the fall. They said that after medical school I should consider a career as a patent attorney. They even kept me on the rolls of the Patent Office as an unpaid employee for one year, expecting me to return to resume a career in patent law.

Years later in working with previously unknown new molecules synthesized from homocysteine thiolactone I realized that these new compounds could be patented because of their potential for treatment of cancer and other diseases. I also knew that no commercial company could invest significant funds in developing these new compounds unless they could license a patent for exclusive use of the invention. My first patent was granted for homocysteine thiolactone perchlorate, the previously unknown salt with unusual solubility in organic solvents and the ability to cause necrosis (cellular death) of transplanted cancers in mice. Since my research program was supported by a grant from the National Institutes of Health, I reported the invention to their legal office. The cost of the patent application process was paid by the National Institutes of Health, and the patent rights of the 1981 patent were assigned to the US Government. This patent was never licensed for development and has since lapsed.

During my period of rejection and ostracism by the medical establishment from 1979 to 1981 I decided to apply for a patent on the new molecules that my associates and I had synthesized from homocysteine thiolactone by reaction with arachidonic acid, maleimide, or oxalyl chloride and rhodium trichloride. All of these new molecules significantly inhibited growth of transplanted cancers in mice. Since my research grant from the National Institutes of Health had terminated before I left the Massachusetts General Hospital in 1979, I asked permission to apply for the patent in my own name and paid for by my own personal funds. The legal department of the National Institutes of Health granted permission, since no scientist was interested in further development of these molecules. My second patent covering these new compounds with anti-cancer effects was granted in 1983 and has since lapsed.

During my years of service at the Providence VA Medical Center, I was able to invent and characterize the new molecules, thioretinamide, thioretinaco, and thioretinaco ozonide. The development work on these molecules was an independent investigation, not supported by research funds from the VA or any other agency. Because this research work was outside of my responsibilities as Staff Pathologist, the legal department of the VA Central Office in Washington granted permission for me to apply for these patents as sole owner, paid for by my own personal funds. The patents on these molecules and processes for delivering them to animals were granted in 1986, 1990 and 1996. These patents described my discovery and development of these new compounds and the theory of their usefulness in treatment of cancer. Another patent was granted in 2004 for use of thioretinaco ozonide delivered in second generation liposomes for treatment and prevention of cancer, viral infections and aging [28]. Despite repeated attempts to approach pharmaceutical corporations, large and small, no company has been willing to invest funds into development and implementation of these patented molecules. As described in Chapter 11, a new development of the application of the patented compound, thioretinamide, for use with pancreatic enzymes and a nutritional-metabolic program for therapy of degenerative diseases of aging formed the basis of my new invention. I filed a patent application for this invention with the US Patent and Trademark Office in June, 2011 [29].

REFERENCES

[1] Miller JA. Carcinogenesis by chemicals: an overview – GHA Clowes Memorial Lecture. *Cancer Research*, 1970;30:559-576. This comprehensive review describes the investigation of the electrophilic properties of carcinogenic chemicals and their role in production of experimental cancer. These studies implicated derivatives of methionine and homocysteine in chemical carcinogenesis by acetylaminofluorene, a highly potent synthetic chemical carcinogen.

[2] DeBaun JR, Miller EC, Miller JA. N-hydroxy 2 acetylaminofluorene sulfotransferase: its probable role in carcinogenesis and in protein-(methion-Syl) binding in rat liver. *Cancer Research*, 1970;30:577-595. This study implicates altered methionine and sulfate metabolism in the process of chemical carcinogenesis.

[3] Ryser HJP. Chemical carcinogenesis. *New England Journal of Medicine*, 1970;30:577-595.

[4] Ames BN. Dietary carcinogens and anticarcinogens. *Science*, 1983;231:1256-1264. This article discusses the many chemical carcinogens in food. The relation between mutagenesis, as detected by the Ames test, and carcinogenesis by dietary mutagens in animals are also analyzed and discussed.

[5] Gross L. *Oncogenic Viruses*. New York: Pergamon Press, 1961. This monograph describes the history of research on oncogenic viruses and the author's discovery of the polyoma virus and induction of leukemia and solid cancers in mice.

[6] ZurHausen H. Viruses in human cancers. *Science*, 1991;254:1167-1173. The author describes the status of understanding of human oncogenic viruses and the particular role of human papilloma viruses in the causation of cervical cancer.

[7] Weinberg RA. *The Biology of Cancer*. New York: Garland Science, 2006. This monumental monograph and textbook describes the status of current understanding of the biology and genetics of cancer. There is no discussion of the Warburg effect on metabolism of cancer cells, and there is no discussion of the role of methionine and homocysteine in carcinogenesis. The emphasis is on a comprehensive understanding of how oncogenes and cellular signaling pathways are involved in carcinogensis.

[8] Warburg O. *Metabolism of Tumors.* London: Constable, 1930. This classic monograph describes the discovery and interpretation of the abnormal production of lactic acid by tumor tissues and embryonic tissues in the presence of oxygen.

[9] Warburg O. On the origin of cancer cells. *Science*, 1956;123:309-314. Warburg explains his concept of injury to respiration during carcinogenesis and the consequent shift in metabolism of carbohydrates to fermentation as a source of ATP for cellular metabolism.

[10] Weinhouse S. Oxidative metabolism of neoplastic tissues. *Advances in Cancer Research*, 1955;3:239-325. This monograph describes the status of understanding of the Warburg effect in 1955. Weinhouse was a leading critic of the Warburg approach to understanding abnormal metabolism in cancer cells.

[11] Watson JD. To fight cancer, know the enemy. *New York Times* Op-Ed editorial. August 6, 2009. James Watson declares that increased understanding of the metabolism of cancer cells is needed before a definitive treatment and prevention of cancer can be developed. He states that genetic aspects of cancer are now well understood. However, scientists need to explain the basis for the Warburg effect before a definitive understanding of the biochemistry of cancer cells can be understood.

[12] VanderHeiden MG, Cantley LC, Thompson CB. Understanding the Warburg effect: the metabolic requirements of cell proliferation. *Science*, 2009;324:1029-1033. This review describes the current status of understanding of the origin of the Warburg effect in cancer cells. They state that a definitive explanation of the Warburg effect "remains elusive."

[13] Copeland DH, Salmon WD. Neoplasms in the liver, lungs and other tissues of rats as a result of prolonged choline deficiency. *American Journal of Pathology*, 1946;22:1059-1079.

[14] Poirier LA. The role of methionine in carcinogenesis in vivo. *Advances in Experimental Medicine and Biology*, 1986;206:269-282. This review summarizes the evidence proving that a chemically defined diet which is deficient in choline is carcinogenic in animals.

[15] Hoffman RM. Altered methionine metabolism, DNA methylation and oncogene expression in carcinogenesis. *Biochimica Biophysica Acta*, 1984;738:49-87.

[16] Boerner P, Racker E. Methionine-sensitive glycolysis in transformed cells. *Proceedings of the National Academy of Sciences USA*, 1985;82:6750-6754.

[17] McCully KS. Chemical Pathology of Homocysteine. II. Carcinogenesis and Homocysteine Thiolactone Metabolism. *Annals of Clinical and Laboratory Science*, 1994;24:27-59. This review explains the detailed molecular processes by which thioretinaco ozonide catalyzes ATP synthesis during oxidative phosphorylation and cellular respiration in normal and in cancer cells.

[18] Wu LL, Wu JT. Hyperhomocysteinemia is a risk factor for cancer and a new potential tumor marker. *Clinica Chimica Acta*, 2002;322:21-28.

[19] Marchand LL, White KK, Nomura AMY, Wilkens LR, Selhub JS, Tiiridainen M, Goldman MT, Murphy SP, Henderson BE, Kolonel LN. Plasma levels of B vitamins and colorectal cancer risk: the Multiethnic Cohort Study. *Cancer Epidemiology and Biomarkers Previews*, 2009;18:2195-2201.

[20] Moss RW. *Free Radical. Albert Szent-Gyorgi and the battle over vitamin C.* New York: Paragon, 1988, pp 184-186, 228-230. This biography of Szent-Gyorgi describes his

efforts to develop a theory of cancer based on inhibitory and stimulatory substances extracted from normal tissues. I attended the Symposium on Search and Discovery in 1975 which was organized by Professor Benjamin Kaminer of Boston University to commemorate Szent-Gyorgi's 82d birthday. At this extraordinary symposium Szent-Gyorgi displayed extracts of his inhibitory substances for cancer growth. Michael Kasha gave a description of Szent-Gyorgi's presentation: "Holding giant test tubes in his hands, first one above his head, then the other, gesturing with each to make his point, his face vividly animated, a brilliant red color sparkled as the liquids mixed...Albert danced about the platform, alternating his attention on the audience and on his test tubes. It was a ballet, the 'Ballet of Albert Szent-Gyorgi,' flushed with energy and scientific drama. The physical chemistry and biochemistry were too tightly knit, too convincingly demonstrated, to be taken lightly. It was an hour of triumph."

[21] Varmus H. *The Art and Politics of Science*. New York: Norton, 2009, pp 68-101. In this memoir Harold Varmus describes his discovery with Michael Bishop of the first proto-ongogene and its activation by the Rous sarcoma oncogenic virus.

[22] McCully KS. Homocysteine thiolactone metabolism in malignant cells. *Cancer Research*, 1976;36:3198-3202. This article describes the discovery of the inability of cancer cells to convert homocysteine thiolactone to sulfate. Excess homocysteine thiolactone becomes attached to proteins by peptide bonds. I suggest that normal cells contain a substance containing homocysteine thiolactone that prevents its accumulation by metabolism from methionine.

[23] McCully KS, Tzanakakis GN, Vezeridis MP. Inhibition of neoplastic growth by N-homocysteine thiolactonyl retinamido cobalamin. *Research Communications in Chemical Pathology and Pharmacology*, 1989;66:117-122.

[24] Kazmir M, Wilson FR. Prevention of homocysteine thiolactone-induced atherogenesis in rats. *Research Communications in Molecular Pathology and Pharmacology*, 2002;111:179-198. This article describes an improved method for synthesis of thioretinamide and thioretinaco. The results show that these molecules prevent arteriosclerotic plaques caused by injection of homocysteine thiolactone in rats.

[25] Jakubowski H, Goldman E. Synthesis of homocysteine thiolactone by methionyl tRNA synthetase in cultured mammalian cells. *FEBS Letters*, 1993;317:237-240. This study shows that cultured malignant cells produce homocysteine thiolactone by an error-editing reaction involving the enzymatic activation of methionyl transfer RNA.

[26] Mintz B, Illmensee K. Normal genetically mosaic mice produced from malignant teratocarcinoma cells. *Proceedings of the National Academy of Sciences USA*, 1975;72:3585-3589.

[27] Weaver VM, Petersen OW, Wang F, Larabell CA, Briand P, Dansky C, Bissell MJ. Reversion of the malignant phenotype of human breast cancer cells in three-dimensional culture and in vivo by integrin blocking antibodies. *Journal of Cell Biology*, 1997;137:231-245.

[28] McCully KS. Enhanced liposomal thioretinaco ozonide compositions and liposomal carrier. *US Patent* 6,696,082. February 24, 2004.

[29] McCully KS. Compositions and method for utilization of thioretinamide in therapy of degenerative diseases of aging. US Patent Application 13/067,504. Filed June 6, 2011.

Chapter 11

STEM CELLS, PAPRIKA AND APRICOTS: EFFECT ON THE CANCER INDUSTRY

In 1902 John Beard, lecturer in embryology at the University of Edinburgh, published a remarkable article entitled "Embryological aspects and etiology of carcinoma" in the medical journal *Lancet* [1]. This article announced the startling conclusion that the behavior and appearance of cancer cells resemble that of the trophoblastic cells of the early human embryo. Having studied the embryology of invertebrate parasites for his PhD degree in 1884 at the University of Freiburg, Germany, Beard came to this realization after 14 years of study of the alternation of sexual and asexual cycles in broadbill fish. In his studies of fish embryos in Black Lake, New York and at Edinburgh, Beard identified an obscure structure within the early yolk sac of the fish blastoderm that possessed its own nervous system, separate from that of the developing embryo. When the nervous system of the embryo develops, the nervous system with the yolk sac disappears. From these studies he suspected that an alternation of generations between sexual forms and asexual forms occurs in vertebrates, including humans, as well as in plants and in invertebrates, contrary to the accepted knowledge of the day. He then proposed that germ cells of the embryo originated from trophoblastic cells, one of which is selected to become the definitive embryo that develops into the vertebrate organism. This embryonic germ cell differentiates into all of the tissues of the adult organism. Beard also traced embryonic germ cells as they migrated into the tissues of the developing embryo and considered them to be cells from which malignant tumors develop in older organisms. With this concept he anticipated rather accurately the existence of somatic stem cells within tissues of the human adult.

Beard's concepts about alternation of sexual and asexual generations in vertebrates, the trophoblast as the asexual generation, the embryological development from a single germ cell, and the existence of trophoblastic stem cells in the tissues of the sexual generation were not taken seriously in his day. In his study of billfish, Beard observed that the primitive collection of nerves in the blastoderm began to disappear after appearance of the embryo body. This timing was also observed in many other species that he studied in detail, meaning that the growing embryo somehow suppresses the asexual generation represented by the trophoblast. Beard observed that the critical period during which the trophoblastic cells begin to degenerate is closely timed with the development of enzymes within the pancreas of the embryo. In the human embryo this critical period corresponds to about 7 weeks after implantation and growth of the embryo. He reasoned that the powerful digestive enzymes of the developing pancreas must have the important function of converting the trophoblastic cells of the early embryo into the differentiated cells of the placenta.

To quote from Gonzalez and Isaacs' book, *The Trophoblast and the Origins of Cancer* [2], "Beard built up his complex thesis on the origins of cancer in a step-wise fashion over a 20 year period. By 1895 he had unraveled what he believed to be an apparent alternation of generations in higher vertebrates, identifying the trophoblast as the asexual generation in mammals, and the primordial germ cell as its spore. By 1902 he had brought together his thoughts of malignancy as a misplaced and uncontrolled trophoblast developing from a vagrant germ cell. In 1904 he reported his findings that embryonic pancreatic enzymes were responsible for the normal degeneration of the sexual generation in vertebrates, including the trophoblast in mammals. The following year, in a January 20, 1905 lecture delivered in Liverpool, he first presented his thesis that since pancreatic enzymes such as trypsin ultimately suppress trophoblastic growth in the uterus, and since cancer was trophoblastic in origin, trypsin must represent the body's main defense against cancer and would be useful as a cancer treatment."

As described in his book *The Enzyme Treatment of Cancer and its Scientific Basis,* Beard's theory made a minor impact on the cancer treatment field when physicians and oncologists began his program of injection of pancreatic enzyme extracts from porcine pancreas into patients with primary and metastatic malignancies [3]. In a few cases, dramatic regression of advanced cancers and long term survival were observed. However, in other cases the treatment was ineffective, as reported in medical journals at the time. Beard realized that the extraction of active enzyme preparations from hog pancreas was fraught with difficulties, resulting in enzyme preparations of widely varying potency. He attributed treatment failures to use of these poorly characterized preparations. During Beard's lifetime, the treatment of cancer by radium became a celebrated cause espoused by two time Nobel Prize winner Marie Skladowska Curie, and his concepts fell into oblivion prior to his death in 1924.

In Chapter 10 the efforts of Albert Szent-Gyorgi to characterize extracts of normal tissues that retard cancer growth in animals were described. Szent-Gyorgi arrived at this line of investigation in an interesting manner [4]. He was born in Budapest in 1893 into a family of land-owners and scientists. Albert's uncle Mihaly Lenhossek was a Professor of Physiology at the medical school and influenced him to finish his medical degree, whereupon he announced his intention to become a medical investigator. While working in Groningen after the First World War in a physiology laboratory, Szent-Gyorgi published several important articles on oxidation reactions in biochemistry, later leading to discovery of the tricarboxylic acid cycle in cellular respiration. Searching for examples of oxidation reactions, he happened upon the browning of potatoes and other vegetables when exposed to air. When studying the oxidation of benzidene with peroxides, he discovered a reducing substance in cabbage and citrus juice that slowed the oxidation of benzidine by peroxides. Based on an erroneous assumption about the color of the skin in Addison's disease, Szent-Gyorgi decided to test adrenal glands for hormones that would modify these oxidation reactions. He found that adding silver nitrate to a mince of adrenal gland yielded an intense black color, indicating the presence of a strong reducing agent, possibly related to the existence of a previously unrecognized adrenal hormone.

Through his publications and connections in the scientific world, Szent-Gyorgi was introduced to Professor Henry H. Dale of Cambridge University and later to Professor Frederick Gowland Hopkins, who became interested in the isolation of this new hormone from adrenal gland and offered Szent-Gyorgi a post doctoral position. Working in Hopkin's laboratory at Cambridge, he succeeded in isolating a sugar-like substance from adrenal cortex that he crystallized and identified as "hexuronic acid." On the strength of 55 articles and a PhD dissertation written about this substance, Szent-Gyorgi was offered a professorship in Szeged in his native Hungary, supported by a major grant from the Rockefeller Foundation. Adrenal glands proved to be a difficult source of "hexuronic acid" for further study, and by chance he discovered that Hungarian paprika contains large quantities of this substance, providing enough for isolation, crystallization, and determination of its chemical structure. An American physiologist from Pittsburg, Joseph Svirbely, came to Szeged to help Szent-Gyorgi establish ascorbic acid as vitamin C, the substance isolated from paprika that cures experimental scurvy in guinea pigs.

In the 1930s ascorbic acid, vitamin C, was found to influence the growth of cancer in animals, mainly acting to extend their life span [5]. Moreover, the amount of ascorbic acid in the tissues of animals with cancer is decreased, further suggesting the possibility of a therapeutic action in human patients with cancer. As discussed in Chapter 10, the German biochemist, Otto Warburg discovered the role of cytochrome enzymes in cellular respiration. Later he demonstrated that cancer cells and embryonic cells have a characteristic mode of cellular respiration, aerobic glycolyis, in which glucose is converted to lactic acid instead of conversion to carbon dioxide, as seen in normal cells. These observations seemed to suggest that ascorbic acid was able in some way to affect cellular respiration of cancer cells.

Controversial studies were published in the 1970s by Cameron and Campbell in Scotland, showing that massive doses of ascorbic acid cause regression of human cancers and extended the life span of patients with terminal malignancy. Linus Pauling became involved in these studies, and he helped to have them published in the *Proceedings of the National Academy of Sciences of the USA* in 1975 and 1976. Later in the 1980s controlled studies showed that massive doses of vitamin C have minor effects on the side effects of chemotherapy and radiation, and they caused a slight increase in survival times in human patients [5].

As described in Chapter 4, I published an article in *Nature* concerning homocysteine metabolism in guinea pigs with experimental scurvy, showing that ascorbic acid is required for oxidation of the sulfur atom of homocysteine thiolactone to sulfate. In the 1980s Linus Pauling sent me a copy of his book on vitamin C and cancer, and he sent me a letter commenting on my discoveries regarding homocysteine and arteriosclerosis. In his later years Szent-Gyorgi worked in his laboratory at Woods Hole, isolating extracts of normal tissues that would promote growth of tumors in animals, which he called "promine," or retard growth of tumors, which he called "retine." These efforts were inspired by the death of his beloved wife Nellie from cancer and from his collaboration with F.B. Straub resulting in the discovery of the important muscle proteins, actin and actomyosin. Szent-Gyorgi was not able to characterize the molecular nature of these "retine" extracts with anti-cancer activity.

As described in Chapter 7, in 1930 Weston A. Price retired from a brilliant career as a leading dentist in Cleveland, Ohio. Price was born in 1870 to parents of Welsh ancestry on the pioneer family farm, known as Eagle Rock Farm, in southern Ontario. After completing undergraduate studies at the University of Toronto, he enrolled in the University Of Michigan School Of Dentistry and was awarded the M.S. and D.M.D. degrees. In addition to his career as a highly successful practitioner of dentistry, Price was a teacher and author of many scientific articles and textbooks. After his retirement from dental practice at the age of 60, he decided to travel with his wife Florence, visiting primitive peoples around the world and studying their dentition and general health in relation to their dietary practices. The result of 9 years of travel was summarized in his great book *Nutrition and Physical Degeneration*, originally published in 1939, and republished as a 50th Anniversary Edition in 1989 [6].

As described in Chapter 7, Weston and Florence visited primitive peoples consuming traditional diets in remote areas of Switzerland, Scotland, Alaska, Northern Canada, Florida, Melanesian and Peloponnesian Islands of the Pacific, Central and East Africa, Peru, Ecuador, Australia and New Zealand. In each case they compared the dental and general health of these primitive peoples with closely related groups that had become "modernized" by exposure to processed, canned, and packaged foods containing sugar, flour, powdered milk, and other refined ingredients. Price's great discovery is that exposure to the "Westernized" diet resulted in deterioration of the dental and physical health of primitive peoples within one generation. The dental arches became narrowed, the teeth became carious, and susceptibility to a wide variety of degenerative diseases increased. To quote Price, "Associated with a fine physical condition, the isolated primitive groups have a high level of immunity to many of our modern degenerative processes, including tuberculosis, arthritis, heart disease, and affections of the internal organs. When, however, these individuals have lost this high level of physical excellence, a definite lowering in their resistance to the modern degenerative processes takes place." Price's book is richly illustrated with photographs and radiographs of the primitive peoples and their "modernized" counterparts, showing the dramatic differences in the teeth, bones, and general appearance of health between the two groups.

Price's great discovery was substantiated by other epidemiologists, explorers, and physicians like Albert Schweitzer, Dennis Burkitt, Colonel Cleave, and Robert McCarrison. These observers noted a remarkable lack of cancer, heart disease, diverticulosis, arthritis, mental illness, hearing loss, appendicitis, ulcerative colitis, and colonic polyps among primitive peoples consuming traditional diets around the world. It was the English physician McCarrison who first studied the people of the isolated Hunza valley in the Himalayan region between Pakistan, India and China in 1922. He reported in the *Journal of the American Medical Association* [7] that "The Hunza has no known incidence of cancer. They have an abundant crop of apricots, which they dry in the sun and use very largely in their food." The Hunza are known for their longevity and lack of disease, many elders reaching the century mark. Their most prized food is the apricot seed, and modern analysis shows that the Hunza diet contains 200 times the quantity of the important nitriloside nutrients in comparison with the modern American diet.

In 1952 Ernest Krebs Jr, a biochemist from San Francisco, advanced the theory that susceptibility to cancer is related to dietary deficiency of nitrilosides [8]. These substances contain a nitrile group, related to cyanide, and are found to be widely distributed in foods, especially in fruit seeds, berries, legumes, grasses, and grains. The nitriloside amygdalin was discovered by Justus von Leibig in 1830, and its chemical nature was later determined to be mandelonitrile diglucuronide. According to the Merck Index, amygdalin is also known as laetrile, "a toxic drug that is not effective as a cancer treatment." According to Krebs, primitive peoples such as the Kakorum of West Pakistan, aboriginal Eskimos, North American Indians in the native state, and tribes of South Africa and South America living on native foods consume 250 to 3000 milligrams of nitrilosides per day, in comparison with "civilized man" consuming 2 milligrams per day. How is consumption of these appreciable amounts of nitrilosides in foods by populations protected from disease reconciled with the statement in the Merck Index that "amygdalin is a toxic drug?"

In cellular metabolism the nitrilosides, amygdalin, dhurrin, linamarin and lotaustralin, are hydrolyzed by glucosidase to the free nitrile compound, which decomposes to cyanide, benzaldehyde, and other products [9]. In normal cells the cyanide is quickly converted to thiocyanate by reaction with hydrogen sulfide and other sulfur compounds, catalyzed by rodanese, a sulfo-transferase enzyme. In contrast to the highly toxic cyanide, thiocyanate is relatively non-toxic except for a mild anti-thyroid action. Malignant cells contain abundant glucosidase to hydrolyze nitrilosides, but they contain little rhodanese, exposing them to high concentrations of the cytotoxic cyanide molecule. Thus the toxicity of cyanide generated from nitrilosides is targeted selectively to malignant cells, a form of chemical surveillance to eliminate malignant cells that arise continually within normal tissues. In support of this concept, experiments show that exposure to the toxic gas, hydrogen cyanide, completely eliminates transplanted cancers in animals. Theoretically cyanide reacts with the cobalt atom of thioretinaco ozonide, inactivating its diminished concentration in malignant cells [10].

It is worth mentioning that hydrogen sulfide is a toxic gas produced from the sulfur atom of homocysteine by the action of two enzymes, cystathionine synthase and cystathionase. Hydrogen sulfide has recently been identified as a "gasotransmitter" that mediates and controls oxidation reactions within cells [11]. My 1976 article in *Cancer Research* showed that cancer cells are unable to metabolize the sulfur atom of homocysteine thiolactone to sulfate [12]. Recent studies have implicated the heme group of the enzyme cystathionine synthase as the catalyst for formation of thioretinamide from retinol (vitamin A) by oxidation with superoxide and activation by dehydroascorbate, the oxidized form of vitamin C [13]. Thioretinamide combines with cobalamin (vitamin B_{12}) to form thioretinaco, the catalyst for oxidative metabolism and ATP synthesis by formation of a complex with ozone and oxygen (Figure 15). Cyanide combines with thioretinaco ozonide to inactivate the complex and prevent cellular oxidation, effectively poisoning the cell by preventing cellular respiration [10]. The inability of cancer cells to convert the sulfur atom of homocysteine thiolactone to sulfate is related to the decreased ability of malignant cells to synthesize thioretinamide and thioretinaco, leading to decreased formation of thioretinaco ozonide and thereby increasing their susceptibility to killing by the cyanide released from dietary nitrilosides.

The synthesis of thioretinaco from thioretinamide is facilitated by the thyroxine that is transported by plasma transthyretin, explaining how oxidative metabolism is stimulated by thyroxine [13]. Only higher eukaryotes, such as mammals and humans, contain cystathionine synthase with a heme functional group, and the cystathionine synthase of prokaryotes, such as yeast and flagellates, contains no heme functional group [14]. Embryonic and malignant cells are deficient in activity of cystathionine synthase [15]. Thus malignant cells are deficient in oxidation of homocysteine thiolactone to sulfate, since they lack the heme oxygenase function of cystathionine synthase.

Biosynthesis of thioretinamide from retinol and homocysteine thiolactone

- Retinol is bound to Retinol Binding Protein-4 and transported to cells by transthyretin
- Retinol is oxidized to enzyme-bound retinoic acid by superoxide produced by the heme oxygenase function of cystathionine synthase.
- Retinoic acid reacts with homocysteine thiolactone to produce thioretinamide.
- Ascorbic acid is necessary for oxidation of sulfur atom of homocysteine thiolactone to sulfate, as shown in scorbutic guinea pigs (McCully KS, NATURE 1971;231:391-392)

Retinol + superoxide radical + dehydroascorbate → retinoic acid + semidehydroascorbate + water

Retinoic acid + homocysteine thiolactone →thioretinamide + water

Thioretinamide + cobalamin + ozone + oxygen → thioretinaco ozonide oxygen

Figure 15. The sequence of steps involved in the biosynthesis of thioretinamide from retinol, superoxide, dehydroascorbate and homocysteine thiolactone is followed by formation of thioretinaco ozonide from thioretinaco, cobalamin, ozone and oxygen.

Human embryonic and malignant cells produce small quantities of the hormone, chorionic gonadotrophin [16]. This hormone is produced by the placenta in large quantities in pregnancy. Chorionic gonadotrophin is also produced in large quantities by the highly malignant tumor of placenta, choriocarcinoma. These observations provide evidence for the trophoblastic origin of cancer, as predicted by Beard in 1902. Although the origin of adult stem cells is currently poorly understood, Beard's concept of sensitivity of malignant tumor cells to the effects of pancreatic enzymes and pro-enzymes forms the theoretical basis for this approach to cancer therapy.

The sensitivity of malignant cells to pancreatic enzyme therapy may be related to the accumulation of proteins, nucleic acids, and glycosaminoglycans with homocysteine molecules attached to these macromolecules by peptide bonds [13]. The homocysteinylated macromolecules are produced from excessive synthesis of homocysteine thiolactone from methionine by malignant cells. The accumulation of excessive homocysteine thiolactone in malignant cells is caused by deficiency of thioretinamide and thioretinaco synthesis, leading to a metabolic block in the conversion of the sulfur atom of homocysteine thiolactone to sulfate, as previously discussed.

Pancreatic extracts contain active trypsin, chymotrypsin, hyaluronidase, elastase, amylase, lipase, ribonuclease, and deoxyribonuclease, as well as pro-enzyme precursors of these digestive enzymes. These powerful enzymes are capable of hydrolyzing the homocysteinylated proteins, nucleic acids, and glycosaminoglycans that accumulate in malignant tissues and in the tissues of aging persons. The enzymatic therapy of cancer by injected pancreatic enzymes failed to realize its potential because of difficulties in preparation of pancreatic extracts of consistent potency, potential problems with immunological rejection of foreign enzyme proteins, and disapproval of the use of parenteral preparations of pancreatic enzymes by governmental authorities [2].

Instead of development of metabolic and nutritional methods to cancer therapy, the mainstays of conventional cancer therapy during the past century have been methods of radical surgery, radiation therapy and chemotherapy. Recent studies have demonstrated that oral pancreatic enzymes are absorbed by the intestinal tract, producing an internal circulation of these enzyme proteins, caused by their absorption into the blood stream and re-secretion by the pancreas of the animal or person with cancer. Some success has recently been claimed by Nicholas Gonzalez and Linda Isaacs, based on the pioneering studies of William Donald Kelley, Max Gerson, and other investigators, using pancreatic extracts containing a high concentration of pro-enzymes [2].

With all of this promising chemistry and nutritional evidence at hand, what happened when Krebs and other investigators advocated use of nitrilosides and pancreatic enzymes for cancer chemotherapy? In his extraordinary book *World without Cancer*, G. Edward Griffin, describes how the experiments to demonstrate the efficacy of laetrile against growth of cancer in animals were deliberately sabotaged [9]. Dr. Kanematsu Sugiura was a senior investigator at the Sloan-Kettering Cancer Institute in New York who conducted intensive studies of laetrile from 1972 to 1977. The official report of these experiments states "the results show that amygdalin significantly inhibits the appearance of lung metastasis in animals bearing spontaneous mammary carcinoma and increases significantly the inhibition of growth of the primary tumors." Other investigators at the Institute found that addition of pancreatic enzymes to the laetrile protocol produced a 100% cure rate in their mice.

The Rockefeller family became intimately involved with the Sloan-Kettering Institute in 1927. Later they donated the land for construction of a new Institute in the 1930s. The Board of Directors is controlled by members of the pharmaceutical industry and by the Rockefeller brothers. When the Board found out about the promising results of the laetrile experiments, they arranged for a protocol designed for failure to be conducted by another scientist, Dr. Daniel Martin of Catholic Medical Center in Queens. At a confrontation between Dr. Sugiura and Dr. Martin held at a press conference in 1977, Dr. Sugiura repeated his insistence that laetrile was effective. When the writer Ralph Moss, who was assistant public affairs director of the Institute, threatened to expose the machinations about the failed experiments, he was fired the next day. Several years earlier in 1974 the Institute had become embroiled in the William Summerlin affair, a scientific scandal involving fraudulent experiments on skin graft rejection. One of my classmates who worked for many years at the Institute told me that Laurance Rockefeller and the Board of Directors were responsible for the abrupt dismissal in 1981 of the esteemed immunologist, Robert Good, who was Director of the Institute during this period. Good was blamed for the Summerlin affair, and his support of the laetrile experiments by Dr. Sugiura undoubtedly contributed to his dismissal.

The book by Griffin describes at great length the efforts of the Rockefeller family, the drug cartels, and the cancer industry to conceal the truth about the efficacy of laetrile in cancer therapy. The upshot of this episode was a hearing in 1977 by the US Senate Subcommittee on Health and Scientific Research chaired by Senator Ted Kennedy, ultimately resulting in a ban of the compound laetrile from interstate commerce by the US Food and Drug Administration.

In 1981 a Cornell University Medical School student, Nicholas Gonzalez, became interested in the enzyme treatment of cancer and approached Dr. Robert Good, then Director of the Sloan-Kettering Institute, to guide his investigation of an obscure practitioner who claimed success with this method. Gonzalez investigated 400 cases of advanced human cancer that had been treated with enzyme therapy and nutritional manipulations by William Donald Kelley DDS of Fort Worth, Texas. His success rate with this complex nutritional protocol varied from about 25% to over 75%, depending upon the severity and stage of the cancer under treatment.

Kelley was a successful orthodontist with an interest in nutrition when he developed advanced pancreatic cancer himself in his mid-30s. In desperation to maintain his health with a family of four children to support, Kelley devised a complex nutritional program composed of organic raw vegetables, a variety of supplements, filtered water, and coffee enemas. He added large doses of oral pancreatic enzymes to relieve severe digestive distress and excruciating pain. With this regimen his tolerance for food improved, and his abdominal tumors regressed. Searching the medical literature, Kelley later came upon Beard's book from 1911 and his earlier articles about the trophoblastic origin of cancer.

After surviving this serious threat to his life by use of his nutritional protocol, Kelley decided to become an alternative practitioner in nutritional cancer therapeutics. In 1969 he self published a book *One Answer to Cancer*, securing his position as a leading alternative cancer therapist and exposing himself to criticism by the mainstream cancer industry [17]. In the late 1980s Kelley's success with cancer patients declined, possibly because of his delegation of therapy to over 1000 "Kelley Counselors" and because of use of a different enzyme preparation.

For his efforts and the nationwide publicity engendered by his book and appearances on television, Kelley was investigated by the Texas State Board of Medical Examiners and the U.S. Congress. He was denounced as a quack by the American Cancer Society and the National Cancer Institute in connection with the death of the actor Steve McQueen, who died in 1980 of mesothelioma while under alternative treatment with laetrile in Mexico. Eventually Kelley became discouraged and paranoid, lashing out at his critics and his supporters alike, until his death from heart failure in 2005 at the age of 80.

Today Nicholas Gonzalez and other alternative medical practitioners are using the discoveries of Beard, Szent-Gyorgi, Krebs, and Kelley in treatment of human cancer. In her recent book *Knockout Interviews with Doctors who are Curing Cancer*, Suzanne Somers describes her 11 year survival from breast cancer, which she attributes to alternative cancer therapy [18]. She also relates interviews with medical practitioners like Stanislaw Burzynski and Nicholas Gonzalez who are continuing to offer therapy to cancer patients, despite harassment from the U.S. Food and Drug Administration and the cancer industry.

REFERENCES

[1] Beard J. Embryological aspects and etiology of cancer. *Lancet*, 1902;159(4112):1758-1761.

[2] Gonzalez N, Isaacs L. *The Trophoblast and the Origins of Cancer*. New York: New Spring Press, 2009.

[3] Beard J. *The Enzyme Treatment of Cancer and its Scientific Basis.* London: Chatto & Windus, 1911. Republished in New York: New Spring Press, 2010.

[4] Moss RW. *Free Radical. Albert Szent-Gyorgi and the Battle over Vitamin C.* New York, Paragon House, 1988.

[5] Meyskens FL Jr, Prasad KN. *Vitamins and Cancer. Human Cancer Prevention by Vitamins and Micronutrients.* Clifton NJ: Humana Press, 1986.

[6] Price WA. *Nutrition and Physical Degeneration. 50th Anniversary Edition.* New Caanan CT: Keats Publishing, 1989.

[7] McCarrison R. Faulty food in relation to gastro-intestinal disorder. *Journal of the American Medical Association,* 1922;78:1-8.

[8] Krebs ET Jr. The nitrilosides in plants and animals. In: *The Laetriles—Nitrilosides—in the Prevention and Control of Cancer.* Los Angeles: Cancer Book House, 1965.

[9] Griffin GE. *World without Cancer. The Story of Vitamin* B_{17}. Second Edition. Westlake Village CA: American Media, 2009. This remarkable book describes the saga of laetrile from its discovery by Krebs in the 1950s, to testing in animals at the Sloan-Kettering Cancer Institute, and to its banning in interstate commerce by the Food and Drug Administration in 1977. The second half of the book is devoted to the politics of cancer research and the influence of the Rockefeller family, the chemical cartel I.G. Farben, and Federal agencies on medical research, medical education, and protection of radical surgery, radiation therapy, and chemotherapy by the cancer industry.

[10] McCully KS. Chemical Pathology of Homocysteine. IV. Excitotoxicity, oxidative stress, endothelial dysfunction and inflammation. *Annals of Clinical and Laboratory Science,* 2009;39:219-232. This fourth installment of my monograph on the Chemical Pathology of Homocysteine discusses the potent toxicity of homocysteine, glutamate, and other amino acids for nerve cells. The toxicity of fluoride is attributed to effects on oxidative metabolism catalyzed by thioretinaco ozonide and effects of fluoride on hydrogen bonding of enzyme proteins. The discussion explains the role of infections on creation of vulnerable plaques, endothelial dysfunction and inflammation in arteriosclerosis.

[11] Wang R. Two's company, three's a crowd: can H2S be the third endogenous gasotransmitter? FASEB J 2002;16:1792-1798.

[12] McCully KS. Homocysteine thiolactone metabolism in malignant cells. *Cancer Research,* 1976;36:3198-3202.

[13] McCully KS. Chemical Pathology of Homocysteine. V. Thioretinamide, thioretinaco, and cystathionine synthase function in degenerative diseases. *Annals of Clinical and Laboratory Science*, 2011;41:301-314. This fifth installment of my monograph on the Chemical Pathology of Homocysteine discusses the synthesis of thioretinamide from retinol by its oxidation to retinoic acid by superoxide synthesized by the heme oxygenase of cystathionine synthase and homocysteine thiolactone. The review discusses the enzymatic therapy of cancer by pancreatic enzymes, glycolysis, nitrilosides, and hydrogen sulfide in malignant cells, and the use of these concepts in the metabolic and nutritional therapy of degenerative diseases of aging.

[14] Miles EW, Kraus JP. Cystathionine β-synthase: structure, function, regulation, and location of homocystinuria-causing mutations. *Journal of Biological Chemistry,* 2004;279:29871-29874.

[15] Kim J, Hong SJ, Park JH, Park SY, Kim SW, Cho EY, Do IG, Joh JW, Kim DS. Expression of cystathionine β-synthase is downregulated in hepatocellular carcinoma and associated with poor prognosis. *Oncology Reports,* 2009;21:1449-1454.

[16] Acevedo HF, Tong JY, Hartsock RJ. Human chorionic gonadotropin-beta subunit gene expression in cultured fetal and cancer cells of different types and origins. *Cancer,* 1995;76:1467-1475.

[17] Kelley WD. *One Answer to Cancer.* Los Angeles CA: Cancer Book House, 1969.

[18] Somers S. *Knockout Interviews with Doctors who are Curing Cancer.* New York: Three Rivers Press, 2009.

Chapter 12

HOMOCYSTEINE AND AGING

The biochemical, cellular, and metabolic processes involved in aging have intrigued medical scientists for many years. Within the past century there has occurred a major change in life expectancy in the United States and other developed countries, increasing by 25 years or more and reaching 78 years for males and 80 years for females in many countries. This spectacular increase in life expectancy has been attributed to prevention and treatment of infectious diseases, improved sanitation, and improved nutrition. And yet the underlying process of aging leading to senescence seems largely unchanged, despite this improvement. The leading causes of death and disability today are from vascular diseases and cancer. The incidence of these diseases is each closely correlated with the aging process. Other conditions associated with the aging process, such as kidney failure, autoimmune diseases, diabetes, dementia, osteoporosis and cataract, are considered to be degenerative diseases of aging.

With the discovery of the disease homocystinuria in 1962, it became apparent that some features of accelerated aging are observed in these individuals. The decreased lifespan of untreated subjects with homocystinuria is closely tied to the occurrence of vascular disease, including heart attack, stroke, and thrombosis of arteries and veins to the major organs of the body [1]. In addition, many persons with homocystinuria exhibit other prominent features of aging, especially osteoporosis, graying of hair, dementia, cataract, loss of skin elasticity, and joint stiffness due to osteoarthrosis. Some subjects with homocystinuria have decreased glucose tolerance and insulin resistance, important features of the aging process in the general population. Increased susceptibility to cancer, however, is not found in homocystinuria, in contrast to the association of cancer with aging in the general population.

After introduction of automated methods for determination of blood homocysteine levels 20 years ago, it became apparent that a gradual elevation of blood homocysteine is associated with the aging process. In untreated normal persons in populations without folic acid fortification of the food supply, the blood homocysteine level gradually increases by about 1 micromole per liter for each decade over the age of 60. Although this change is correlated with aging, insufficiency of dietary vitamin B6, folate and vitamin B12 is also related to aging, both through decreased food consumption and also through decreased absorption of these B vitamins.

In the Framingham Heart Study about two thirds of elderly participants over the age of 67 were found to have deficient blood levels of these three B vitamins [2]. In the case of vitamin B6 and folate, the source of the deficiency is loss of these sensitive vitamins by their destruction by traditional methods of food processing, such as milling of grains, commercial canning and freezing methods, extraction of oils and sugars from whole foods, and addition of chemical oxidizing and stabilizing agents. In the case of vitamin B12, the deficiency of this vitamin in a significant fraction of the elderly is caused by poor absorption from the gastrointestinal tract because of loss of stomach acid needed for release of B12 from food and loss of intrinsic factor needed for absorption of B12 from the distal small intestine (ileum). The elevation of blood homocysteine levels in these elderly Framingham participants is directly related to dietary deficiency of vitamin B6 and folate and deficient absorption of vitamin B12.

Following early observations on growth retardation by caloric restriction in experimental animals (rats) by Osborn in 1915, McCay and his team demonstrated in 1935 that significant restriction of dietary calories in albino rats not only retarded growth, but the life span of the animals was increased about 20% [3]. They also observed a decrease in age-related pathological changes in hair structure. Over the years since these original investigations, caloric restriction has been observed to prolong life span in a wide variety of organisms, including worms, fruit flies, yeasts, rats and mice.

A recent report demonstrates that a 20 year period of caloric restriction increased the life span of Rhesus monkeys, showing that among 76 animals in the experiment 80% of animals on the reduced calorie diet survived, compared with 50% survival among animals consuming the normal diet [4]. Furthermore, caloric restriction delayed the onset of degenerative diseases of aging, including diabetes, cancer, vascular disease and brain atrophy. The incidence of colon cancer in monkeys consuming the caloric restricted diet was 50% of the incidence in animals consuming the normal diet. Cardiovascular disease was 50% of controls, and diabetes and pre-diabetes were completely prevented by caloric restriction. Another striking finding was that caloric restriction in monkeys significantly preserved brain size and weight, involving cerebral cortex and basal ganglia, compared with the brain shrinkage (atrophy) observed in control animals. Because of its consistent effect on prolongation of life span in a great variety of species, from yeast to worms to fruit flies, rodents and primates, caloric restriction has become an important scientific model for study of the aging process.

Another important approach to understanding the aging process is the comparison of aging in different species, an approach promoted by Caleb Finch, among many other investigators. Finch's extraordinary monograph, *Longevity, Senescence and the Genome*, summarizes the evidence for genomic influences on the aging process [5]. Each species generally possesses a characteristic and defined life span, as determined by the evolutionary process. The maximum life span for the human species is approximately 110 years, domestic dogs 20 years, laboratory mice and rats 4-6 years, herring gull 49 years, fruit fly 0.3 years, and soil roundworms 0.15 years. Finch points out that the Mortality Rate Doubling Time (MRDT) is slowest for the human species and most rapid for short-lived flies, nematodes (worms) and rotifers (microscopic marine invertebrates), about a thousand fold greater.

According to Finch "A widely discussed hypothesis proposes that senescence is caused by an accumulation of somatic mutations or other informational errors ... but there is little evidence that accumulated point mutations or other types of errors in genomic information flow are a basic mechanism of senescence." And Finch concludes that "the diverse but characteristic species differences in the pathophysiological mechanisms of senescence restrict the generalizability of random genomic damage as a major mechanism of senescence."

As described in Chapter 3, my encounter with Francis Crick in 1962 during my interview for the Harvard Society of Fellows revolved about his question about theories of aging. My studies of transfer RNA structure and function in Cantoni's laboratory gave me the appropriate scientific knowledge and background for pursuing the informational error theory of aging [6]. However, my subsequent considerations about the molecular basis for aging led me away from this hypothesis, as summarized by the previous quote from Finch's monograph. Thus the powerful theories and conclusions of the "central dogma" of molecular biology, the translation of genomic information from nucleotide sequences in DNA to the structure of proteins, failed to provide a coherent or persuasive theory of aging.

The robust effect of caloric restriction on extension of life span in a wide variety of species, from yeast to worms, insects, rodents and primates, suggests that a basic change in metabolism of food in some way underlies the aging process. It has been known for many years that oxygen consumption and basal metabolic rate decline gradually with aging. In 1954 Denham Harman proposed the "free radical theory of aging" in order to explain the relationship of the life span of mammalian species to their basal metabolic rate [7]. According to Harman, "the free radical theory of aging assumes that there is a single basic cause of aging, modified by genetic and environmental factors, and postulates that free radical reactions are involved in aging and age-related disorders."

Free radicals are highly reactive chemicals arising within the tissues of the body during metabolism because of the reaction of the carbon and hydrogen atoms of foods with the oxygen of air inspired during breathing. Harman called attention to the production of free radicals within the body by ionizing radiation, such as X-rays, gamma rays, and decay of radioactive elements, as factors known to accelerate the aging process and degenerative diseases of aging [8]. As described in previous chapters, oxidative reactions involving free radicals are known to be essential components of the process by which carcinogenic chemicals lead to cancer and by which oxidation of cholesterol and lipoproteins participate in production of arteriosclerotic plaques. Moreover, free radical reactions are known to participate in breakdown of chemical constituents of cells during aging, leading to oxidative damage to proteins, DNA, fats and proteoglycans and deposition of the inert age-related pigment lipofuscin. Antioxidants derived from foods or from synthetic chemicals increase the life span of mice, rats, fruit flies, nematodes, yeast, fungi and rotifers, presumably by counteracting the age-promoting effects of free radicals that arise during the metabolism of food constituents by oxygen.

An important aspect of the free radical theory of aging is that over 90% of oxygen inspired into animals, including human beings is processed in the mitochondria of cells during cellular respiration. Mitochondria are cellular organelles, originally derived from symbiotic microbes during evolution, that function as the energy power plants of cells, generating ATP from the reduction of oxygen atoms to water by the electrons of carbon, hydrogen, nitrogen, sulfur and other atoms of foods. The accumulation of free radicals within mitochondria during cellular respiration causes changes in the number of mitochondria, their morphological abnormalities, and enzymatic activities during aging. It is noteworthy that many of the mitochondrial abnormalities found in senescent cells are also observed in liver cells and aortic cells in cases of human homocystinuria and in experimental animals subjected to high blood levels of homocysteine.

In his review Bruce Ames points out that ten-fold more oxidative damage occurs in mitochondrial DNA, compared with nuclear DNA, during the aging process [9]. In an interesting experiment Ames found that feeding old rats the normal mitochondrial metabolites acetyl carnitine and lipoic acid for several weeks restores mitochondrial function, lowers oxidants to the level of a young rat, and increases ambulatory activity. He also points out that deficiencies in vitamins B12, folic acid, B6, niacin, vitamin C, vitamin E, iron or zinc appear to mimic radiation effects in damaging DNA by causing single stranded or double stranded chromosomal breaks and incorporation of the nucleotide base uracil in place of thymine into DNA. Thus deficiencies in micronutrients cause damage to human DNA and chromosomes similar to the damage to DNA observed in the aging process.

Further evidence for the importance of oxidation and free radical damage during aging is provided by Earl Stadtman and his team, who showed that proteins and enzymes become oxidized and contain increased carbonyl groups in place of amino groups during the aging process [10]. They found that the activity of proteolytic enzymes that hydrolyze oxidized proteins is not sufficient to prevent the age-associated increase in oxidized proteins in tissues of aged animals. During my two years as a research associate at the National Institutes of Health from 1960-1962, I met Bruce Ames and his wife who were working with Maxine Singer on nucleotide metabolism. I also attended Earl Stadtman's legendary course on microbial biochemistry before he became interested in the biochemistry of aging.

My colleague Andrzej Olszewski and I published a hypothesis article in *Free Radical Biology and Medicine* in 1993, calling attention to the biochemical oxidation of homocysteine thiolactone to sulfate, the auto-oxidation of homocysteine to hydrogen peroxide, oxygen radicals and homocysteinyl radicals, and the theoretical participation of thioretinaco ozonide in mitochondrial oxidative phosphorylation and ATP production during cellular respiration [12]. We pointed out that these free radical oxidation reactions involving homocysteine may underlie the free radical reactions observed in aging, carcinogenesis, and atherogenesis.

Because of the many profound hormonal changes associated with aging and because of the function of the central nervous system in controlling and coordinating endocrine secretions, the neuroendocrine theory of aging ascribes primacy to these physiological changes in aging. As it happens, I met one of the earliest proponents of the neuroendocrine theory of aging, V. M. Dilman, while he was being evaluated at the Providence VA Medical Center for symptoms of cancer. In 1971 Dilman discovered that there is an age-associated increase in the threshold for hypothalamic feedback control of endocrine secretions. The hypothalamus is the part of the brain responsible for coordinating and controlling hormonal secretions of adrenal glands, thyroid gland, ovaries or testes, and for controlling secretion of growth hormone. In 1984 Dilman proposed a comprehensive theory of aging in which declining hypothalamic control of gonadotropin secretion, depression of immunity, declining insulin secretion and insulin resistance, obesity, stress and over-nutrition are viewed as the primary causes of the aging process [13].

Certainly many hormonal changes accompany the aging process. Some prominent examples are declining levels of dehydroepiandrosterone (DHEA), an androgenic hormone produced by the adrenal gland, decreased secretion of gonadotropic hormones, growth hormone, testosterone, estrogen, and increased insulin resistance. In contrast, secretion of pituitary adrenocorticotropic hormone (ACTH) and levels of adrenocortical hormones like corticosterone are not impaired in aging, either in animals or in humans. The degree to which loss of neurons from the hypothalamus or other parts of the brain affects these hormonal changes is uncertain. An example of another prominent hormonal change associated with aging is calcification of the pineal gland associated with decreased secretion of melatonin, the hormone that controls the circadian rhythm and stimulates melanin pigment formation in melanocytes of the skin. Many theories have been proposed relating the pineal gland and melatonin secretion to aging, but their exact role in the aging process is unclear.

In the populations of many developed nations, women consistently live longer lives than men. One of the reasons for this disparity is the earlier onset of cardiovascular disease in men compared with women. After menopause, mortality from cardiovascular disease accelerates in women, and mortality from heart disease is the leading cause of death in women, because of this rapid increase. Studies of plasma homocysteine levels have consistently shown that men have higher levels than women of the same age. After menopause, however, plasma homocysteine levels in women increase until they approach the levels found in older men. The exact role of ovarian hormones in preventing increased homocysteine levels in pre-menopausal women, however, is unclear. There is some evidence that estrogenic hormones produced by the ovary are associated with slightly increased plasma homocysteine levels during the first 14 days of the menstrual cycle, and progestational hormones secreted during the second 14 days of the cycle are associated with decreased levels of plasma homocysteine. This evidence fits with the earlier finding that high dose contraceptive hormones lead to increased arterial plaques and risk of thrombosis in younger women. I discussed the relation of oral contraceptive hormones to homocysteine levels and risk of vascular disease at a symposium held by the National Institutes of Health in Mobile, Alabama, in 1975 [14].

Another important connection between neuroendocrine physiology and homocysteine metabolism is the observation that experimental mental stress, hostility and anger lead to a rapid increase in blood levels of homocysteine [15]. These changes in homocysteine levels are correlated with increases in heart rate and blood pressure, and participants with a family history of heart disease have higher levels of plasma homocysteine following experimental psychological stress. These observations were discussed by Catherine Stoney at the 4th World Congress of Cellular and Molecular Biology at a symposium organized by Lesley Klevay and Kilmer McCully on homocysteine in health and disease held in Poitiers, France in October 2005.

An important advance in understanding the cellular basis of aging was the observation by Leonard Hayflick that cultured human diploid fibroblast-like cells can only be passaged about 50 times in culture, after which the cells fail to divide further, a process called clonal senescence [16]. In addition, cultured fibroblasts from embryos have a greater capacity to divide under culture conditions, compared with fibroblasts from adult animals or humans. Cells cultured from the skin of children and adolescents, for example, have the capacity for about 45 doublings in culture, whereas cells taken from adults over age 70 have the capacity for about 30 doublings.

A possible clue to the biochemical and cellular control of clonal senescence is the observation that homocysteine thiolactone greatly reduces the growth of cultured skin cells from a child with homocystinuria from cystathionine synthase deficiency. Vitamin B6 reverses this inhibition of cellular growth by homocysteine thiolactone in cell cultures taken from a child with pyridoxine-responsive homocystinuria. The accumulation of granular highly sulfated proteoglycans (ground substance) resembles the changes in cell cultures from normal human donors observed in the process of clonal senescence [17]. These observations suggest the possibility that homocysteine thiolactone reduces the concentration of an unknown substance needed to support cell doubling in cell culture conditions. Thus it seems possible that clonal senescence in cultured human diploid cells may be related to loss of a critical substance related to homocysteine, such as thioretinaco ozonide, during repeated cell divisions.

Telomeres have long been known to cytologists and geneticists as the cap structure on the end of each chromosome. Telomeres are specialized regions of DNA consisting of a loop structure of nucleotides with associated nucleoproteins. During the aging process in all cells of the body and with each cell division, the telomeres of chromosomes become progressively shortened, and chromosomes fuse together, triggering arrest of cell division, senescence and cell death [18]. The enzyme telomerase is a ribonucleoprotein that elongates the DNA of telomeres by copying the sequences of nucleotides of RNA to restore the DNA sequence by a reverse transcriptase activity. In cancer cells, telomeres become shorted, but telomerase activity is characteristically increased to compensate for this loss of telomere length [19]. High telomerase activity is associated with increased risk of recurrence and decreased survival in human breast, prostate, colon and lung cancer cases.

In genetic premature aging syndromes, like Werner's syndrome, Bloom's syndrome, and dyskeratosis congenita, there is a predisposition to malignancy, and the mutations of these disorders may interfere with maintenance of telomere length by telomerase. Insertion of the gene for activating telomerase synthesis into normal human cells in culture overcomes clonal senescence and leads to a greatly expanded life span in cell cultures. The relation of telomeres and telomerase to the anti-cancer effects of thioretinamide and thioretinaco, as described in Chapter 10, is presently unknown. The loss of telomeres by normal cultured human cells is believed to determine the life span of these cells in culture. However, the accumulation of double strand breaks of DNA of senescent cells involved both telomeric and non-telomeric DNA.

A recent innovative approach to understanding cellular senescence involves the study of aging in the common yeast *Saccharomyces cerevisiae*. Caloric restriction of cultures of this yeast extends the life span by increasing the activity of sirtuin deacetylases, enzymes that remove acetyl groups from the histone proteins of chromosomes [20]. In aging yeast cells toxic forms of non-chromosomal DNA coding for ribosomal RNA accumulate. These toxic DNA by-products have been identified as extra-chromosomal DNA circles. Notably, the sirtuin enzymes are dependent upon nicotinamide adenosine dinucleotide (NAD), an important coenzyme of energy metabolism. Recently the immunosuppressive anticancer drug rapamycin has been found to extend the life span of yeast, round worms and fruit flies by suppressing a signaling pathway protein kinase called target of rapamycin (TOR). David Sinclair and his team at Harvard Medical School have recently found that TOR inhibition extends life span of yeast by the same process as caloric restriction, namely to increase sirtuin activity and to stabilize the ribosomal DNA locus, promoting genomic stability during aging.

In his analysis of theories of aging, Sinclair cites evidence for and against earlier hypotheses regarding caloric restriction and life span extension in experimental animals [21]. Certain point mutations in the DNA of flies, yeast, mice and worms extend lifespan of these organisms. In some studies genetic analysis revealed a dramatic extension of life span associated with impairment of the insulin signaling pathway or with increased expression of sirtuins, which are inhibited by the insulin signaling cascade.

According to Sinclair, certain molecules originally derived from plants, such as metformin from lilac and resveratrol from grapes, nuts and herbs extend the life span of yeast, worms and flies by stimulating the activity of sirtuins. To explain the influences of caloric restriction, heat and salt stress on yeast life span, Sinclair advances the concept of hormesis, namely that these phytochemicals deplete nicotinamide and activate sirtuins, thereby increasing life span. Whether the hormesis concept explains aspects of aging in mammals and humans is currently under active investigation by scientists in the field of aging research [22].

A possible connection between homocysteine metabolism and insulin signaling is our 1976 observation in *Science* that homocysteic acid promotes growth of hypophysectomized rats treated with thyroxine by release of the insulin signaling molecule, insulin-like growth factor, from liver of these animals [23]. Homocysteic acid is the fully oxidized form of homocysteine, showing a connection between oxidation and formation of a molecule that activates the insulin signaling pathway. In aging animals, homocysteine becomes oxidized more readily, activating insulin signaling and affecting metabolism of glucose, as commonly observed in human aging.

Several lines of evidence support a close correlation between altered homocysteine metabolism and the aging process. The decreased life span of subjects with homocystinuria is attributable mainly to increased risk of vascular disease. In addition, degenerative diseases of aging, especially osteoporosis, osteoarthrosis, graying of hair, dementia, cataract, renal failure, and pre-diabetes are observed with increased frequency in these subjects.

In studies with young and old animals, a basic alteration in methionine and homocysteine metabolism was demonstrated by study of metabolites of these amino acids in liver [24]. Older animals were found to accumulate more homocysteine thiolactone in liver than in liver of younger animals. Conversion of homocysteine thiolactone to cystathionine is greater in older than in younger animals. Young animals accumulate homocysteine, the reduced sulfhydryl form of the molecule, whereas older animals accumulate homocystine, the oxidized, disulfide form of homocysteine. This declining efficiency of homocysteine metabolism and increased oxidation of homocysteine with aging may be explained by decreased concentrations of thioretinaco ozonide in mitochondria and microsomal membranes in aging animals. Studies with cell cultures show that homocysteine accumulation within cells leads to defective repair of DNA molecules and decreased methylation of DNA, both characteristic features of senescent cells.

The important metabolic regulator of homocysteine metabolism, adenosyl methionine, also known as SAMe, is formed by reaction of methionine with ATP. Adenosyl methionine concentrations in plasma and tissues decline with aging. Yet no decrease in the activity of the enzyme catalyzing adenosyl methionine synthesis was found in aging cells and tissues to explain this decline in adenosyl methionine. In my second monograph "Chemical Pathology of Homocysteine" I suggested that thioretinaco may participate in the synthesis of adenosyl methionine and that age-related loss of thioretinaco ozonide from cellular membranes may explain the decline in adenosyl methionine concentrations with aging [25].

Adenosyl methionine is the methylating coenzyme for more than 100 different reactions involving neurotransmitters, hormones, proteins and nucleic acids. As previously discussed, melatonin is the pineal hormone, which functions as a regulator of the internal biological clock and as a controller of melanin pigment formation by skin cells. In aging the pineal gland becomes calcified and gradually loses the ability to secrete melatonin. This aging change may be explained by decreased methylation of N-acetyl serotonin to form melatonin because of decreased formation of adenosyl methionine, the methylating coenzyme. Another example of decreased methylation is the reduced methylation of DNA found in senescent cells and tissues, which is also explained by decreased formation of adenosyl methionine in aging. These lines of evidence support the suggestion that increased homocysteine thiolactone synthesis from methionine and elevated blood levels of homocysteine are caused by loss of thioretinaco ozonide from cellular membranes.

In 1986 while working at the Providence VA Medical Center, I received an unsolicited article from Yves Ingenbleek, of University Louis Pasteur, Strasbourg, France concerning elevation of blood homocysteine in protein energy malnutrition [26]. His research team determined that the indigenous population in Senegal, West Africa, which consumes a mainly vegetarian diet, is characterized by varying degrees of protein energy malnutrition and hypothyroidism. By studying the amino acids of plasma in these malnourished subjects, his team observed that the concentration of essential amino acids declined with severity of malnutrition. Thus tryptophan, phenylalanine, threonine, leucine, isoleucine, valine and phenylalanine declined to about 60% of the concentration observed in the well nourished control group. The exception was methionine, the concentration of which was maintained at or above the control value except in the most severe stage of malnutrition. To their surprise, Ingenbleek and his team discovered that plasma homocysteine became progressively more elevated, reaching 168% of control values, as malnutrition became more severe.

Ingenbleek had previously established plasma transthyretin as a sensitive marker of protein energy malnutrition, and their studies established a relationship between decreased transthyretin and elevated homocysteine levels in these malnourished populations. Transthyretin, formerly known as prealbumin, is a plasma protein that transports thyroid hormone, retinol binding protein, and retinol in plasma. Transthyretin is a sensitive indicator of malnutrition because it contains a high concentration of tryptophan and rapidly turns over in the plasma. In protein energy malnutrition, there is increased susceptibility to hypothyroidism and vitamin A deficiency because of diminished transthyretin levels in plasma.

In subsequent studies Ingenbleek and his collaborators at Massachusetts Institute of Technology, lead by Vernon Young, studied sub-clinical protein energy malnutrition and hypothyroidism as a cause of hyperhomocysteinemia [27]. They suggested that this abnormal metabolic pattern resembled the findings in homocystinuria, namely elevated homocysteine, decreased cystathionine, and decreased sulfate excretion, because of an acquired deficiency of cystathionine synthase. Ingenbleek points out that those populations at risk of vascular disease from elevated homocysteine have hidden protein energy malnutrition as a cause. Furthermore, independent studies have shown that only about 30% of the variance of homocysteine concentrations in populations can be explained by deficiency of the B vitamins, folate, pyridoxal, and cobalamin. This concept helps to explain why high dose B vitamin trials in subjects with advanced vascular disease fail to prevent secondary development of heart attack, stroke and amputation. In a recent study from Chad, vegetarianism was found to produce elevation of blood homocysteine by down-regulation of cystathionine synthase, the enzyme that is deficient in many cases of homocystinuria, confirming Ingenbleek's earlier interpretation [28].

The concept of hidden protein energy malnutrition as a cause of elevated homocysteine was nicely supported by a study of retired school teachers from the Baltimore area [29]. Those teachers consuming a low protein diet were found to have significantly higher homocysteine levels than teachers consuming a higher protein diet. Transthyretin is known to decline in aging, paralleling the loss of skeletal muscle with aging, particularly in elderly men. The known decrease in adenosyl methionine with aging may explain why homocysteine levels increase with age, because of decreased activation of cystathionine synthase. The finding of constant methionine levels in aging and protein energy malnutrition, however, suggests that another pathway for synthesis of adenosyl methionine is impaired in the aging process. In my monograph, "Chemical Pathology of Homocysteine," I suggest that thioretinamide and thioretinaco may catalyze formation of adenosyl methionine from methionine [25]. Loss of thioretinamide and thioretinaco from cell membranes during the aging process, therefore, would explain the decreased activity of cystathionine synthase from decreased adenosyl methionine synthesis, explaining the elevation of homocysteine in aging.

REFERENCES

[1] Mudd SH, Skovby F, Levy HL, Pettigrew KD, Wilcken B, Pyeritz RE, Andria G, Boers GHJ, Bromberg IL, Cerone R, Fowler B, Grobe H, Schmidt H, Schweitzer L. The natural history of homocystinuria due to cystathionine beta synthase deficiency. *American Journal of Human G*enetics, 1985;37:1-31. This study describes the clinical and epidemiological findings in 629 world wide cases of homocystinuria. About 75% of patients survived to the age of 50, and most deaths were caused by thromboembolism.

[2] Selhub J, Jacques PF, Wilson PWF, Rush D, Rosenberg IH. Vitamin status and intake as primary determinants of homocysteinemia in an elderly population. *Journal of the American Medical Association*, 1993;270:2693-2698. This study of 1160 adult survivors of the Framingham Heart Study original cohort, aged 67 to 96 years, showed that 30% of participants had high levels of blood homocysteine, and two thirds of cases were deficient in one or more B vitamins, including folic acid, vitamin B6 or vitamin B12.

[3] McCay CM, Crowell MF. The effect of retarded growth upon the length of life span and upon the ultimate body size. *Journal of Nutrition*, 1935;10:63-79. McCay CM, Maynard LA, Sperling G, Barnes LL. Retarded growth, life span, ultimate body size and age changes in the albino rat after feeding diets restricted in calories. *Journal of Nutrition*, 1939;18:1-25.

[4] Colman RJ, Anderson RM, Johnson SC, Kastman EK, Kosmatka KJ, Beasley TM, Allison DB, Cruzen C, Simmons HA, Kemnitz JW, Weindruch R. Caloric restriction delays disease onset and mortality in Rhesus monkeys. *Science*, 2009;325:201-204.

[5] Finch CE. *Longevity, Senescence and the Genome*. Chicago: Unversity of Chicago Press, 1990.

[6] Orgel LE. The maintenance of the accuracy of protein synthesis and its relevance to aging. *Proceedings of the National Academy of Sciences USA* 1963;49:512-517.

[7] Harman D. Aging: a theory based on free radical and radiation chemistry. *Journal of Gerontology*, 1956;11:298-300.

[8] Harman D. The aging process. *Proceedings of the National Academy of Sciences USA*, 1981;78:7124-7128.

[9] Ames BN, Shigenaga MK, Hagen TM. Oxidants, antioxidants, and the degenerative diseases of aging. *Proceedings of the National Academy of Sciences USA*, 1993;90:7915-7922.

[10] Ames BN. Micronutrients prevent cancer and delay aging. *Toxicology Letters*, 1998;102-103:5-18.

[11] Stadtman ER. Protein oxidation and aging. *Science*, 1992;257:1220-1224.

[12] Olszewski AJ, McCully KS. Homocysteine metabolism and the oxidative modification of proteins and lipids. *Free Radicals in Biology and Medicine*, 1993;14:683-693.

[13] Dilman VM, Dean W. *The Neuroendocrine Theory of Aging and Degenerative Disease.* Pensacola FL: Center for Bio-Gerontology, 1992:93-96. Dilman VM. Three models of medicine. An integrated theory of aging and age-associated diseases. *Medical Hypotheses*, 1984;15:185-208.

[14] McCully KS. Homocystine, atherosclerosis and thrombosis: implications for oral contraceptive users. *American Journal of Clinical Nutrition*, 1975;28:542-549.

[15] Stoney CM. Plasma homocysteine levels increase in women during psychological stress. *Life Sciences*, 1999;64:2359-2365. Stoney CM, Engebretson TO. Plasma homocysteine concentrations are positively associated with hostility and anger. *Life Sciences*, 2000;66:2267-2275.

[16] Hayflick L. Moorhead P. The serial cultivation of human diploid cell strains. *Experimental Cell Research*, 1961;25:585-621.

[17] McCully KS. Macromolecular basis for homocysteine-induced changes in proteoglycan structure in growth and arteriosclerosis. *American Journal of Pathology*, 1972;66:83-96.

[18] Shay JR. Wright WE. Senescence and immortalization: role of telomeres and telomerase. *Carcinogenesis,* 2005;26:867-874.

[19] Shin J-S, Hong A. Solomon MJ, Lee CS. The role of telomeres and telomerase in the pathology of human cancer and aging. *Pathology*, 2006;38:103-113.

[20] Medvedik O, Lamming DW, Kim KD, Sinclair DA. MSN2 and MSN4 link caloric restriction and TOR to sirtuin-mediated lifespan extension in Saccharomyces cerevisiae. *PLOS Biology*, 2007;5:2330-2341.

[21] Sinclair DA. Toward a unifed theory of caloric restriction and longevity regulation. *Mechanisms of Ageing and Development*, 2005;126:987-1002.

[22] Droge W, Shipper HM. Oxidative stress and aberrant signaling in aging and cognitive decline. *Aging Cell*, 2007;6:361-370.

[23] Clopath P, Smith VC, McCully KS. Growth promotion by homocysteic acid. *Science,* 1976;192:372-374.

[24] McCully KS. Growth disorders and homocysteine metabolism. *Annals of Clinical and Laboratory Science*, 1975;5:147-152.

[25] McCully KS. Chemical Pathology of Homocysteine. III. Cellular function and aging. *Annals of Clinical and Laboratory Science*, 1994;24:134-152.

[26] Ingenbleek Y, Barclay D, Dirren H. Nutritional significance of alterations in serum amino acid patterns in goitrous patients. *American Journal of Clinical Nutrition*, 1986;43:310-319.

[27] Ingenbleek Y, Young V. Transthyretin (prealbumin) in health and disease. Nutritional implications. Annu Rev Nutr 1994;14:495-533.

[28] Ingenbleek Y, McCully KS. Vegetarianism produces subclinical malnutrition, hyperhomocysteinemia and atherogenesis. *Nutrition*, 2012;28:148-153.

[29] Stolzenberg-Solomon RZ, Miller ER, Maguire MG, Selhub J, Appel LJ. Association of dietary protein intake and coffee consumption with serum homocysteine concentrations in an older population. *American Journal of Clinical Nutrition,* 1999;69:467-475.

Chapter 13

CONCLUSION: LEGACY OF A NEW UNDERSTANDING OF DISEASE

The story of my career in medical science illustrates the experience of other pioneers whose discoveries in years past advanced understanding of the origin of disease through introduction of novel concepts. Despite criticism and ridicule, only those investigators, who pursue the ramifications of their discoveries, overcoming rejection and opposition, are able to arrive at a new paradigm which overturns obsolete and disproven theories. The essential ingredients to success in medical science, as in other human enterprises, are persistence and confidence.

As Calvin Coolidge, the 30th President of the United States once said: "Nothing in this world can take the place of persistence. Persistence and determination alone are omnipotent." A corollary of persistence in science is the pursuit of truth. The persistent scientific pioneer who is confident of the significance of his discovery will be rewarded with the truth of new understanding of the origin of disease. The motto on the emblem of Harvard University is "Veritas" which means "truth" in Latin. Persistence in the pursuit of truth is essential to the advancement of all human enterprise including medical science.

Having experienced an arduous, interesting and stimulating educational and practical preparation for a career in medical science, I was indeed fortunate to have been able to make a critical observation that opened an entire new field of investigation. My background and experience in medicine, pathology, biochemistry, molecular biology and genetics prepared me for innovative advances in homocysteine research, based on this discovery. The many novel discoveries and developments that I experienced during my medical research career were extraordinary. My years of apprenticeship in medical science illustrated to me the difficulty that the investigator encounters in identifying a promising and significant question, the answer to which will open a productive new field of knowledge. Many, if not most, experiments and studies fail to achieve significant results if the underlying assumptions are incompletely understood by the investigator. On the other hand, positive results in multiple endeavors reward the investigator with hard evidence that his concepts and theories have a basis in reality.

My observation of accelerated arteriosclerosis in children with homocystinuria caused by different inherited enzymatic deficiencies of methionine metabolism was the key to a new understanding of the metabolic origin of degenerative diseases of aging. By discovering the ability of homocysteine to cause arterial plaques in children and experimental animals and to convert normal skin cells to cancer cells in experimental animals, I was able to relate these diseases of aging to fundamental abnormalities of methionine metabolism.

Through my discovery of a new pathway for conversion of the sulfur atom of homocysteine to sulfate in cultured cells from a child with cystathionine synthase deficiency and homocystinuria, I was able to implicate this metabolic pathway in the pathogenesis of arteriosclerosis and cancer. My discovery of the abnormal blockade of conversion of homocysteine to sulfate in malignant cells led to invention of synthetic derivatives of homocysteine that prevent arterial plaques in animals, decrease the growth of malignant tumors in animals, and decrease the action of carcinogenic chemicals in animals with cancer. The most important of these new compounds are thioretinamide, synthesized from retinoic acid and homocysteine thiolactone, and thioretinaco, synthesized from thioretinamide and cobalamin.

Our discovery of the growth hormone-like effects of homocysteic acid in normal and hypophysectomized animals led to the demonstration that insulin-like growth factor causes this growth response. Our discovery of abnormal homocysteine metabolism in guinea pigs with experimental scurvy led to new understanding of the important function of ascorbic acid in the synthesis of thioretinamide from retinoic acid and homocysteine thiolactone by cystathionine synthase.

My discovery that thioretinamide forms a complex with cobalamin to produce thioretinaco was the key to developing a new theory of oxidative phosphorylation that offers a new explanation of the origin of oxidative stress in aging and degenerative diseases. The realization that ozone and oxygen activate the binding of ATP with the sulfonium sulfur atoms of thioretinaco ozonide was the critical insight that was responsible for establishing the molecular basis for this theory.

As discussed in Chapter 12, the African studies with Yves Ingenbleek concerning the down regulation of cystathionine synthase function in protein energy malnutrition led to a new appreciation of the function of transthyretin and thyroid hormone in control of oxidative metabolism. The recent discovery of synthesis of superoxide by the heme oxygenase group of cystathionine synthase led to elucidation of the function of this enzyme in biosynthesis of thioretinamide from the retinol of transthyretin, dehydroascorbate, and homocysteine.

As presented in Chapter 11, the re-discovery of the amazing observations of John Beard in 1902 in his development of the trophoblastic theory of cancer led to a new explanation of the efficacy of digestive pancreatic enzymes in control of neoplastic growth and cancer. This new understanding of the anti-cancer function of pancreatic enzymes relates degradation of homocysteinylated proteins, nucleic acids, and glycosaminoglycans to the oncolytic properties of these enzymes. Of course, the origin of homocysteinylated macromolecules in aging tissues, in arteriosclerosis, and in cancer is the excessive production of homocysteine thiolactone from methionine because of the cellular deficiency of thioretinaco ozonide in these diseases.

As discussed in Chapter 11, the recent demonstration of production of chorionic gonadotrophic hormone by cancer cells and the discovery of abnormal cystathionine synthase function in cancer cells supports Beard's trophoblastic theory of cancer. His demonstration of the migration of trophoblastic cells into the tissues of the developing embryo anticipated the discovery of stem cells, supporting his suggestion that these trophoblastic cells give rise to malignant cells of the adult, under the influence of carcinogenic chemicals, microbes, and radiation.

These new developments in homocysteine research are crucial to understanding the origin of degenerative diseases of aging. For many years these diseases have been understood by medical scientists to result from the interaction of nutrition, life style, and environmental toxins with the genetic endowment of individuals and populations.

Beginning in the early 20th century, with the observations of arteriosclerosis in experimental animals by Ignatowsky and by Antischkow and with the observations of heart disease by DeLangen in human populations, arteriosclerosis and heart disease have long been attributed to abnormalities of diet and nutrition [1]. The results of homocysteine research have clarified the role of cholesterol in arteriosclerosis as a factor that inactivates bacteria and viruses in the production of vulnerable plaques of the arteries by forming complexes with lipoproteins containing homocysteine groups. For many years the myth of the origin of arterial plaques from dietary cholesterol and fats has been a barrier to progress in understanding the cause of arteriosclerosis.

In contrast to the cholesterol hypothesis, the homocysteine theory of arteriosclerosis implicates deficiencies of folate, pyridoxal and cobalamin, resulting from methods of food processing, as important factors in the catastrophic increase in coronary heart disease in mid 20th century America. Similarly, the impressive decline in heart disease in the US since the 1960s is partly attributable to restoration of deficiencies of folate and pyridoxal through dietary supplementation and fortification of the food supply.

The more recent understanding of the importance of dietary sulfur deficiency and methionine inadequacy in vegetarians has called attention to the importance of adequate protein nutrition in controlling arteriosclerosis in these populations. This new understanding outlines a potential strategy for prevention of mortality in vegetarian populations, which suffer one half of deaths from heart disease worldwide. Thus the homocysteine theory of arteriosclerosis places sub-optimal nutrition, food processing, suppressed immunity, and susceptibility to infections as the cause of vulnerable plaques which directly produce the mortality and morbidity from heart disease, stroke, and generalized arteriosclerosis.

The conventional wisdom in contemporary cancer research places the origin of this disease in altered expression of the genetic information of DNA through mutation, the action of oncogenic viruses and bacteria, and the interaction of radiation energy and carcinogenic chemicals with the integrity and function of DNA. As explained in Chapter 10, the nutritional origin of cancer first implicated altered methionine metabolism as cause of cancer by demonstration of the cancer-inducing effects in animals of experimental diets that are deficient in choline, folate, and other methylating nutrients.

With our discovery of the blockade in conversion of the sulfur atom of homocysteine to sulfate in cultured malignant cells, a precise area of metabolism was identified to be critical in the carcinogenic process. The result of this metabolic blockade is over-production of homocysteine thiolactone from methionine in malignant cells. Thus the excessive production of homocysteine thiolactone induces the cancer profile in malignant cells by homocysteinylation of free amino groups of nucleic acids, proteins and glycosaminoglycans. These reactions produce genetic mutations and chromosomal abnormalities by reaction with DNA and altered expression of DNA genetic information by reaction with small inhibitory RNA molecules. The reactions of homocysteine thiolactone with nucleic acids cause aggregation and aneuploidy of chromosomes. Similar reactions alter protein structure and function, degrade cellular membranes, and alter connective tissues through overproduction of collagen, angiogenesis, inflammation, all through homocysteinylation of free amino groups of these macromolecules. The result is the malignant cell, as demonstrated by the characteristic pathological abnormalities in cancer that have been known since the 19th Century.

The carcinogenic effect of homocysteine thiolactone free base was directly demonstrated in the skin of mice, where application of this amino acid causes invasive squamous cell carcinoma of the skin cells of the epithelium. As described in Chapter 10, investigation of the anti-cancer effects of synthetic model compounds containing homocysteine thiolactone led to the discovery of thioretinamide, synthesized from retinoic acid and homocysteine thiolactone, and its complex with cobalamin to produce thioretinaco. The novel concept of oxidative metabolism catalyzing ATP synthesis by thioretinaco ozonide offers a new explanation of the origin of aerobic glycolysis of malignant cells, explaining the Warburg effect in molecular detail.

The recent elucidation of the molecular basis for biosynthesis of thioretinamide by cystathionine synthase from the retinol of transthyretin, and from dehydroascorbate led to the concept of deficient heme oxygenase function as the basis for selection and proliferation of malignant cells under the influence of carcinogens [2]. Some evidence for this concept is the recent discovery of deficiency of cystathionine synthase in malignant cells. In addition, demonstration of synthesis of chorionic gonadotrophic hormone by malignant cells supports their theoretical origin from trophoblastic cells.

These findings explain how decreased synthesis of retinoic acid from retinol and decreased synthesis of thioretinamide from retinoic acid, dehydroascorbate, and homocysteine thiolactone lead to deficiency of thioretinaco ozonide in malignant tissues. This deficiency is the cause of overproduction of homocysteine thiolactone from methionine in cancer cells. The effects of excess homocysteine thiolactone on DNA and RNA structure and function explain the origin of genetic changes, chromosomal abnormalities, and expression of altered genetic information in cancer cells.

As explained in Chapter 11, consumption of amygdalin and other plant nitrilosides is believed to have protective and therapeutic actions against human malignancies. The cyanide from these plant compounds is believed preferentially to inhibit growth of malignant cells by combining with thioretinaco ozonide, further reducing its concentration and making cancer cells non-viable [3]. Methionine and homocysteine are the principal source of sulfide, which reacts with cyanide to produce relatively non-toxic thiocyanate. Unlike normal cells, malignant cells accumulate cyanide from nitrilosides because they lack sufficient sulfotransferase enzyme rhodanese to catalyze normal thiocyanate synthesis from cyanide and thiosulfate. The presence of this enzyme in normal cells explains the preferential therapeutic action of nitrolosides in malignant tissues. Accumulation of cyanide is thereby prevented in normal cells, and cyanide production from nitrilosides in malignant cells explains the preferential therapeutic action of these dietary constituents in malignant tissues.

The dream of mankind since antiquity has been to delay inevitable death by slowing the aging process. Ancient Egyptians of the Sinai Peninsula and occupants of the Qumran settlement in ancient Judea operated metallurgical laboratories for the production of "white powder gold." This substance was fed to Egyptian Pharaohs and Judean Kings because of its supposed anti-aging properties. The archeological history of these discoveries is described in the recent book by Laurence Gardner, *Lost Secrets of the Sacred Ark. Amazing Revelations of the Incredible Power of Gold* [4].

The independent investigator David Radius Hudson claims to have discovered a form of precious metals, including gold that has unusual chemical and physical properties and resists analysis by conventional methods [5]. He claims that transition metals of the precious metal series, ruthenium, rhodium, palladium, silver, osmium, platinum and gold exist in a monoatomic form containing superdeformed nuclei in a high spin state with orbitally rearranged structures and superconductive properties. He furthermore claims that these substances have anti-AIDS, anti-cancer, and anti-aging activities in human subjects. Although Hudson was awarded a British patent for his process of producing "monoatomic precious metals," his claims have not been substantiated by physicists, chemists, or medical scientists [6]. Whether these substances are present in seawater, plants and animals, as some have claimed, has not been established by conventional scientists, leaving the ancient dreams of anti-aging by "white powder gold" unsubstantiated.

It is worth pointing out that the transitional metal cobalt is a constituent of cobalamin and its complex with thioretinamide, thioretinaco. For many years the precious metal complex, cis-diamminodichloro platinum (cisplatin) has been utilized as a critical component of several chemotherapy protocols for cancer therapy. Whether such complexes with other precious metal transition elements exist in tissues is presently unknown. Our investigation of anti-neoplastic compounds containing homocysteine thiolactone, as described in Chapter 10, showed that the transition metal element, rhodium, forms a complex with oxalyl chloride, and this complex has powerful anti-cancer properties.

In my monograph,"Chemical Pathology of Homocysteine. III. Cellular function and aging," I suggest that the aging process is related to gradual loss of thioretinaco ozonide from cellular membranes [7]. This original proposal is a novel concept that explains many features of the aging process, as described in Chapter 12. The features of accelerated aging, as observed in patients with homocystinuria, including arteriosclerosis, osteoporosis, osteoarthrosis, graying of hair, dementia, cataract, kidney failure, and pre-diabetes are explained as a result of decreased efficiency of homocysteine metabolism and increased oxidation of homocysteine with aging, secondary to loss of thioretinaco ozonide from membranes of mitochondria and other cellular organelles.

The lack of increased risk of cancer in subjects with homocystinuria may be explained by preservation of the heme oxygenase component of cystathionine synthase, allowing oxidation of retinol to retinoic acid, biosynthesis of thioretinamide, and formation of thioretinaco from thioretinamide and cobalamin. The decline in adenosyl methionine with aging is also attributable to loss of thioretinaco ozonide from cellular membranes, explaining the reduced methylation of DNA and N-acetyl serotonin, a precursor of melatonin, found in aging tissues.

Radiation energy, whether from radioactive elements like radium, uranium, or thorium, from external radiation sources like X-rays, cosmic rays, gamma rays from therapeutic radioactive nuclides like cobalt-60, or from exposure to ingested radionuclides, has long been known to shorten life span of humans and experimental animals. Some causes of shortened life span from radiation are leukemia and other malignancies, accelerated aging, infant mortality, and coronary heart disease.

A recent comprehensive monograph documents the effects of radionuclide contamination of the environment from the Chernobyl disaster on plants, animals, and human victims. The extraordinary book, *Chernobyl, consequences of the catastrophe for people and the environment,* by AV Yablokov, UB Nesterenko, and AV Nesterenko, was recently published in English translation by the New York Academy of Sciences [8]. This multi-authored study documents the effect of fallout from the Chernobyl nuclear power station meltdown in April 1986 on Ukraine, surrounding countries of Eastern Europe, and other countries of the Northern hemisphere. The technique of the studies, carried out by Eastern European scientists and physicians, is to compare the incidence and severity of disease, congenital abnormalities, mortality, and genetic effects in heavily contaminated areas, compared to less contaminated areas, providing an accurate estimate of the effect of radionuclides on health, disease, and mortality. According to this report, "No fewer than 3 billion persons inhabit areas contaminated by Chernobyl's radionuclides. More than 50% of the surface of 13 European countries and 30% of eight other countries [in the Northern hemisphere] have been contaminated." As it happened, my wife Annina and I were guests of the National Institute of Food and Nutrition in Warsaw, Poland in September 1986 for 10 days. The medical scientists at the Institute were gravely concerned about the adverse health effects of Chernobyl fallout on affected areas of Poland and adjacent countries.

In populations exposed to Chernobyl fallout, many features of accelerated aging were observed, including arteriosclerosis, osteoporosis, dementia, kidney failure, infections, inflammation of major organs, senile cataracts, presbyopia (far sightedness), hearing loss, diabetes, and balding. A wide variety of non-malignant diseases and conditions were demonstrated in areas of heavy contamination, especially brain damage, neuro-psychiatric disorders, cataracts, tooth decay, endocrine abnormalities like decreased thyroid function, decreased fertility, congenital abnormalities, increases in bacterial, viral and parasitic diseases, and many more.

Important increases in malignant diseases, especially leukemia, thyroid cancer, breast cancer, lung cancer, stomach cancer, skin cancer and rectal cancer were documented in heavily contaminated areas. Cancer mortality from Chernobyl was estimated at 245,000 deaths in Europe and 19,000 deaths in the rest of the Northern hemisphere. The overall death toll was conservatively estimated at 1 million victims in the 26 years since the disaster. Mortality was found to be especially high in newborns, and increased stillbirths, perinatal mortality, infant mortality, and total mortality were documented in heavily contaminated areas.

Closer to home, the contamination of the environment by radionuclides from production of nuclear weapons was described in the moving autobiography of Karl Z. Morgan, *The Angry Genie* [9]. Morgan was a founder of the field of health physics, the study of the effect of radiation on human health. During his dramatic career on the Manhattan Project, he witnessed the production of the atomic bomb, beginning with construction of the atomic pile at the University of Chicago to the construction of the Oak Ridge National Laboratory in Tennessee. Morgan was the first health physicist in the world, devoting his career to measurement of radiation exposure and development of methods to assess the damage of radiation on the human body.

Among his many achievements, Morgan directed the first system of monitoring of radiation exposure with film badges, analysis of workers' urine samples, a whole body counter, and a neutron dosimeter. He describes "the biggest mistake of my life" as his failure to advocate more strongly for the molten salt breeder reactor as a safer alternative to the liquid metal fast breeder reactor, because of political pressure from higher-ups at Oak Ridge National Laboratory. The problem of storage of waste fission products from nuclear power plants would be much less hazardous with his original design rather than the adopted design which "would allow billions of curies of fission products to remain in the reactor for the fuel lifetime, essentially waiting for an explosion (like those that later occurred at Three Mile Island and Chernobyl) to smear them around the world." The price of Morgan's mistake was creation of nuclear power reactors that created "rivers of radioactive waste."

While working in my position as Chief Pathologist and Director of Pathology and Laboratory Medicine at the VA Medical Center in Boston, I received an unsolicited shipment of a recently published book, *Radiation from medical procedures in the pathogenesis of cancer and ischemic heart disease,* by John W. Gofman, MD, PhD [10]. According to Karl Morgan, Gofman was "one of the leading scientists of the 20th Century. Along with Glenn Seaborg, Gofman co-discovered uranium-233, and he was also the first one to isolate plutonium." In the medical field Gofman is recognized as the scientist who discovered the correlation between the lipoprotein classes, LDL and HDL, and susceptibility to heart disease and arteriosclerosis. Through epidemiological and statistical studies of radiation exposure by medical procedures – X-rays, CT scans, radionuclide scans – Gofman's extensive studies show that cumulative radiation exposure from medical sources increases the risk of developing cancer and heart disease.

The Nobel Prize in Medicine was awarded to Herman J. Muller in 1946 for his discovery of the production of mutations by means of X-ray irradiation. In his lecture, he called attention to the random nature of radiation-induced mutations, the high frequency of recessive lethal mutations, and the frequency of chromosomal aberrations, such as translocations, inversion, and aneuploidy, from the genetic effects of radiation [11]. He also commented on the similarity of these abnormalities to those found in cells of malignant neoplasms. Because of his important work on the genetic effects of radiation, Muller served as a consultant to the Oak Ridge National Laboratory during development of the atomic bomb in the 1940s. Muller also collaborated with Guido Pontecorvo, the prominent geneticist with whom I studied microbial genetics and amino acid metabolism at Glasgow University from 1963-1964.

The effects of ionizing radiation or ultraviolet radiation on DNA, causing mutations and chromosomal abnormalities, have generally been attributed to alterations in the nucleotide sequence of DNA. These alterations are nucleotide substitutions affecting expression of genetic information of DNA, often associated with single strand breaks or double strand breaks of DNA molecules. In addition, the effects of radiation have been found to activate an extensive system of repair enzymes that correct the nucleotide substitutions or reconstitute single strand breaks of DNA. Double strand breaks are associated with chromosomal aberrations that cannot be repaired by the system of DNA repair enzymes, resulting in translocation of chromosomal fragments. It is noteworthy that elevation of plasma homocysteine from dietary folate vitamin B12 deficiency causes decreased DNA methylation and uracil incorporation, leading to genomic instability in human cells [12]. The effect of ionizing radiation is to flood the cells and tissues with reactive oxygen radical compounds and other free radicals which are counteracted by reaction with reduced glutathione and other cellular anti-oxidants.

Our discovery of thioretinamide and thioretinaco, the complex of thioretinamide with cobalamin, suggests the possibility that the genetic and chromosomal effects of ionizing radiation on DNA may be mediated by decomposition of cellular thioretinaco ozonide from absorption of radiation energy by the cobalt atom of this complex. The thermal neutron cross section of cobalt is several orders of magnitude higher than other common cellular elements, making thioretinaco particularly susceptible to decomposition by capture of radiation energy within target cells. Loss of thioretinaco ozonide cannot readily be replaced by biosynthesis, so cellular loss of this key compound from irradiated cells will result in production of excessive homocysteine thiolactone from methionine. The excessive homocysteine thiolactone produced within target cells will react with free amino groups of DNA, resulting in homocysteinylation of adenine and cytosine. The increased reaction of homocysteine with these nucleotides to produce peptide bonds will result in mutation in the case of single strand breakage, and chromosomal aberrations in the case of double strand breakage of DNA. Thus the mutational and chromosomal effects of radiation are attributable to cellular effects of homocysteine thiolactone production in cells with depletion of thioretinaco ozonide from cellular membranes. This formulation explains why the effects of radiation on cellular DNA mimic the mutational and chromosomal abnormalities found in malignant cells, since they are also depleted of thioretinaco ozonide during chemical, microbial and radiation carcinogenesis.

In his book, *Ignore the Awkward!* Uffe Ravnskov explains "how the cholesterol myth is kept alive [13]." In an extensively referenced and carefully argued exposition of the 100 year history of the cholesterol myth, he explains how proponents of this obsolete hypothesis "ignore contradictory evidence, exaggerate insignificant results, explain away awkward results, lie convincingly, ignore alternative explanations, ignore or humiliate the critics, and resort to industrial tricks."

According to another critic of the drug industry, Marcia Angell, the manipulation of clinical trials and the sponsorship of medical journals, medical research, and medical education by industry "makes a mockery of the traditional role of researchers as independent and impartial scientists [14]." The litany of industrial tricks to brainwash the public and the medical profession concerning the cholesterol myth includes direct financial payments to "opinion leaders" in the medical field, false advertisements, fake medical journals, and threats to reputable medical journals to withdraw income from advertising and reprints by the drug industry. The net result is a medical system that wastes untold billions of dollars on disproven and ineffective therapies, driving up the cost of US health care to the highest in the world by far.

Through lobbying and influence peddling in the US federal government, the mission of the Food and Drug Administration, the Department of Agriculture, the National Institutes of Health and others has been subverted by drug company lobbyists and insiders. To quote Ravnskov "The pharmaceutical industry has by far the largest lobby in Washington. In 2002 the number was 675 lobbyists, more than one for each member of Congress. They also knew how to exert an influence because 26 of the lobbyists were former Congress members, and 342 had been otherwise connected with government officials."

Industrial and medical influence peddling are not confined to supporters of the cholesterol myth. The cancer industry assiduously defends its turf against incursions by practitioners of nutritional and metabolic medicine. Chapter 11 describes how experimental demonstration of the efficacy of amygdalin against cancer growth in animals was deliberately sabotaged in order to cast doubt on the efficacy of this approach. In his book *World without Cancer. The vitamin B17 story,* Griffin describes in detail how influential medical scientists were mislead, and how government officials and the US Food and Drug Administration were able to ban the use of this plant constituent in cancer therapy and to outlaw its use in interstate commerce through US government legislation and regulations [3].

A contemporary example of the protection of its turf by the cancer industry is the deliberate sabotage of the clinical trial of nutritional and metabolic therapy of pancreatic cancer by officials of the National Cancer Institute, the National Institutes of Health, and

Columbia University. In his recent book, *What Went Wrong* Nicholas Gonzalez painted the picture of sabotage of a clinical trial in excruciating detail [15]. Participants with pancreatic cancer were randomized into a group to be treated by conventional surgery, radiation, and chemotherapy, in comparison with a group to be treated with nutritional and metabolic therapy. By violating the guidelines of the trial protocol, the principal investigator was able to select subjects for the nutritional group with far advanced cancer who could not possibly benefit from nutritional therapy. In addition, the principal investigator was a collaborator on chemotherapy trials, rendering him biased and unqualified to direct the trial because of this conflict of interest.

It was significant that supporters of the pancreatic cancer trial in the US Congress had limited ability to call officials of the National Cancer Institute, the Office of Research Integrity and other governmental bureaucracies on the carpet for the glaring violations of the protocol of this clinical trial. The result was a surreptitious publication of the flawed results favoring traditional cancer chemotherapy over nutritional-metabolic therapy. Tactics like this amount to stone-walling of new ideas that do not fit with the conventional wisdom of the cancer industry and threaten the profits of the pharmaceutical industry.

Abnormal homocysteine metabolism has been demonstrated in an impressive and lengthy list of degenerative diseases and conditions. The more important include arteriosclerosis, stroke, acute coronary syndrome, cancer, osteoporosis and fracture, dementia and other neurodegenerative diseases, autoimmune diseases such as lupus erythematosus, ulcerative colitis, thyroiditis and pernicious anemia, venous thrombosis and pulmonary embolism, retinal vein thrombosis, hypothyroidism, accelerated aging, renal failure and uremia, diabetes mellitus, metabolic syndrome, macular degenerative, severe psoriasis, organ transplantation with therapeutic immune suppression, protein energy malnutrition, familial or spontaneous amyloidosis, dietary vitamin deficiencies of folate, pyridoxal, and cobalamin, complications of pregnancy such as pre-ecclampsia and placenta previa, and congenital birth defects, including neural tube defects, cleft palate, and congenital heart disease.

The etiology of many of these diseases and conditions is incompletely understood. However, many of these chronic degenerative diseases are strongly correlated with the aging process. The importance of deficiencies of thioretinaco ozonide in cells of aging tissues was discussed in Chapter 12. Regardless of etiology, however, elevation of plasma homocysteine levels and homocysteinylation of macromolecules in degenerative diseases are susceptible to therapeutic intervention by preservation of cellular oxidative metabolism through increased production of thioretinaco ozonide and by enhanced catabolism of homocysteine produced through degradation of homocysteinylated macromolecules by pancreatic enzymes.

In order to facilitate the application of homocysteine research to control of these diseases and conditions, I recently applied for a US patent regarding utilization of thioretinamide in therapy of degenerative diseases of aging [16]. My invention consists of administration of thioretinamide and other carefully selected components to enhance synthesis of thioretinaco ozonide by aging cells and tissues, combined with pancreatic enzymes and pro-enzymes to degrade the homocysteinylated macromolecules of these cells and tissues.

Besides thioretinamide and pancreatic enzymes, the other components of the program consist of vitamins, supplements, and foods. The vitamins folate, pyridoxal and cobalamin are used to enhance the activity of cystathionine synthase and methionine synthase. Adenosyl methionine is used to activate cystathionine synthase and suppress methylenetetrahydrofolate reductase by allosteric effects. Essential amino acids including tryptophan are used to enhance synthesis of transthyretin by the liver. Ascorbate with mixed flavonoids is used to catalyze oxidation of retinol to retinoic acid by superoxide. Nitrilosides such as amygdalin are used to provide cyanide to combine with hydrogen sulfide produced by the actions of cystathionine synthase and cystathionase on homocysteine and cystathionine, respectively. Retinol is employed as a precursor to retinoic acid and thioretinamide, synthesized by cystathionine synthase in aging cells and tissues. Unsaturated n-3 oils from fish or seeds are employed to lower homocysteine levels; menaquinone is used to prevent dystrophic calcification; and vitamin D3 is used to stabilize mitochondrial thioretinaco ozonide.

This metabolic program of thioretinamide, enhanced biosynthesis of thioretinaco ozonide, and enhanced homocysteine catabolism by pancreatic enzymes will decrease accumulation of homocysteinylated macromolecules in aging cells and tissues. The program will also decrease the oxidative stress associated with accumulation of homocysteine and inhibition of oxidative metabolism found in human degenerative diseases through increased biosynthesis of thioretinaco ozonide. In diseases exacerbated by a microbial etiology, such as arteriosclerosis and dementia, use of appropriate antibiotics and saturated medium chain triglycerides counteracts microbial growth and inflammation. This strategy will facilitate resolution of pathological lesions by catabolism of homocysteinylated macromolecules by enzyme and metabolic therapy.

Comprehensive dietary improvement will provide an essential component of nutritional and metabolic therapy. Dietary improvement, as described in Chapter 9 and in *The Heart Revolution,* consists of elimination of processed industrial foods, additives like sugar, fructose, alcohol and glutamate, combined with fresh, raw or lightly cooked vegetables and fruits, ample fresh seafoods, dairy products and fresh meats to provide dietary methionine, and foods containing nitrilosides to catabolize hydrogen sulfide. This diet of real, nutritious food will form the basis for prevention and treatment of degenerative diseases.

The impact of this nutritional and metabolic program upon patients with arteriosclerosis or cancer will be studied in a recently approved clinical trial, the Saudi Arabia Homocysteine Arteriosclerosis Cancer Trial (SAHACT) to be conducted at the Prince Sultan Cardiac Care Hospital in Al Hasa, Saudi Arabia. I was privileged to attend and present lectures at the 2010 King of Organs Conference on Heart Disease at this state-of-the-art ultra modern facility with a talented staff of clinicians and medical investigators. Such a trial could not be conducted in the USA because of objections and criticisms of the cholesterol cartel and the cancer industry.

In reflecting upon the lessons learned from the vicissitudes of my career in medical science, it is apparent to me that scientists, doctors, and industrialists in the biomedical field adhere to outmoded and disproven theories because of intellectual and commercial self interest. The scientist is unwilling to part with a pet theory that was nurtured by a life time of investigation and publication, even when contradictory facts invalidate his assumptions and convictions. The doctor is unwilling to attempt new approaches to therapy of disease, even though his present convictions about the validity of his approach conflict with mounting evidence of toxicity or ineffectiveness of conventional therapy. The industrialist rejects new theories and new treatments of disease that threaten to cut his profits because of rejection of his obsolete pharmaceutical agents by the marketplace. Only when productive new theories, improved treatment, and more effective drugs become available, does the younger generation reject outmoded conventional wisdom and disproved theories.

The pace of advancement of medical is often painfully slow because of the years needed for the older generation of medical scientists to be replaced by the younger generation, who understand the new paradigm and are no longer attached to the outmoded and disproven theories and assumptions of the past. As expressed by the physicist, Max Planck, "A new scientific truth does not triumph by convincing its opponents and making them see the light, but rather because its opponents eventually die, and a new generation grows up that is familiar with it." My experiences in medical science are an apt illustration of Arthur Schopenhauer's analysis of the search for truth, "All truth passes through three stages. First, it is ridiculed. Second, it is violently opposed. Third, it is accepted as being self-evident."

What is the legacy of the new understanding of the cause of disease revealed by homocysteine research? My belief is that prevention and treatment of degenerative diseases of aging must be accomplished through metabolic and nutritional control, based on discoveries and concepts regarding the fundamental role of homocysteine metabolism in the aging process. Pharmaceutical agents that are designed to minimize symptoms or suppress manifestations of degenerative disease are doomed to failure. These agents do not address or correct the underlying causes of these diseases or conditions and thus remain ineffective and disappointing in their control. Only a rational system of metabolic and nutritional control of the disease process will be effective in prevention and treatment of these diseases. Homocysteine research provides a rationale of efficacy because of the increased understanding of the pathogenesis of degenerative diseases.

REFERENCES

[1] McCully KS. Hyperhomocysteinemia and arteriosclerosis: historical perspectives. *Clinical Chemistry and Laboratory Medicine*, 2005;43:980-986.

[2] McCully KS. Chemical Pathology of Homocysteine. V. Thioretinamide, thioretinaco, and cystathionine synthase function in degenerative diseases. *Annals of Clinical and Laboratory Science*, 2011;41:301-314.

[3] Griffin GE. *World without Cancer. The Story of Vitamin B17*. 2d Ed. Westlake Village CA: American Media, 2009.

[4] Gardner L. *Lost Secrets of the Sacred Ark. Amazing Revelations of the Incredible Powers of Gold.* London: HarperCollins, 2003.

[5] Hudson DR. Lecture to the International Forum on New Science, Ft. Collins CO, 1995. www.halexandria.org/dward467.htm

[6] Hudson DR. Non-metallic monoatomic forms of transition elements. British Patent GB 2,219,995A, December 28, 1989.

[7] McCully KS. Chemical Pathology of Homocysteine. III. Cellular function and aging. *Annals of Clinical and Laboratory Science*, 1994;24:134-152.

[8] Yablokov AV, Nesterenko VB, Nesterenko AV. *Chernobyl. Consequences of the Catastrophe for People and the Environment.* New York: New York Academy of Sciences, 2009. Vassily B. Nesterenko was the Director of the Byelorussian Nuclear Center, who died in 2008. He and his son, Alexy V. Nesterenko have the same name as my grandmother Maria Litwinenco's maiden name: Nesterenko. My grandmother was originally from a family living in Odessa, Ukraine before her emigration with my grandfather to the pioneer farm in South Dakota in 1890.

[9] Morgan KZ, Peterson KM. *The Angry Genie. One Man's Walk through the Nuclear Age*. Norman OK: University of Oklahoma Press, 1999.
[10] Gofman JW. *Radiation from Medical Procedures in the Pathogenesis of Cancer and Ischemic Heart Disease*. San Francisco CA: Committee for Nuclear Responsibility, Inc., 1999.
[11] Muller HJ. The production of mutations. *Nobel Lecture*, December 12, 1946.
[12] Fenech M. The role of folic acid and vitamin B12 in genomic stability of human cells. *Mutation Research,* 2001;475:57-57.
[13] Ravnskov U. *Ignore the Awkward! How the Cholesterol Myths are Kept Alive*. Lexington KY, 2010.
[14] Angell M. *The Truth about the Drug Companies. How They Deceive Us and What To Do About It.* New York: Random House, 2004.
[15] Gonzalez N. *What Went Wrong*. New York: New Spring Press, 2012. The book explains in excruciating detail how a promising clinical trial of nutritional and enzymatic therapy of human pancreatic cancer was systematically sabotaged by the National Cancer Institute, the National Institutes of Health, the National Center for Complementary and Alternative Medicine, and Columbia University.
[16] McCully KS. Compositions and method for utilization of thioretinamide in therapy of degenerative diseases of aging. US Patent Application S.N. 13/067,504. Filed June, 2011.

GLOSSARY

Acetate: A two carbon acid produced by metabolism of carbohydrates and proteins of foods and used for synthesis of cholesterol and fatty acids by liver and other organs.

Acetyl choline: An important neurotransmitter compound formed from acetate and choline.

Acute coronary syndrome: Heart disease caused by narrowing of coronary arteries and producing myocardial infarct or angina pectoris.

Adenocarcinoma: A malignant tumor originating in glandular or ductal epithelial cells.

Adenosyl methionine: A coenzyme formed from adenosine and methionine by the reaction of ATP and methionine, catalyzed by the methionine activating enzyme of Cantoni, responsible for transmethylation reactions and allosteric regulation of enzymes that metabolize homocysteine.

Adenosyl cobalamin. The coenzyme form of vitamin B12 responsible for methyl malonic acid synthesis.

Aflatoxin: A toxin produced by *Aspergillus* molds, a common contaminant of peanuts.

Amide: A chemical group consisting of nitrogen and hydrogen atoms adjacent to a carbonyl group.

Amino acid: The building block constituents of proteins, each containing an amino group, a carboxyl group, and another group confering specific properties on the amino acid.

Aneuploidy: An abnormal number of chromosomes within dividing cells.

Angina pectoris: Chest pain caused by insufficient blood circulation within coronary arteries of the heart, related to narrowing of arteries by arteriosclerosis or low blood perfusion of heart muscle.

Angiogenesis: The process by which malignant tumors or inflammation causes formation of new blood vessels within tissues of the body.

Anti-atherogenic: A substance that prevents or diminishes atherosclerosis.

Anti-neoplastic: A substance that prevents or diminishes tumors.

Aorta: The major artery of the body carrying blood from the heart to the major arterial branches and supplying the organs of the body.

Arachidonic acid: A highly unsaturated n-6 essential fatty acid used for synthesis of the cytokines, prostaglandins, thromboxanes and leukotrienes.

Arginine: The essential amino acid that forms nitric oxide by the action of nitric oxide synthase and participates in metabolism of nitrogen compounds.

Arteriosclerosis: Hardening and narrowing of the arteries caused by fibrous arterial plaques or fibro-calcific arterial plaques.

Ascorbic acid: The acid form of vitamin C which forms ascorbate when neutralized.

Aspergillus nidulans: A common mold used in experimental genetic analysis.

Atherosclerosis: A form of arteriosclerosis characterized by fibrolipid arterial plaques.

ATP: Adenosine triphosphate, the coenzyme produced by oxidative metabolism in mitochondria that provides energy for cellular enzyme reactions. **ADP** contains one fewer phosphate groups than ATP and combines with phosphate to produce ATP in oxidative metabolism.

Auto-antibody: An antibody directed against an antigen arising from constituent macromolecules of body tissues.

Autoimmune disease: A disease arising by immune reaction against antigens of body tissues.

Betaine: A form of the amino acid glycine containing methyl groups that convert homocysteine to methionine by the enzyme betaine methyl transferase.

Bleomycin hydrolase: A cellular enzyme that hydrolyzes homocysteine thiolactone to homocysteine and hydrolyzes the chemotherapeutic antibiotic drug bleomycin.

C-reactive protein: Protein synthesized by liver in response to inflammation capable of binding to oxidized LDL enhancing phagocytosis of LDL aggregates by macrophages.

Calcium: Element deposited in arterial plaques forming fibrocalcific plaques.

Cancer: Malignant cells tissues derived from normal cells and capable of invading and spreading through normal organs and tissues of the body.

Carotid artery: Artery in the neck that supplies blood to the brain.

Carbon 14: C14 is a radioactive isotope of carbon used in investigation of metabolism.

Carbonyl: Chemical group containing carbon and oxygen derived from carboxyl group.

Carcinogen: Chemical, microbial or physical agent capable of converting normal cells to malignant cells.

Carpal tunnel syndrome: Painful condition of hand fingers and wrist caused by compression of blood vessels and nerves by the carpal ligament of the wrist.

Cataract: Opacification of the optic lens of the eye caused by ultraviolet radiation, free radicals, and the aging process.

Cellular respiration: Metabolic process by which cells combine electrons of acetyl-coenzyme A of carbohydrates with oxygen to produce ATP, water and carbon dioxide.

Charge transfer complex: Combination of two different molecules that share electrons in overlapping orbitals, causing a shift in the wavelength of light absorption.

Chelation therapy: Controversial intravenous therapy for removal of heavy metals and calcium of arterial plaques by sodium ethylenediaminetetracetate (EDTA).

Chlamydia pneumoniae: Intracellular microbe infecting lungs and arterial plaques.

Cholesterol: Polycyclic hydrocarbon alcohol contained in all cell membranes and lipoproteins of animals and humans.

Cholesterol oxides: Oxidized forms of cholesterol such as cholesterol triol, hydroxyl-cholesterol, and cholestanone formed by oxidative metabolism of cholesterol.

Choline: Constituent of lecithin containing methyl groups for transfer to homocysteine to form methionine and to prevent fat accumulation in liver.

Chondrocyte: The constituent cell of cartilage tissues.

Chorionic gonadotropin: Hormone formed by placental cells that stimulate the ovaries to produce progesterone. Produced by malignant cells and choriocarcinoma cells.

Chromosome: Nucleoprotein structures of the nucleus containing genetic information of DNA.

Circadian rhythm: The cycle of brain function and metabolism related to waking and sleeping, controlled by melatonin secretion of the pineal gland.

Cirrhosis: A fibrotic disease of liver caused by toxins or infections.

Cisplatin: A chemotherapeutic drug containing platinum complexed with ammonia and chloride groups.

Clonal senescence: Process by which cells stop growing after multiple passages in cell culture.

Cobalamin: Vitamin B12 containing cobalt atom responsible for methylation reactions and methyl malonate synthesis in mammalian cells.

Cobalamin C disease: Inherited metabolic disease characterized by elevated homocysteine and cystathionine and decreased methionine in plasma, caused by intracellular deficiency of methionine synthase function.

Column chromatography: A method for separating chemicals by adherence from solutions when applied to columns of resins or adsorbents.

Contact inhibition: Process by which cultured cells stop growing when in contact with adjacent cells.

Coronary heart disease: Disease of the heart caused by narrowing of the coronary arteries by arterial plaques.

Cyanide: Toxic molecule containing carbon and nitrogen capable of combining with metal atoms such as the iron of hemoglobin or respiratory enzymes and the cobalt atom of thioretinaco ozonide to inhibit oxidative phosphorylation.

Cystathionine: Sulfur compound discovered by Vincent DuVigneaud formed by enzymatic combination of homocysteine and serine.

Cystathionine synthase: Enzyme that catalyzes synthesis of cystathionine from homocysteine and serine.

Cysteine: Sulfur amino acid containing three carbon atoms, sulfhydryl group, amino group and carboxyl group. Forms a mixed disulfide with homocysteine by oxidation.

Cytomegalovirus: A ubiquitous virus infecting cells and causing very large intranuclear inclusions.

Cytoplasm: The portion of the cell within the plasma membrane and excluding the nucleus, containing specialized organelles which support function of the cell.

Degenerative disease of aging: Diseases related to the aging process, including cancer, arteriosclerosis, osteoporosis, dementia, autoimmune disease, and other diseases.

Dehydroepiandrosterone: An androgen produced by the adrenal gland that is diminished during aging.

Dementia: Loss of cognitive function of the brain caused by arteriosclerosis, Alzheimer's disease, infections, and neurodegenerative diseases.

Diabetes mellitus: A disease of glucose metabolism caused by insufficient secretion of insulin by the pancreas (Type I) or resistance to the effect of insulin (Type II).

Dialysis: A process for separating large and small molecules in solution by a membrane.

Diploid: Cell containing two sets of chromosomes, one from each parent.

Dislocated lenses: Displacement of optic lens of the eye found in homocystinuria and in Marfan's syndrome.

DNA Deoxyribonucleotide polymer containing genetic code in the sequence of its nucleotides.

Dyslipidemia: A condition in which LDL is elevated and HDL is depressed in plasma, related to infection or to progression of atherosclerosis.

Dysplasia: An abnormality of cells characterized by irregular chromatin of nucleus, enlarged nucleus and nucleolus, loss of cytoplasm and displacement from normal location within tissues. Dysplasia may progress to malignancy under the influence of carcinogens.

Elastin: Elastic tissue layers giving elasticity to arteries, veins, lungs and other tissues.

Embryogenesis: Process by which the embryo is produced from a fertilized ovum.

Endothelial dysfunction: Swelling and abnormal function of endothelial cells that line the interior surface of arteries and veins, produced by homocysteine and other factors, generally considered to be the earliest manifestation of arteriosclerosis.

Epidermal growth factor: A protein that stimulates growth of epidermal cells and other epithelial cells, involved in stimulation of cancer cell growth.

Erythropoiesis: Production of red blood cells by bone marrow.

Esterase: An enzyme that hydrolyzes esters. Esterases convert homocysteine thiolactone to homocysteine.

Estrogen: Female sex hormone produced by the ovary responsible for endometrial growth and secondary sex characteristics of tissues.

Ethyl carbamate (urethane): A chemical carcinogen that produces lung tumors in strain A mice.

Excitotoxin: Amino acids including cysteine, homocysteine, aspartate, and glutamate that excite nerve activity and cause necrosis of nerve cells.

Extracellular matrix: Proteinaceous substance produced by cells and released into surrounding connective tissues.

Fibrin thrombus: A mass of polymerized fibrin protein derived from prothrombin by the blood coagulation process, causing obstruction of arteries and veins.

Fibrolipid plaque: Arterial plaque of atherosclerosis containing fibrous tissue and lipid deposits.

Fibrous histiocytoma: A benign tumor of connective tissues consisting of fibrous tissue and histiocytes, also exists as a malignant version in rare cases.

Flouride: Toxic anion derived from the element fluorine and produced by dissolving fluoride salts or fluosilicic acid in water.

Fluoroacetate: Gifblaar poison derived from poisonous South African plants inactivating aconitase, one of the enzymes of the tricarboxylic acid cycle of metabolism.

Fluosilicic acid: Toxic byproduct of the fertilizer industry commonly used for fluoridation of drinking water.

Folate: Vitamin B9 required for transfer of methyl groups to cobalamin and homocysteine to produce methionine, also required for synthesis of the nucleotide bases of DNA.

Folic acid: The synthetic form of vitamin B9 that is converted to folate in the body, used for fortification of flour and other refined grain foods in the US and Canada since 1998.

Free radical: Reactive form of a molecule containing an unpaired electron, arising from oxidative metabolism.

Gallstone: Calculus of gall bladder consisting of free cholesterol or the degraded blood pigment bilirubin.

Gangrene: Death of tissues of toes or legs or other parts of the body caused by obstruction of blood flow in arteries affected by arteriosclerosis and thrombosis.

Gene: The part of DNA coding for production of a specific protein.

Genetic polymorphism: Occurrence of different types of mutations of a single gene, occurring in individuals of populations.

Glutamate and aspartate: Excitotoxic anion forms of the amino acids glutamic acid and aspartic acid.

Glutathione: Intracellular tripeptide containing cysteine, glycine and glutamine and providing the major cellular defense against oxidation and oxidative stress.

Glycolysis: Form of metabolism of carbohydrates that produces lactate.

Glycosaminoglycans: Polymerized carbohydrate substances of extracellular matrix containing free amino groups, and sulfate groups.

Growth hormone: Pituitary hormone causes growth of cartilage, bone, and other tissues during growth and development.

Haploid: Cell containing one set of chromosomes from one parent.

Heart disease: Abnormal function of the heart most commonly produced by narrowing of coronary arteries by arteriosclerotic plaques.

Heme oxygenase: An enzyme containing an iron heme group capable of producing oxygenation of metabolic products. The constituent of cystathionine synthase that produces superoxide.

Hemorrhage: Leakage of blood from within blood vessels into surrounding tissues.

Herpesvirus: A type of virus causing ubiquitous infections like cold sores.

Heterozygous: A type of cell containing different alleles of a gene, one from each parent.

Homocysteine: Amino acid containing four carbon atoms, a sulfhydryl group, an amino group and a carboxyl group. **Homocystine** is dimerized homocysteine produced by oxidation of the sulfhydryl groups. **Homocysteine thiolactone** is the reactive cyclic anhydride of homocysteine. **Homocysteic acid** is the fully oxidized sulfonic acid form derived from homocysteine. **Homocysteine diketopiperazine** is a cyclic form of two molecules of homocysteine formed by hydrolysis of homocysteine thiolactone by weak alkali, containing free sulfhydryl groups and forming insoluble polymers with oxidation.

Homocysteinylation: Combination of homocysteine with a macromolecule by reaction of homocysteine thiolactone with free amino group to form a peptide bond. The homocysteinylation process results in a free sulfhydryl group, thus termed **thiolation.**

Homocystinuria: The inherited metabolic disease most commonly resulting from abnormality of cystathionine synthase, causing urinary excretion of homocystine.

Hydrocarbon: Molecule containing carbon and hydrogen. **Polycyclic hydrocarbon** is a complex form of carbon and hydrogen, some of which are carcinogenic.

Hyperlipemia: Elevate plasma levels of lipoproteins, also called **hyperlipidemia.**

Hydrolysis: Introduction of a water molecule into a molecule, catalyzed by acid, base, or enzymes.

Hyperhomocysteinemia: Elevation of blood homocysteine levels in the plasma.

Hypertension: Elevated blood pressure affecting arteries of the general circulation or the pulmonary circulation.

Hypothalamus: A specialized area of the diencephalon that controls secretion of hormones, regulation of vascular tone, water balance, sleep and other functions.

Hypothyroidism: Condition of decreased metabolic activity caused by decreased secretion of thyroid hormone, secondary to decreased thyrotropic hormone, thiouracil, isoflavones, thiocyanate, and other toxins or by destruction of the thyroid gland.

Indole acetic acid: An amino acid that functions as a plant growth hormone.

Inflammation: A pathologic process by which cells, blood vessels, and cytokines respond to microbes invading cells and tissues of the body.

Insulin: A polypeptide hormone produced by the beta cells of the pancreatic islets that controls glucose metabolism by lowering plasma glucose and transporting glucose into cells.

Insulin-like growth factor: A polypeptide hormone produced by liver under the influence of growth hormone, increasing sulfate binding to cartilage cells, previously known as **sulfation factor** or **somatomedin.**

Ionizing radiation: A form of radiation energy that splits molecules into charged ions.

Keratin: Specialized protein produced by skin epidermal cells and containing sulfur. **Keratinization:** Conversion of glandular cells into cells producing keratin by the process of metaplasia.

Kidney failure: Loss of function of the kidneys producing uremia, oxidative stress, and hyperhomocysteinemia.

Lactate: The neutralized form of lactic acid, a product of glycolysis of glucose by carbohydrate metabolism.

Laetrile: A synthetic form of **amygdalin**, a cyanogenic component of fruits, grasses, and seeds containing a cyanide group, benzaldehyde and glucosides.

Lanosterol: A steroid component of wool fat that is a precursor in the biosynthesis of cholesterol.

Lathyrism: An experimental disease of connective tissues produced by beta propionitrile, a toxic constituent of sweet peas, *Lathyrus odoratus.*

Lecithin: A phospholipid containing choline, found in egg yolk and soybeans, used for emulsification and preservation.

Leiomyosarcoma: A malignant tumor arising from smooth muscle cells.

Leukemia: A cancer of the white blood cells originating in the bone marrow. Closely related diseases are **aplastic anemia** affecting red blood cells of bone marrow and **mycosis fungoides** affecting epidermis and superficial layers of the skin.

Lipid: A fatty substance containg fatty acids, triglycerides, or steroids that is insoluble in water.

Lipoprotein: A plasma particle containing protein and lipid. **Low-density lipoprotein (LDL)** has increased bouancy and **high-density lipoproteine (HDL)** has decreased bouancy in ultracentrifuge preparations of plasma.

Liposome: A particle containing lipids that encloses a non-lipid in an emulsion, used to transport drugs into cells, may contain fatty acids, cholesterol esters, phospholipids, and polyglycols.

Lymphatics: Thin walled vessels of tissues, lined by endothelial cells, which transport lymph from the extracellular fluid to the venous circulation.

Macrophages: Cells derived from **monocytes** form **foam cells** by phagocytosis of lipoprotein aggregates containing microbes during formation of arterial plaques.

Maleic anhydride: A chemical used in the synthesis of **maleyl homocysteine thiolactone imide**, an active anti-neoplastic compound activated by liposomes.

Marfan's syndrome: An abnormality of growth causing long arms and legs with increased elasticity and dislocated lenses of the eye, originally confused with **homocystinuria** because of dislocated lenses and elongated extremities.

Megaloblastosis: Red cell forming cells of bone marrow assuming a characteristic abnormality of maturation, caused by dietary deficiency of vitamin B12 or folate.

Melanin: The dark brown skin pigment produced by melanocytes of skin, stimulated by the hormone melatonin produced by the pineal gland.

Messenger RNA: The ribonucleic acid polymer that copies the genetic code and directs the synthesis of protein molecules by binding to ribosomes to form polyribosomes.

Metabolic syndrome: A common abnormality of human metabolism consisting of insulin resistance, obesity and hypertension, related to consumption of processed carbohydrates, including high fructose corn syrup.

Metabolism: The chemical processing of foods by cellular enzymes.

Metachromasia: A shift of wavelength of absorption of light caused by a charge-transfer complex between molecules.

Methionine: An essential four carbon amino acid containing a methyl group attached to the sulfur atom which produces homocysteine by metabolic removal of the methyl group.

Methionine synthase: An enzyme that catalyzes transfer of a methyl group from methylcobalamin (vitamin B12) to homocysteine to produce methionine.

Methionyl acyl synthase: An enzyme that attaches methionine to transfer RNA and produces homocysteine thiolactone by an error editing reaction.

Methylenetetrahydrofolate reductase: An enzyme that reduces methylenetetrahydrofolate to methyltetrahydrofolate, which gives a methyl group to cobalamin for the synthesis of methylcobalamin, required for conversion of homocysteine to methionine by transmethylation.

Methyl group: A chemical group containing one carbon atom and three hydrogen atoms, transferred to different metabolites by transmethylation from adenosyl methionine.

Methylmalonic acid: A metabolite excreted in the urine associated with dietary deficiency of vitamin B12 or with cobalamin C disease and other inherited diseases.

Monolaurin: A triglyceride fat formed from the medium chain fatty acid lauric acid that has anti-microbial properties.

Mutation: An abnormality of a specific gene causing an abnormality of an enzyme or other protein, caused by **mutagenesis.**

Myelocyte: An immature bone marrow cell that produces white cells of the granulocytic series.

Myocardial infarct: Death of part of the heart muscle caused by obstruction of coronary artery by arterial plaques and thrombosis.

Necrosis: Cellular or tissue death caused by lack of blood and oxygen or by toxins.

Neural tube: The part of the embryo that forms the spinal cord and brain during embryogenesis, abnormality of which is caused by homocysteine related to dietary deficiency of folate.

Neutrophil: A white blood cell with a multilobated nucleus that kills microbes by phagocytosis and secretion of reactive oxygen species.

Nitric oxide: A gas consisting of nitrogen and oxygen produced from arginine by nitric oxide synthase, causing relaxation of smooth muscle, decreased blood pressure, and decreased blood clotting from decreased activation of platelets.

Nitrilosides: Components of grasses, fruits, seeds, containing cyanide groups and glucoside groups, consisting of **amygdalin, dhurrin, lotaustralin, and linamarin.**

NMDA (N-methyl-D-aspartate) receptor: A neurotransmitter receptor activated by NMDA or homocysteine, causing excitotoxicity.

NNT (number needed to treat): A statistical number relating the number of subjects required by drug treatment to produce a positive outcome in one subject.

Nucleotides: The components of ribonucleic acid (RNA) and deoxyribonucleic acid (DNA) consisting of four bases, adenine, guanine, cytosine, uracil (RNA) or thymine (DNA) attached to a sugar phosphate polymer backbone, transmitting the genetic code by nucleotide sequences within DNA and RNA.

Nucleus: The portion of a cell containing nucleoprotein surrounded by the nuclear membrane and containing a nucleolus, responsible for production of RNA.

Oncolytic: Property of suppression of cancer growth.

Oleic acid: Monounsaturated fatty acid. **Linoleic acid**: Diunsaturated fatty acid.

Osteoarthrosis: Degenerative disease of joints consisting of thinning of cartilage and destruction of joint function, a comparable term to **osteoarthritis.**

Osteoporosis: Loss of minerals, thinning and weakening of bones related to aging, as found in subjects with homocystinuria.

Oxalyl chloride: Reactive bifunctional chemical that produces oxalyl homocysteine thiolactone by reaction with homocysteine and forms a complex with rhodium trichloride with anti-neoplastic properties.

Oxidative phosphorylation: Metabolic process of mitochondria by which ADP and phosphate are linked to form ATP from energy produced by reduction of oxygen by electrons from foods, as supplied by electron transport and catalyzed by thioretinaco ozonide.

Oxidative stress: Reaction of radicals with cellular constituents caused by excess production of oxygen radicals by metabolism, radiation, aging and various diseases.

Oxygen: Compound formed from two atoms of oxygen.

Oxygen difluoride: Highly toxic gas that inhibits oxidative metabolism by displacing ozone from thioretinaco ozonide, sensitive to decomposition by water vapor.

Oxygen radicals: Highly reactive oxygen compounds containing unpaired electrons.

Ozone: Highly reactive oxidizing gas formed from three atoms of oxygen.

Pancreatic enzymes: Digestive enzymes of pancreatic secretions containing amylase, trypsin, chymotrypsin, lipase, ribonuclease, deoxyribonuclease, elastase, hyaluronidase, and other enzymes.

Papilloma: Tumor caused by infection with papilloma virus, causing cervical cancer, warts of skin, and venereal warts in humans.

Paraoxonase: The esterase enzyme constituent of HDL that hydrolyzes the insecticide paraoxane and hydrolyzes homocysteine thiolactone to homocysteine.

Pellagra: Vitamin deficiency disease consisting of dermatitis, dementia and diarrhea, caused by lack of dietary niacin.

Peritonitis: Inflammation of the lining of the abdominal cavity caused by infection or chemical irritation.

Peroxide: Reactive form of compounds containing excess oxygen atoms.

Phagocytosis: Process by which microbes are engulfed within the cytoplasm of white blood cells.

Phenotype: The expression of genetic characteristics in an organism. **Genotype** is the genetic composition that directs formation of the phenotype of an organism.

Phosphoadenosine phosphosulfate: The sulfating coenzyme formed from sulfate and ATP responsible for transfer of sulfate groups to glycosaminoglycans, steroid hormones, and toxins in the liver. Also formed from thioretinamide by oxidation with superoxide.

Phlebothrombosis: Obstruction of veins by thrombi from blood coagulation.

Phytates: Phosphorus polymers of soybeans and other plant foods that chelate minerals and inhibit their absorption by the intestine.

Phytochemicals: Complex constituents of plant foods that function as anti-oxidants and other functions when consumed in the diet.

Phytoestrogens: Constituents of soybeans and other legumes consisting of genestein, diadzin, isoflavones, causing precocious puberty and decreased fertility.

Pineal gland: A gland located within the brain that secretes melatonin and regulates diurnal cycles and melanin synthesis in the skin.

Pituitary gland: The endocrine master gland located at the base of the brain responsible for secretion of thyrotropic hormone, growth hormone, prolactin, follicle stimulating hormone, pitressin, oxytocin and other hormones.

Platelet: The cellular fragments in blood responsible for activation of blood coagulation and formation of thrombi.

Polyribosomes: Polymers of messenger RNA and ribosomes that provide the template for protein synthesis from transfer RNA molecules containing amino acids.

Polyterpenes: Polymers of 5 carbon unsaturated terpenoid units from **mevalonate, squalene, geranyl phosphate** and other intermediates in the biosynthesis of cholesterol from acetate in liver and other tissues.

Polyunsaturated fatty acids: Long chain essential fatty acids containing conjugated double bonds starting at the n-3 or n-6 positions.

Porphyomonas gingivalis: An infectious microbe of the oral cavity found in arterial plaques.

Progesterone: The steroid hormone that supports pregnancy, synthesized from **pregnenolone** and **hydroxypregnenolone** in the ovary.

Proline and hydroxyproline: Amino acid constituents of collagen and other proteins.

Pronase: A bacterial enzyme that hydrolyzes proteins.

Proteins: Polymers of amino acids forming enzymes and membranes of cells.

Protein synthesis: The process by which messenger RNA of polyribosomes directs the sequence of amino acids of proteins from individual transfer RNA molecules, according to the sequence of codons contained within the genetic code of DNA.

Proteoglycan: A glycosaminoglycan macromolecule containing protein.

Proto-oncogenes: Constituents of normal DNA of cells containing genes activated by oncogenic viruses. The cellular enzyme c-src is converted to the activated form v-src that causes protein phosphorylation and promotes tumor growth.

Protozoan: Unicellular infectious microbe.

Pulmonary embolism: Obstruction of the pulmonary artery by thrombi originating from veins.

Pulmonary infarction: Death of lung tissue caused by obstruction of circulation of blood within pulmonary artery.

Pustule: Collection of white blood cells within tissues caused by inflammation.

Pyridoxal homocysteine thiolactone enamine: The compound formed from vitamin B6 and homocysteine thiolactone that inhibits tumor growth by pre-treatment prior to tumor transplantation in experimental animals.

Pyridoxal phosphate: The coenzyme form of vitamin B6 that catalyzes enzymatic reactions in amino acid metabolism, including cystathionine synthase and cystathionase.

Reducing agent: A chemical that supplies electrons to reduce the state of oxidation of a molecule.

Restenosis: The gradual narrowing of an artery following dilation by angioplasty.

Resveratrol: An anti-oxidant pigment produced by grape vines and other plants.

Retinol: Vitamin A, a fat-soluble vitamin that is transported in plasma by transthyretin.

Retinoic acid: The oxidized form of vitamin A combines with homocysteine thiolactone to produce thioretinamide, catalyzed by cystathionine synthase.

Revascularization: Surgical procedure to re-establish arterial circulation by angioplasty or by-pass grafting, used to relieve symptoms of angina pectoris from coronary heart disease or to restore arterial circulation to an organ or extremity affected by arteriosclerosis.

Reverse transcriptase: The enzyme of viruses which uses RNA as a template for synthesis of DNA for transmitting the genetic code.

Rhodium trichloride: The salt of a transition metal complex of rhodium combined with chloride ions that react with oxalyl homocysteine thiolactone to produce a complex with anti-neoplastic activity in animals with transplanted tumors.

Riboflavin: Vitamin B2 is used in metabolism as a co-enzyme for methylenetetrahydrofolate reductase and other flavin enzymes.

Ribonuclease: An enzyme found in pancreatic secretions that hydrolyzes RNA to its component nucleotides.

Risk reduction, absolute: The statistic indicating the reduction in absolute risk in a clinical trial which considers the difference between the percentages of events observed in the treated and untreated groups. The total number of participants in the trial is included in this calculation.

Risk reduction, relative: The statistic indicating the reduction in relative risk in a clinical trial which considers the percentage of events observed in the treated group compared with the events in the untreated group. The total number of participants in the trial is excluded from this calculation.

Rotavirus: An infectious virus produces gastro-intestinal disease, fragments of which are demonstrated in arterial plaques.

***Salmonella*:** A gram negative bacterium causes gastro-intestinal infections, fragments of which are demonstrated in arterial plaques.

Sarcoma: A malignant tumor arising from connective tissues cells, such as muscle cells, fibroblast cells, or adipocytes.

Scurvy: The human disease or experimental disease of guinea pigs caused by dietary deficiency of vitamin C, characterized by fragility of capillaries, hemorrhages, thinning of blood vessels, growth inhibition, and death.

Sirtuin: An enzyme that removes acetyl groups from nucleoproteins of chromatin, believed to be of importance in the aging process.

Small inhibitory RNA: A short chain ribonucleic acid nucleotide capable of reacting with a specific area of DNA to regulate gene expression.

Smooth muscle cell: A cell of artery wall or intestinal wall that contracts to control blood pressure or to control propulsion of food in stomach and intestine during digestion.

Squamous cell carcinoma: A malignant tumor arising from the skin epidermis or from other organs in the body, characterized by flattened cells containing keratin.

Squamous metaplasia: The conversion of a glandular or ductal epithelium to a squamous epithelium, found in dietary or experimental deficiency of vitamin A.

Stem cells: Primitive cells of embryos or tissues that are capable of producing a full embryo or fully developed tissues of an organ.

Staphylococcus: A gram positive bacterium that causes skin infections, pneumonia, and other infections, fragments of which are demonstrated in arterial plaques.

Stroke: Damage to part of the brain caused by obstruction of cerebral artery by thrombus or by hemorrhage from a cerebral artery.

Sulfate: The fully oxidized form of sulfur in tissues, attached to glycosaminoglycans, steroid hormones, drugs and other components.

Sulfide: A reduced form of sulfur that forms hydrogen sulfide with hydrogen atoms.

Sulfonium group: A fully oxidized sulfur group within a molecule, found in thioretinaco ozonide complexing with ATP during oxidative phosphorylation.

Sulfur 35: S35 is a radioactive isotope of sulfur used in studies of metabolism of sulfur compounds, including methionine, homocysteine, and homocysteine thiolactone.

Superoxide: A highly reactive oxygen radical containing an unpaired electron, capable of oxidation of retinol to retinoic acid, conversion of thioretinamide to sulfite and alpha butyric acid, and other oxidation reactions, causing oxidative stress of cells and tissues.

SV40 polyoma virus: An ongogenic virus capable of inducing malignant tumors in different tissues of experimental animals, originally derived from simian (monkey) virus 40 and capable of causing a perpetual growth pattern of cultured cells.

Telomerase: The nuclear enzyme containing RNA that elongates telomeres of chromosomes.

Telomere: The end fragment of chromosomes that is gradually lost during cellular senescence.

Testosterone: The androgenic steroid hormone produced by testis, responsible for maintaining male secondary sex characteristics and libido.

Teratocarcinoma: A malignant tumor that arises from germ cells of the ovary or testis and produces multiple differentiated tissues. Experimental teratocarcinoma can be serially passaged by injection of ascitic fluid in the abdominal cavity of mice.

Thiamine: Vitamin B1 containing sulfur and producing the disease beri-beri when lacking in the diet.

Thioco: A complex formed from cobalamin and homocysteine thiolactone.

Thiocyanate: A non-toxic compound containing sulfur, carbon and nitrogen with a mild inhibitory effect on formation of thyroxine by the thyroid gland.

Thioretinamide: A compound formed from retinoic acid and homocysteine thiolactone, catalyzed by cystathionine synthase.

Thioretinaco: A complex formed from one molecule of cobalamin and two molecules of thioretinamide.

Thioretinaco ozonide: A complex formed from thioretinaco and ozone, capable of binding the phosphate groups of ATP to the sulfonium centers of thioretinamide groups during the process of oxidative phosphorylation.

Thrombosis: Obstruction of blood flow in an artery or vein by a thrombus (blood clot) that obstructs the lumen.

Thrombus: A mass of coagulated blood containing platelets, fibrin, and cells, capable of obstructing the lumen of an artery or vein.

Thymoma: A malignant tumor derived from cells of the thymus gland.

Thyroid hormone: An amino acid hormone containing iodine produced by the thyroid gland that regulates oxygen metabolism of cells.

Thyrotropic hormone: A polypeptide hormone produced by the pituitary gland that stimulates production of thyroid hormones by the thyroid gland.

Thyroxine: A form of thyroid hormone containing four iodine atoms.

Transfats: Saturated fatty acids produced by reaction of hydrogen with unsaturated fatty acids, catalyzed by nickel and implicated in increased risk of vascular disease.

Transfer RNA: A small RNA molecule in the shape of a cloverleaf capable of recognizing and binding a specific amino acid and functioning in protein synthesis by binding of its anti-codon to the codon of messenger RNA.

Transition metal: A metal ion capable of assuming multiple states of oxidation and functioning in biochemistry as reactive centers for enzyme activation or binding of oxygen and other gases, found in the iron of hemoglobin, copper of ceruloplasmin, mangnanese of superoxide dismutase, cobalt of cobalamin, and many other constituents of tissues.

Transformed cell: A cell produced by an oncogenic virus in cell culture, capable of indefinite passages in culture without clonal senescence.

Transmethylation: The biochemical process by which methyl groups are transferred from adenosyl methionine, methyl folate, choline, betaine and other compounds to acceptor molecules, associated with mobilization of fat by liver and conversion of homocysteine to methionine.

Transthyretin: The plasma protein that transports thyroid hormone and retinol to tissues by forming a complex with retinol-binding protein.

Tricarboxylic acid cycle: The metabolic series of enzymes that convert glucose to acetate, providing electrons for oxidative phosphorylation in mitochondria.

Trichloroacetic acid: A form of acetate containing three chloride atoms and used for precipitation of proteins from plasma or other fluids.

Trophoblast cells: Cells of the early embryo capable of forming cells of the placenta or a fully developed embryo, as studied by John Beard in 1902.

Troxerutin: A potent anti-oxidant nutrient derived from orange peel.

Tyrosine kinase: An enzyme that catalyzes phosphorylation of the hydroxyl group of the amino acid tyrosine, important in regulation of multiple cellular functions.

Ultraviolet radiation: Light energy of short wavelength causes damage to DNA of skin epidermal cells and produces malignant tumors by a carcinogenic effect. Also responsible for biosynthesis of vitamin D3 from cholesterol in skin cells.

Vasa vasorum: Small blood vessels supply the smooth muscle layers of arterial wall, can become obstructed by lipoprotein aggregates, causing hypoxia, cell death, and hemorrhage, leading to formation of vulnerable plaques.

Vascular disease: Narrowing of arteries by arterial plaques from atherogenesis.

Vasodilation: Increase in diameter of artery caused by relaxation of smooth muscle cells of arterial wall.

Veins: Thin walled blood vessels that transport blood from the tissues to the heart.

Vena cava: The major vein of the abdomen and thorax that transports blood from the veins of the organs and extremities to the heart.

Vulnerable plaque: An intimal fibrolipid arterial plaque resembling a pustule that causes thrombosis when ruptured, leading to myocardial infarct, stroke, or gangrene.

Yolk sac: A transient structure of the early embryo containing trophoblastic cells, according to John Beard's studies of 1902.

INDEX

A

B

C

D

E

F

G

H

I

J

K

L

M

Q

R

S

V

W

X

Y

Z